T0296782

Essentials of Neuroanesthesia and Neurointensive Care

Essentials of Neuroanesthesia and Neurointensive Care

Arun K. Gupta, MBBS, MA, PhD, FRCA
Consultant in Anaesthesia and Neurointensive Care
Director of Postgraduate Medical Education
Addenbrooke's Hospital
Cambridge University Hospitals
NHS Foundation Trust
Associate Lecturer
University of Cambridge
Cambridge, United Kingdom

Adrian W. Gelb, MBChB, DA, FRCPC
Professor
Department of Anesthesia and Perioperative Care
University of California–San Francisco
San Francisco, California

SAUNDERS
ELSEVIER

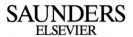

1600 John F. Kennedy Blvd., Suite 1800
Philadelphia, PA 19103-2899

Essentials of Neuroanesthesia and Neurointensive Care   ISBN: 978-1-4160-4653-0

Library of Congress Cataloging-in-Publication Data
Essentials of neuroanesthesia and neurointensive care / [edited by] Arun K. Gupta, Adrian W. Gelb. – 1st ed.
   p. ; cm. – (Essentials of anesthesia and critical care series)
  Includes bibliographical references.
  ISBN 978-1-4160-4653-0
  1. Anesthesia in neurology. 2. Neurological intensive care. 3. Nervous system–Surgery.
I. Gupta, Arun K. II. Gelb, Adrian W. III. Series.
  [DNLM: 1. Anesthesia–methods. 2. Neurosurgical Procedures.
3. Brain–drug effects. 4. Intensive Care. 5. Perioperative Care. WL 368 E775 2008]
  RD87.3.N47E87 2008
  617.9′6748–dc22
                                 2007038047

Executive Publisher: Natasha Andjelkovic
Developmental Editor: Isabel Trudeau
Publishing Services Manager: Joan Sinclair
Project Manager: Lawrence Shanmugaraj
Text Designer: Karen O'Keefe Owens

Working together to grow
libraries in developing countries

www.elsevier.com | www.bookaid.org | www.sabre.org

ELSEVIER   BOOK AID International   Sabre Foundation

Printed in China
Last digit is the print number: 9 8 7 6 5 4 3 2 1

Dedication

I would like to dedicate this book to my family, whose understanding and patience
have made this book possible.
AKG

With thanks and love for those who matter most —
Lola, Megan, Karen, and Julia.
AWG

Contributors

Anthony Absalom, MBChB, MD, FRCA, ILTM
Consultant in Anaesthesia
Addenbrooke's Hospital
Cambridge University Hospitals
NHS Foundation Trust
Cambridge, UK

Ram Adapa, FRCA
Specialist Registrar in Anaesthesia
and Intensive Care
Addenbrooke's Hospital
Cambridge University Hospitals
NHS Foundation Trust
Cambridge, UK

Olga N. Afonin, MD
Assistant Clinical Professor
Department of Anesthesia
and Perioperative Care
University of California–San Francisco
San Francisco, California

Arnab Banerjee, FRCA
Specialist Registrar in Anaesthesia
and Intensive Care
Addenbrooke's Hospital
Cambridge University Hospitals
NHS Foundation Trust
Cambridge, UK

Anuj Bhatia, MBBS, MD, MNAMS, FRCA
Clinical Fellow
Anaesthesia and Pain Management
Wasser Pain Management Centre
Mount Sinai Hospital
Toronto, Ontario
Canada

Claire Brett, MD
Professor
Department of Anesthesia
and Perioperative Care
University of California–San Francisco
San Francisco, California

Rowan Burnstein, MBBS, FRCA, PhD
Consultant in Anaesthesia
and Intensive Care
SDU Director of Neurocritical Care
Addenbrooke's Hospital
Cambridge University Hospitals
NHS Foundation Trust
Cambridge, UK

Ian Calder, MB, ChB, DRCOG, FRCA
Consultant in Neuroanaesthesia
and Neurocritical Care
The National Hospital for Neurology
and Neurosurgery
University College London Hospitals
London, UK

James E. Caldwell, MD
Professor and Vice Chair
Department of Anesthesia
and Perioperative Care
Director of Clinical Anesthesia Services
University of California–San Francisco
San Francisco, California

Randall M. Chesnut, MD, FACS, FCCM
Director of Cranial and Spinal
Trauma Center
Harborview Medical Center
Associate Professor of Neurological
Surgery
University of Washington School
of Medicine
Seattle, Washington

Jonathan P. Coles, MBChB, PhD, DA, FRCA
Honorary Consultant
Academy of Medical Sciences/Health
Foundation Clinician Scientist
University Department of Anaesthesia
Addenbrooke's Hospital
Cambridge University Hospitals
NHS Foundation Trust
Cambridge, UK

Rosemary Ann Craen, MBBS, FRCPC
Associate Professor
Department of Anaesthesia
and Perioperative Medicine
London Health Sciences Centre
London, Ontario
Canada

Marek Czosnyka, MSc, PhD, DSC
Reader in Brain Physics
Department of Clinical Neurosciences
University of Cambridge
Neurosurgical Unit
Addenbrooke's Hospital
Cambridge University Hospitals
NHS Foundation Trust
Cambridge, UK

Rose Du, MD, PhD
Instructor
Department of Neurosurgery
Brigham and Women's Hospital
Harvard Medical School
Boston, Massachusetts

Derek T. Duane, FRCA, MSc, MPhil
Consultant in Neuroanaesthesia
and Neurointensive Care
University Department of Anaesthesia
Addenbrooke's Hospital
Cambridge University Hospitals
NHS Foundation Trust
Cambridge, UK

Adrian W. Gelb, MBChB, DA, FRCPC
Professor
Department of Anesthesia
and Perioperative Care
University of California–San Francisco
San Francisco, California

Jonathan H. Gillard, FRCR
Reader in Neuroradiology
University of Cambridge
Honorary Consultant
University Department of Radiology
Addenbrooke's Hospital
Cambridge University Hospitals
NHS Foundation Trust
Cambridge, UK

Arun K. Gupta, MBBS, MA, PhD, FRCA
Consultant in Anaesthesia
and Neurointensive Care
Director of Postgraduate Medical
Education
Addenbrooke's Hospital
Cambridge University Hospitals
NHS Foundation Trust
Associate Lecturer
University of Cambridge
Cambridge, UK

Nicolas P. Hirsch, MBBS, FRCA
Consultant in Neuroanesthesia
and Neurocritical Care
The National Hospital for Neurology
and Neurosurgery
University College London Hospitals
London, UK

Katharine Hunt, FRCA
Consultant in Neuroanesthesia
and Neurocritical Care
The National Hospital for Neurology
and Neurosurgery
University College London Hospitals
London, UK

Peter Hutchinson, BSc, MBBS, PhD, FRCS
Senior Academy Fellow
Honorary Consultant Neurosurgeon
Addenbrooke's Hospital
Cambridge University Hospitals
NHS Foundation Trust
Cambridge, UK

Alexander Kopelnik, MD
Fellow, Division of Cardiology
Department of Medicine
University of California–San Diego
San Diego, California

Rodney J. C. Laing, MA, MB, BChir, MD, FRCS(SN)
Consultant Neurosurgeon
Addenbrooke's Hospital
Cambridge University Hospitals
NHS Foundation Trust
Cambridge, UK

Chanhung Z. Lee, MD, PhD
Assistant Professor
Department of Anesthesia
and Perioperative Care
University of California–San Francisco
San Francisco, California

Jeremy A. Lieberman, MD
Associate Professor
Department of Anesthesia
and Perioperative Care
University of California–San Francisco
San Francisco, California

Daniel A. Lim, PhD
Assistant Professor
Department of Neurological Surgery
University of California–San Francisco
San Francisco, California

Lawrence Litt, PhD, MD
Professor
Department of Anesthesia
and Perioperative Care
University of California–San Francisco
San Francisco, California

Balachandra Maiya, FRCA, MD, MBBS
Specialist Registrar in Anaesthesia
and Intensive Care
Addenbrooke's Hospital
Cambridge University Hospitals
NHS Foundation Trust
Cambridge, UK

Pirjo H. Manninen, MD, FRCPC
Associate Professor
Department of Anaesthesia
University of Toronto
Director of Neuroanaesthesia
Toronto Western Hospital
University Health Network
Toronto, Ontario, Canada

Basil F. Matta, MA, FRCA
Clinical Director
Perioperative Care Services
Department of Anaesthesia
Addenbrooke's Hospital
Cambridge University Hospitals
NHS Foundation Trust
Cambridge, UK

Michael W. McDermott, MD
Professor
Department of Neurological Surgery
University of California–San Francisco
San Francisco, California

David K. Menon, MBBS, MD, PhD, FRCP, FRCA, FMedSci
Professor and Head
Division of Anesthesia
University of Cambridge
Honorary Consultant in
Neuroanaesthesia and
Neurocritical Care
Addenbrooke's Hospital
Cambridge University Hospitals
NHS Foundation Trust
Cambridge, UK

Virginia Newcombe, BSc, MPhil, MBBS
Clinical Research Fellow
Division of Anaesthesia
Wolfson College
Cambridge University
Cambridge, UK

Mary C. Newton, MBBS
Consultant in Neuroanaesthesia
and Neurocritical Care
Department of Neuroanesthesia
The National Hospital for Neurology
and Neurosurgery
University College London Hospitals
London, UK

Jurgens Nortje, FRCA
Consultant in Anaesthesia
and Intensive Care
Critical Care Unit
Norfolk and Norwich University
Hospital
Norwich, UK

Piyush M. Patel, MD, FRCPC
Professor of Anesthesiology
University of California–San Diego
Anesthesia Service
Veterans Affairs Medical Center
San Diego, Califonia

Vinodkumar Patil, MBBS, DA, DNB, FRCA
Specialist Registrar in Anaesthesia
and Intensive Care
Addenbrooke's Hospital
Cambridge University Hospitals
NHS Foundation Trust
Cambridge, UK

Adam D. Peets, MD, MSc
Clinical Assistant Professor
Department of Critical Care Medicine
University of Calgary
Foothills Medical Centre
Calgary, Alberta, Canada

Hélène G. Pellerin, MD, FRCPC
Assistant Professor
Department of Anaesthesia
and Intensive Care
Hôpital de l'Enfant-Jésus
Université Laval
Québec, Canada

Tamsin Poole, FRCA
Specialist Registrar in Anaesthesia
and Intensive Care
Addenbrooke's Hospital
Cambridge University Hospitals
NHS Foundation Trust
Cambridge, UK

Amit Prakash, MD, FRCA
Specialist Registrar in Anaesthesia
and Intensive Care
Addenbrooke's Hospital
Cambridge University Hospitals
NHS Foundation Trust
Cambridge, UK

Jane E. Risdall, MBBS, MA(cantab), DA(UK), FFARCSI
Surgeon Commander, Royal Navy
Consultant in Anaesthesia
and Intensive Care
University Department of Anesthesia
Addenbrooke's Hospital
Cambridge University Hospitals
NHS Foundation Trust
Cambridge, UK

Mark A. Rosen, MD
Professor
Department of Anesthesia
and Perioperative Care
University of California–San Francisco
San Francisco, California

Keith J. Ruskin, MD
Professor
Department of Anesthesiology
Yale University School of Medicine
New Haven, Connecticut

Susan Ryan, MD, PhD
Associate Professor
Department of Anesthesia
and Perioperative Care
University of California–San Francisco
San Francisco, California

Peter M. Schulman, MD
Assistant Clinical Professor
Department of Anesthesia
and Perioperative Care
University of California–San Francisco
San Francisco, California

Daniel Scoffings, MRCP, FRCR
Specialist Registrar in Neuroradiology
Department of Radiology
Addenbrooke's Hospital
Cambridge University Hospitals
NHS Foundation Trust
Cambridge, UK

Martin Smith, MBBS, FRCA
Consultant in Neuroanaesthesia
and Neurocritical Care
Honorary Senior Lecturer
in Anaesthesia
Department of Neuroanaesthesia
The National Hospital for Neurology
and Neurosurgery
University College London Hospitals
London, UK

James Stimpson, FRCA
Specialist Registrar in Anaesthesia
and Intensive Care
Addenbrooke's Hospital
Cambridge University Hospitals
NHS Foundation Trust
Cambridge, UK

Jane Sturgess, FRCA
Specialist Registrar in Anaesthesia
and Intensive Care
Addenbrooke's Hospital
Cambridge University Hospitals
NHS Foundation Trust
Cambridge, UK

Michael Sughrue, MD
Resident
Department of Neurological Surgery
University of California–San Francisco
San Francisco, California

Pekka O. Talke, MD
Chief of Neuroanesthesia
Department of Anesthesia
and Perioperative Care
University of California–San Francisco
San Francisco, California

John M. Taylor, MD
Assistant Professor
Department of Anesthesia
and Perioperative Care
University of California–San Francisco
San Francisco, California

Ivan Timofeev, MD

Specialist Registrar in Neurosurgery
Addenbrooke's Hospital
Cambridge University Hospitals
NHS Foundation Trust
Cambridge, UK

Monica S. Vavilala, MD

Associate Professor of Anesthesiology
and Pediatrics
Adjunct Professor of Neurological
Surgery
University of Washington School
of Medicine
Associate Director
Injury Prevention and Research Center
Harborview Medical Center
Seattle, Washington

Daniel M. Wong, MBBS, FANZCA

Staff Anaesthetist
St. Vincent's Hospital
Melbourne, Victoria, Australia

Peter Wright, MD

Professor
Department of Anesthesia
and Perioperative Care
University of California–San Francisco
San Francisco, California

Sarah Yarham, FRCA

Specialist Registrar in Anaesthesia
Addenbrooke's Hospital
Cambridge University Hospitals
NHS Foundation Trust
Cambridge, UK

William L. Young, MD

James P. Livingston Professor
and Vice Chair
Department of Anesthesia
and Perioperative Care
Professor of Neurological
Surgery and Neurology
University of California–San Francisco
San Francisco, California

Jonathan Zaroff, MD

Assistant Professor
Division of Cardiology
Department of Medicine
University of California–San Francisco
San Francisco, California

David Zygun, MD, MSc, FRCPC

Assistant Professor
Department of Critical Care Medicine
University of Calgary
Intensivist
Foothills Medical Centre
Calgary, Alberta, Canada

Preface

The subspecialty of neuroanesthesia and neurointensive care has become established in many centers around the world. Accordingly, our understanding of the neurosciences has continued to grow, inevitably leading to modifications and changes in neuroanesthesia, intensive care, and neurosurgical practice. Although the complexity of the knowledge base is rapidly expanding, there is an expectation that all caregivers have a grasp of the physiology, pharmacology, and anatomy of the central nervous system. *Essentials of Neuroanesthesia and Neurointensive Care* aims to provide the essential information required to enable understanding of the basic principles of a particular subject prior to the reader's applying them in clinical practice. In keeping with essential information, the chapters are brief and easily read in a short period of time. This book is therefore likely to be of most use to residents and specialist trainees in anesthesia who either are undertaking a training module in neuroanesthesia or neurointensive care or have finished their training and may be doing ad hoc or occasional work in neuroanesthetic practice. Other health care professionals who are associated with the neuroscience patient will also find this book useful.

In many centers, health care providers other than neuroanesthesiologists have responsibilities in neurointensive care. In recognizing this, we have categorized the chapters into neuroanesthesia and neurointensive care sections, with a separate section on monitoring techniques. We have attempted to minimize inevitable overlap between the sections with cross referencing. However, certain principles and facts need reemphasizing often in a slightly different context, and we make no apology for this repetition. The "Key Facts" should provide the reader with a rapid reminder of the principles of each subject, and the "Further Reading" section lists a small number of key articles or book chapters where more in-depth information can be obtained. The transatlantic editorship and authorship have allowed us to take into consideration variations in practice on both sides of the Atlantic and to describe current best practice from both perspectives.

We would like to thank all of our colleagues who contributed to this book, in particular Ken Probst, for his skill in preparing many of the illustrations.

Arun K. Gupta • Adrian W. Gelb

Contents

Section V NEUROINTENSIVE CARE

Section VI MONITORING

Section VII MISCELLANEOUS

Section VIII APPENDICES

Index, 329

Section I
Anatomy

Chapter 1

Structure and Function of the Brain and Spinal Cord

Daniel A. Lim • Michael Sughrue • Michael W. McDermott

Spinal Cord	**Infratentorial Compartment**
Supratentorial Compartment	Brainstem
Cerebrum and Neocortices	Cerebellum
Diencephalon	**Extrapyramidal Organs**
	Basal Ganglia

The central nervous system (CNS) can be divided grossly into five bilaterally paired anatomic regions (Fig. 1-1):

1. Spinal cord
2. Cerebral hemispheres
3. Diencephalon
4. Brainstem, including the medulla, pons, and midbrain
5. Cerebellum

For practical purposes, many surgeons divide the intracranial compartment into supratentorial and infratentorial compartments. The *supratentorial* compartment contains the cerebral hemispheres and the diencephalon, whereas the *infratentorial* compartment includes the brainstem and cerebellum.

The CNS is bathed in cerebrospinal fluid (CSF), which is created in the ventricles by the choroid plexus at a rate of about 15 to 20 mL/hr in adults (Fig. 1-2A) and circulates through the ventricular system to the subarachnoid space. The subarachnoid space is found between the pia mater, which is attached to the brain and spinal cord tissue, and the arachnoid mater, a delicate, spider web–like connective tissue (Fig. 1-2B). Outside the arachnoid is the tough dura mater. Collectively, the pia, arachnoid, and dura mater form the meninges.

SPINAL CORD

The spinal cord extends from the base of the skull and tapers down to the conus, where it becomes the filum terminale between T12 and L2 (Fig. 1-3).

The principal functions of the spinal cord are threefold. First, in its central gray matter lies the cellular circuitry underlying the motor function of most of the body (with the exception of the face, tongue, and mouth), including the anterior horn cells and the indirect pathways that regulate them (reflex loops).

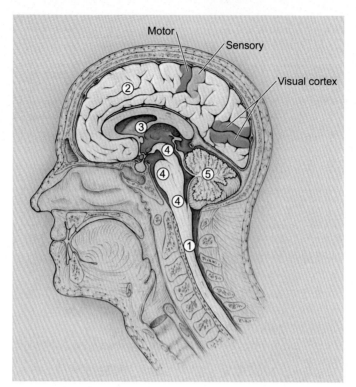

Figure 1-1   Sagittal image showing the relationships of the (1) spinal cord; (2) cerebral hemispheres; (3) diencephalon, (4) brainstem, consisting of the medulla, pons, and midbrain; and (5) cerebellum.

Second, the spinal cord receives sensory input from the peripheral nerves and transmits this input to higher structures. The primary ascending tracts are the posterior columns and the lateral spinothalamic tract (Fig. 1-4). The posterior columns transmit fine touch, vibration, and proprioception. The lateral spino-thalamic tract conveys contralateral pain and temperature. Pain fibers from the dorsal roots ascend or descend one to three segments before synapsing in the spinal cord (Fig. 1-4).

Third, the spinal white matter contains a number of descending tracts that are used by higher CNS structures to regulate spinal cord function either by directly stimulating cells or by regulating interneurons that increase or decrease signaling efficiency. The most clinically important of these tracts is the lateral corticospinal tract (Fig. 1-4), which conveys voluntary, skilled movement from the contralat-eral cerebral hemisphere. Many other motor pathways originate from cortical and brainstem structures to control posture and movement. Additionally, there are descending pathways responsible for the regulation of pain fibers.

Blood is supplied to the spinal cord by paired posterior spinal arteries and a single anterior spinal artery. Whereas the posterior arteries supply the dorsal horns and white matter columns, the anterior spinal artery supplies the anterior two thirds of the cord. Six to eight prominent radicular arteries supply the ante-rior spinal artery network, most numerous in the cervical region and least in the thoracic. The artery of Adamkiewicz, the main thoracolumbar radicular vessel, supplies the spinal cord from T8 to the conus. This artery arises in the T9-L2

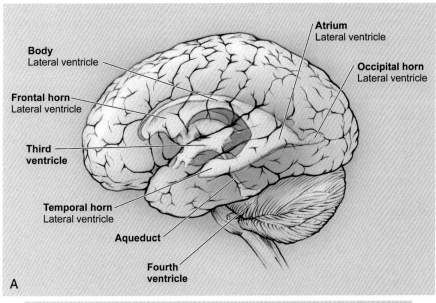

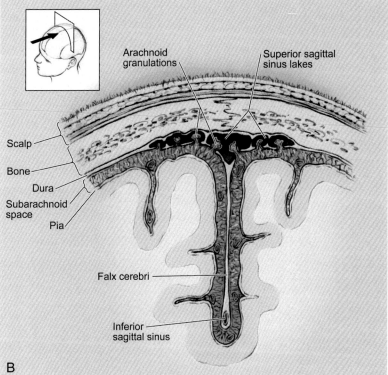

Figure 1-2 **A,** Position of the lateral, third, and fourth ventricles and connection pathways. The lateral ventricle is divided into the frontal horn, body, atrium, and occipital and temporal horns. The choroid plexus is found in the floor of the body of the ventricle, the roof of the temporal horn, and the third and fourth ventricles. **B,** Coronal section showing the relationship of the arachnoid granulations to the superior sagittal sinus.

region and mostly from the left side of the aorta. Spinal artery perfusion pressure is an important consideration, especially in the prone position, where intravenous pressure is elevated.

SUPRATENTORIAL COMPARTMENT

Cerebrum and Neocortices

The cerebral hemispheres consist of the cerebral cortex, white matter projections, and a few deep structures, including the basal ganglia and hippocampus. The cortex is highly convoluted with infoldings called sulci and bumps or ridges called gyri. Each hemisphere is divided into four major lobes: frontal, parietal, temporal, and occipital (Fig. 1-5). The hemispheres are principally defined by the midline interhemispheric fissure, the central sulcus in the posterior frontal lobe, and the large lateral sylvian fissure.

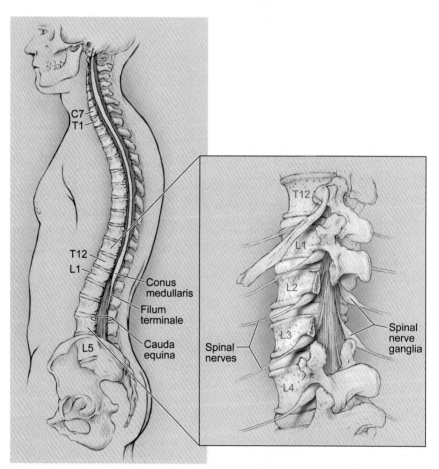

Figure 1-3 Sagittal image of the spine and spinal cord with a close-up of the cauda equina and compound spinal nerves. The spinal cord extends from the base of the skull and tapers down to the conus, at which point it becomes the filum terminale between T12 and L2.

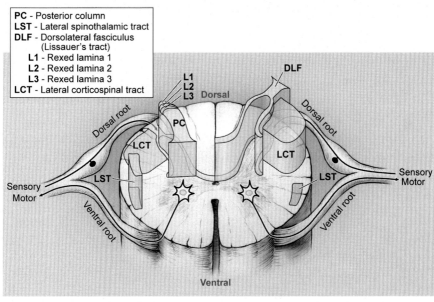

Figure 1-4 Axial schematic representation of the ascending and descending tracts and the dorsal horn.

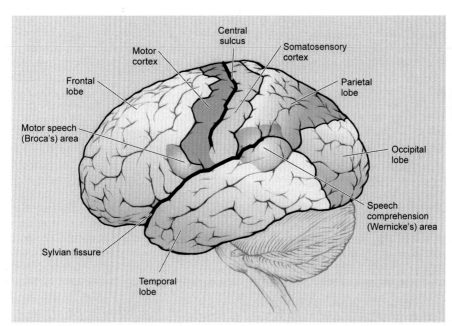

Figure 1-5 The cortex is highly convoluted with infoldings called sulci and bumps or ridges called gyri. Each hemisphere is divided into four major lobes: frontal, parietal, temporal, and occipital. Motor (Broca's) and receptive (Wernicke's) language areas are shown in the frontal and temporal-parietal lobes, respectively.

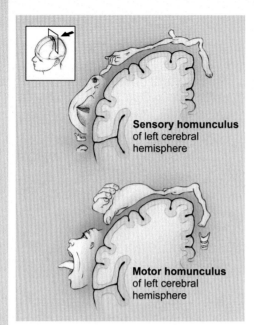

Figure 1-6 Approximate representation of the motor and sensory areas in the precentral and postcentral sulci.

Sensory homunculus of left cerebral hemisphere

Motor homunculus of left cerebral hemisphere

Not all cortex is created equal; some regions can be removed with impunity, whereas others will cause neurologic deficits if injured. Thus, it is essential to understand the location of the so-called eloquent brain regions because noneloquent regions are the preferred operative path for most lesions. Eloquent brain regions include the primary motor and sensory cortices, the speech areas (Broca's and Wernicke's areas), the primary visual cortex, the thalamus, the brainstem reticular activating system, the deep cerebellar nuclei, and to some extent, the anterior parietal lobes. Many of these regions lie near or directly adjacent to the sylvian fissure.

The primary motor cortex and the somatosensory cortex straddle the central sulcus. Both the motor cortex and the sensory cortex represent the opposite side of the body in a precise topologic fashion (Fig. 1-6). The visual cortex is in the occipital lobe, primarily on the medial aspect of the hemisphere above and below the calcarine sulcus.

The left hemisphere is dominant for language in nearly all right-handed patients; about 80% of left-handed people are still left hemisphere language dominant, with bilateral dominance and right-sided dominance in about 15% and 5% of patients, respectively (see Fig. 1-1). Wernicke's area is behind the primary auditory cortex in the posterior superior temporal lobe; lesions in Wernicke's area lead to problems with language comprehension and classically cause fluent aphasia (normal sentence length and intonation, speech devoid of meaning). Broca's area is located in the frontal lobe premotor cortex and is important for word formation; lesions in Broca's area lead to nonfluent aphasia (faltering, broken speech).

Diencephalon

The diencephalon sits above the midbrain and consists of the thalamus and hypothalamus. The thalamus is "an information relay station." All sensory modalities except olfaction pass through the thalamus, and there are many reciprocal connections

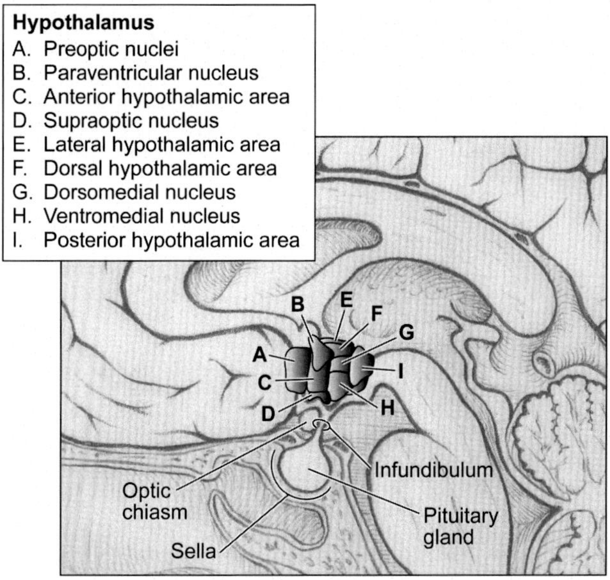

Figure 1-7   Locations of hypothalamic nuclei in the diencephalon.

between the thalamus and the cerebral cortex, as well as with the cerebellum. The thalamus is important for motor control, wakefulness, and processing of sensory information. Thalamic lesion can thus produce coma, tremors and other motor difficulties, and sensory problems, including pain syndromes.

The hypothalamus, located just inferior to the thalamus, controls endocrine, autonomic, and visceral function. The hypothalamus is connected to the pituitary gland by the infundibulum, which continues as the pituitary stalk (Fig. 1-7). The pituitary gland sits within the sella, just behind and inferior to the optic chiasm. Hence, tumors of the pituitary can compress the chiasm and produce visual problems (e.g., bitemporal hemianopia). Hypothalamic releasing and inhibitory factors regulate release of pituitary hormone. Vasopressin (or antidiuretic hormone) is made by hypothalamic cells and transported to the posterior pituitary for release.

The hypothalamus also originates descending fibers that influence the sympathetic and parasympathetic autonomic nervous system. There are discrete nuclei within the hypothalamus that are critical to body homeostasis. Thermoregulation, satiety, and arousal are partially controlled in the hypothalamus, and experimental lesions of the lateral hypothalamus produce anorexia, whereas medial lesions cause overeating.

INFRATENTORIAL COMPARTMENT

Brainstem

The brainstem, a highly complex and clinically critical region of the CNS, consists of the medulla, pons, and midbrain (see Fig. 1-1). Unlike any other region of the brain, it is at the same time the anatomic substrate of consciousness, a regulator

9

Table 1-1 Cranial Nerves and Function

Cranial Nerve	Function	Defined Nucleus Location
I	Smell	Uncus, septal area
II	Vision	Lateral geniculate nucleus
III	Extraocular movement, lid elevation	Midbrain tectum (superior)
IV	Eye movement, down and in	Midbrain tectum (inferior)
V	Sensory to skin of the face Motor to muscles for chewing (V3)	Pons (motor, sensory), medulla, cervical cord (sensory)
VI	Lateral eye movement	Pons (dorsal)
VII	Facial movement Sense of taste (anterior two thirds of the tongue)	Pons (ventral)
VIII	Hearing Balance	Pons (dorsal-lateral)
IX	Palatal movement/sensation Taste in posterior third of the tongue	Medulla
X	Vocal cords Parasympathetic supply to the viscera	Medulla
XI	Trapezius, sternomastoid supply	Medulla
XII	Muscles of the tongue	Medulla

of autonomic function, the origin and target of numerous different descending regulatory fiber tracts and a few ascending ones, a thoroughfare for tracts having no functional relationship to it, the home of 10 of the 12 cranial nerves with their attendant input and output nuclei, and the location of a number of clinically relevant reflexes.

Probably the most clinically important function of the brainstem is its role in maintaining consciousness. Significant injuries to the brainstem lead to stupor and coma because of injury to the reticular activating system. The brainstem reticular formation consists of a set of interconnected nuclei in the core of the brainstem that mediate the level of alertness.

Equally important are the respiratory control centers located in the medulla and pons. Respiratory control neurons are involved in rhythm generation, as well as in processing afferent information from central and peripheral chemoreceptors and various lung receptors. Focal medullary injury or edema can lead to life-threatening respiratory arrest.

Many ascending and descending fiber tracts pass though the brainstem. Other tracts such as the corticobulbar, trigeminothalamic, and central tegmental tracts and the medial longitudinal fasciculus have their origin or termination within brainstem nuclei. For instance, the nuclei for cranial nerves III to XII are in the brainstem (Table 1-1). Importantly, many of these tracts have close analogues in the spinal cord, and lack of concordance of deficits between the face and body (e.g., right facial weakness and left hemiparesis) strongly suggests a lesion in the brainstem.

Brainstem function can be grossly tested in comatose patients by using the pupillary, corneal, and gag/cough reflexes. The pupillary (light) reflex assesses function at the midbrain level, as well as the integrity of the optic and oculomotor nerves. The corneal (blink) reflex assesses brainstem function at the level of the pons. Its afferent limb is the trigeminal nerve and its efferent limb is the facial nerve. The gag reflex tests the lower brainstem, or medulla, as well as the glossopharyngeal and vagus nerves.

The vomiting reflex passes through the medulla. Stimulation of certain neurons of the reticular formation leads to impulses descending down to lower motor neurons that induce contraction of the diaphragm and abdominal muscles.

Cerebellum

The cerebellum is found in the posterior cranial fossa (see Fig. 1-1). It is attached to the brainstem by the three cerebellar peduncles at the level of the fourth ventricle. The tentorium, a transverse fold of dura, stretches over the superior part of the cerebellum and separates it from the occipital lobe of the cerebral hemispheres. This intimate relationship between the cerebellum and brainstem puts the patient's life in danger in cases of acute cerebellar edema.

The oldest part, the archicerebellum, lies in the anteroinferior flocculonodular lobe, receives input from the vestibular nuclei, and regulates control of eye movement. The paleocerebellum consists of the midline vermis and processes proprioceptive input from the ascending spinocerebellar tracts, where it controls axial posture via neocortical projections. The neocerebellum is primarily made up of the lateral hemispheres, which receive neocortical input via the middle peduncle, and sends processed output back to the neocortex via the thalamus.

Lesions of the cerebellum typically produce deficits ipsilateral to the lesion because the output of the cerebellum is crossed, and it affects primarily the descending motor pathways, which are also crossed. Typical symptoms include ataxia and truncal tremor (titubation) with paleocerebellar (medial) lesions or limb ataxia or action tremor with neocerebellar (lateral) lesions.

EXTRAPYRAMIDAL ORGANS

The extrapyramidal organs are structures linked not by spatial proximity but by functional and neuroanatomic similarity. Both structures can be thought of as a form of consultant to the rest of the CNS in that they receive and process input from the neocortex or spinal cord (or both) and relay this processed input back to external targets, commonly the thalamus, where motor, emotional, and cognitive function is modulated. As a result, damage to the extrapyramidal organs classically causes tremor and incoordination (known as extrapyramidal signs), not paralysis.

Basal Ganglia

Within the cerebral hemisphere lie the basal ganglia (Fig. 1-8). The principal components are the caudate nucleus, putamen, globus pallidus, and amygdala.

These organs contain many interconnections, as well as reciprocal connections with other brain regions, including the midbrain, diencephalon, and cerebral cortex. Functionally, these connections can be classified into oculomotor, skeletomotor, limbic, and cognitive circuits, each with different input and targets.

Basal ganglia diseases such as Parkinson's and Huntington's disease lead to abnormal motor control, alterations in muscular tone, and the emergence of irregular, involuntary movements. Moreover, these diseases can cause emotional and cognitive disturbances, depending on the degree of involvement of the emotional and cognitive circuits.

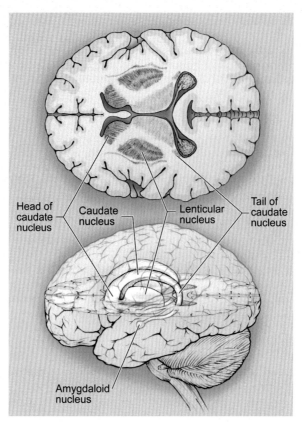

Head of caudate nucleus

Caudate nucleus

Lenticular nucleus

Tail of caudate nucleus

Amygdaloid nucleus

Figure 1-8   Axial and three-dimensional representation of the basal ganglia.

KEY POINTS

- The CNS can be organized into five paired regions: cerebral hemispheres, diencephalon, brainstem, cerebellum, and spinal cord.
- The anterior two thirds of the spinal cord is supplied by the anterior spinal artery. This portion of the spinal cord contains lower motor neurons in the ventral horn, descending corticospinal tracts, and ascending spinothalamic tracts.
- The supratentorial compartment includes the cerebral hemispheres and the diencephalon. More than 80% of people are left hemisphere dominant for speech and language function.
- The infratentorial compartment contains the brainstem, cerebellum, and cranial nerves III to XII.
- The basal ganglia include the caudate, globus pallidus, putamen, and amygdala.

SELECTED READINGS

Kandel ER, Schwartz JH, Jessell TM (eds): Principles of Neural Science, 4th ed. Norwalk, CT, Appleton & Lange, 2000.

Gilman S, Newman S: Manter and Gatz's Essentials of Clinical Neuroanatomy and Neurophysiology, 10th ed. FA Davis, 2002.

Chapter 2

Cerebral Circulation

Rowan Burnstein • Sarah Yarham

Arterial Blood Supply

Venous Drainage

Microcirculation

Blood-Brain Barrier

The brain has the highest metabolic requirements of any organ in the body. It receives 14% of the resting cardiac output in adults ($\approx$700 mL/min) and accounts for 20% of basal oxygen consumption ($\approx$50 mL/min). Blood flow within the brain is variable, with flow in gray matter (80 to 110 mL/100 g tissue/min) being on average five times that in white matter (22 mL/100 g/min).

ARTERIAL BLOOD SUPPLY

The arterial supply to the brain is from (1) both the right and left internal carotid arteries (ICAs) supplying the anterior two thirds of the cerebral hemispheres and (2) the vertebrobasilar system, which supplies the brainstem and posterior regions of the hemispheres.

The *common carotid artery* lies in the neck within the carotid sheath medial to the *internal jugular vein* (IJV), with the *vagus nerve* situated posteriorly between them. The sympathetic trunk runs behind the artery but outside the sheath. At approximately the level of the thyroid cartilage the common carotid artery bifurcates into the ICA and *external carotid artery* (ECA).

Just above the bifurcation, the ECA passes between the ICA and the pharyngeal wall. It supplies the soft tissues of the neck, eye, face, and scalp.

The ICA continues to pass vertically upward in the neck within the carotid sheath and gives off no branches. It is superficial at first in the carotid triangle but then passes deeper, medial to the posterior belly of the digastric muscle. At its origin is a fusiform dilation known as the carotid sinus. The walls of the sinus contain baroreceptors that are stimulated by changes in blood pressure. The carotid chemoreceptor, a small pea-sized structure that is stimulated by hypoxia and metabolic acidosis, sits between the vessels at the bifurcation. The ICA enters the skull through the foramen lacerum and turns anteriorly through the cavernous sinus in the carotid groove on the side of the sphenoid body.

Each ICA gives rise to a *posterior communicating artery* before ending by dividing into the *anterior cerebral artery* (ACA) and *middle cerebral artery* (MCA) (Figs. 2-1 and 2-2). The ACA runs medially and then superiorly and supplies the undersurface of the

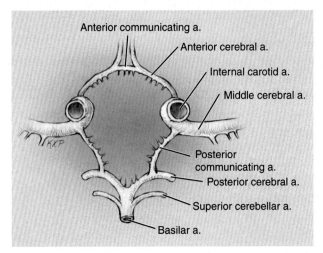

Figure 2-1 Diagrammatic representation of the circle of Willis. This classic polygon is found in less than 50% of brains.

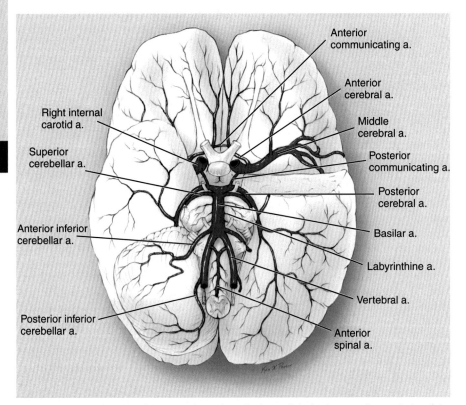

Figure 2-2 Relationship of the arterial supply to the base of the brain. Note the proximity of the circle of Willis to the optic chiasm and pituitary stalk.

14

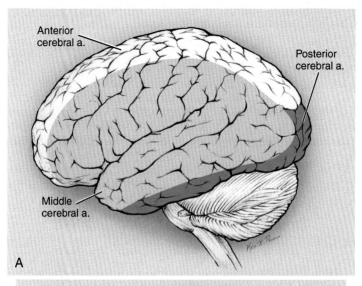

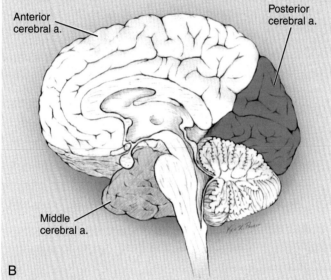

Figure 2-3   **A** and **B,** Areas of the brain supplied by the cerebral arteries.

frontal lobe and the medial neostriatum (Fig. 2-3). The MCA turns laterally from its origin and immediately gives rise to a series of small penetrating branches, the *lenticulo-striate arteries*. These arteries are the only supply to the lateral part of the striatum. The MCA continues to run laterally, where it divides into several major branches carrying blood to the lateral surfaces of the frontal, temporal, and parietal lobes (Fig. 2-3).

The *vertebral arteries* arise from the *subclavian arteries* at the base of the neck. They fuse to form the *basilar artery* at the level of the pontomedullary junction. The *basilar artery* lies on the ventral surface of the brainstem and supplies blood to the pons, midbrain, and cerebellum (see Fig. 2-2). At the level of the midbrain the artery bifurcates to form two large *posterior cerebral arteries* (PCAs), from which several small branches arise, including the small *posterior communicating arteries.*

Anastomoses between the internal carotid system and the vertebrobasilar system form the *circle of Willis* (see Fig. 2-1). It is located in the interpeduncular cistern and encloses the optic chiasm, pituitary stalk, and mammillary bodies. The "classic" polygonal anastomotic ring, however, is found in less than 50% of brains. The vessels of the circle send branches that supply superficial tissue, as well as long penetrating branches that supply deep gray matter structures. These deep penetrating branches are functional end arteries, and although there are anastomoses between distal branches of the cerebral and cerebellar arteries, the concept of boundary zone (i.e., watershed) ischemia is important. Global cerebral ischemia with systemic hypotension (e.g., cardiac arrest) typically produces lesions in areas where the zones of blood supply from two vessels meet—commonly between the cortical areas of distribution of the ACA, MCA, and PCA and between the superior cerebellar and posterior inferior cerebellar arteries (Fig. 2-3). However, the presence of anatomic variations may substantially modify patterns of infarction after large-vessel occlusion.

VENOUS DRAINAGE

Venous drainage (Fig. 2-4) consists of a series of external and internal veins that drain into the *venous sinuses*. The venous sinuses are endothelialized channels continuous with the endothelial surface of the veins, but they lie between folds of dura mater. They have no valves and their walls are devoid of muscular tissue. The sinuses drain into the IJVs, which are continuous with the *sigmoid sinus* at the jugular foramen. The IJV has a "bulb" at its upper end that is an enlargement in the wall of the vein. At the level of the *jugular bulb* the IJVs receive minimal venous return from extracranial tissue, and measurement of oxygen saturation (Sjvo$_2$) at this level can be used as a measure of global cerebral oxygenation. Current evidence suggests that about 70%

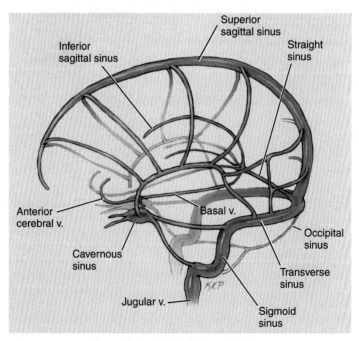

Figure 2-4   Cerebral venous drainage.

of the flow to each vein is from ipsilateral tissue, 3% from extracranial tissue, and the remainder from the contralateral hemisphere.

Many clinicians are concerned that IJV central lines will impair venous drainage from the brain and that this impairment may lead to increased bleeding into the surgical site or increased intracranial pressure in the intact skull of a susceptible patient. However, evidence to support this as being clinically relevant is weak.

MICROCIRCULATION

The architecture of the cerebral microvasculature is highly organized. Pial vessels on the surface of the brain give rise to arterioles that penetrate the brain at right angles. These arterioles give rise to capillaries at all laminar levels. Each arteriole supplies a hexagonal column of tissue, with overlapping boundary zones resulting in columnar patterns of local blood flow. This parallels the columnar arrangement seen within neuronal groups and physiologic functional units. Capillary density in adults is related to the number of synapses and can be closely correlated with the regional level of oxidative metabolism.

BLOOD-BRAIN BARRIER

The endothelial cells in cerebral capillaries contain specialized tight junctions. As a result, cerebral capillary endothelium has high electrical resistance and is relatively impermeable. Passage of substances across an intact blood-brain barrier is predominantly a function of lipid solubility and the presence of active transport systems.

The blood-brain barrier maintains tight control of ionic distribution in the extracellular fluid of the brain. Four areas, the circumventricular organs, which include the posterior pituitary gland, lie outside the blood-brain barrier.

KEY POINTS

- The brain has the highest metabolic requirement of any organ.
- The brain's arterial supply is from the carotid arteries and the vertebrobasilar system.
- The arteries anastomose in the circle of Willis.
- Venous drainage occurs through epithelealized venous sinuses draining into the internal jugular veins.
- The microcirculation is highly organized, with capillary density correlated with functional activity.
- The blood-brain barrier is maintained by the capillary endothelium and is highly impermeable.

FURTHER READING

Menon DK: Cerebral circulation. In Cardiovascular Physiology. London, BMJ Publishing, 1999.
Williams PL, (ed): Gray's Anatomy, 38th ed. Edinburgh, Churchill Livingstone, 1995.

Section II
Physiology

Chapter 3

Cerebral Blood Flow and Its Control

Jurgens Nortje

Despite its relatively small size (about 2% of total body mass), the high metabolic activity of the brain (20% of basal oxygen consumption and 25% of basal glucose consumption) requires reliable and responsive cerebral blood flow (CBF). The brain receives 15% of cardiac output (750 mL/min in adults) at rest, which equates to an *average* CBF of about 50 mL/100 g/min. Mean values for white and gray matter vary between 25 and 80 mL/100 g/min, respectively, as a result of metabolic differences. CBF therefore parallels metabolic activity and varies between 10 and 300 mL/100 g brain/min.

GLOBAL CONTROL OF CEREBRAL BLOOD FLOW

Flow-Metabolism Coupling

Transmission of electrical impulses by the brain is achieved by energy-dependent neuronal membrane ionic gradients. Increases in local neuronal activity, therefore, are accompanied by increases in the regional cerebral metabolic rate. CBF changes parallel these metabolic changes (i.e., flow-metabolism coupling). However, increases in regional CBF during functional activation tend to track the cerebral metabolic rate of glucose utilization (CMR_{gluc}) but may be far in excess of increases in the cerebral metabolic rate of oxygen consumption ($CMRO_2$). The regulatory changes involved in flow-metabolism coupling have a short latency (about 1 second) and may be mediated by regional metabolic or neurogenic pathways. In health, flow and metabolism are closely matched, with remarkably little variation in the oxygen extraction fraction across the brain despite wide regional variations in CBF and $CMRO_2$.

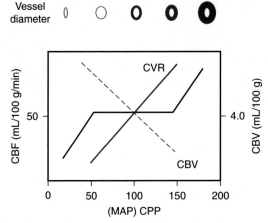

Figure 3-1 Cerebral autoregulation. Cerebrovascular resistance (CVR) changes in response to changes in cerebral perfusion pressure (CPP) to maintain stable cerebral blood flow (CBF). Cerebral vasodilation—and thus a reduction in CVR—maintains CBF during reductions in CPP. This increases cerebral blood volume (CBV), which may result in critical increases in intracranial pressure in patients with poor compliance.

Autoregulation

Autoregulation is the ability of the cerebral circulation to maintain CBF at a relatively constant level by altering cerebrovascular resistance (CVR) despite wide fluctuations in cerebral perfusion pressure (CPP) (Fig. 3-1). The interaction of CPP and CVR with CBF is illustrated by the following equation:

$$CBF = \frac{CPP}{CVR}$$

where CPP = mean arterial pressure (MAP) − (intracranial pressure [ICP] + cerebral venous pressure).

   Autoregulation of cerebral blood flow is a complex process composed of at least two mechanisms operating at different rates; a rapid response sensitive to pressure pulsations (dynamic autoregulation) followed by a slow response to changes in mean pressure (static autoregulation).

Autoregulation has limits (Fig. 3-1), above and below which CBF is directly related to CPP. These limits are usually quoted as 150 and 50 mm Hg, although there is substantial interindividual and regional variation within the brain and more current studies indicate a lower inflection point closer to a mean pressure of 75 to 80 mm Hg. The lower autoregulatory limit is the MAP at which CBF begins to decrease. Symptoms of cerebral ischemia may appear only when MAP falls below 60% of the lower limit. Above the upper limit, the high CPP causes forced dilation of cerebral arterioles with resultant increases in CBV and ICP, disruption of the blood-brain barrier, reversal of hydrostatic gradients, and cerebral edema or hemorrhage (or both).

In contrast to flow-metabolism coupling, autoregulatory responses are slower (5 to 60 seconds). These CVR changes arise as a result of myogenic reflexes in resistance vessels, but neurogenic mechanisms (i.e., sympathetic nervous system activity and metabolic factors) are probably also involved. Thus, chronic hypertension or sympathetic activation shifts the autoregulatory curve to the right, whereas sympathetic withdrawal shifts it to the left. Intracranial pathology and anesthetic agents, especially inhalational agents, may alter autoregulation.

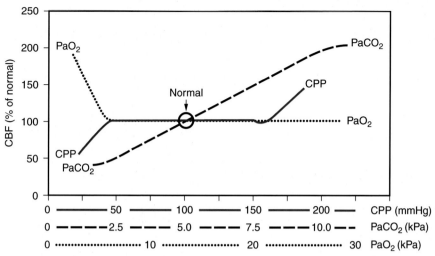

Figure 3-2 Effect of changes in gas tension on cerebral blood flow (CBF). CPP, cerebral perfusion pressure; Pa_{O_2}, arterial oxygen partial pressure; Pa_{CO_2}, arterial carbon dioxide partial pressure.

Arterial Carbon Dioxide Tension

CBF is proportional to arterial carbon dioxide tension (Pa_{CO_2}), subject to a lower limit, below which vasoconstriction results in tissue hypoxia and reflex vasodilation, and an upper limit of maximal vasodilation (Fig. 3-2).

On average, in the midphysiologic range, each 1-kPa (7.5 mm Hg) change in Pa_{CO_2} produces a change of about 15 mL/100 g/min in CBF (about 25%), which corresponds to a change of about 0.3 mL/100 g in CBV (i.e., change in CBF of 2 mL/100 g/min per 1 mm Hg Pa_{CO_2} and a change in CBV of 0.04 mL/100 g per 1mm Hg change in $PaCO_2$). In patients with low intracranial compliance, this small decrease in CBV can result in dramatic reductions in ICP. Caution should, however, be exercised when using hypocapnia (Pa_{CO_2} <4.3 kPa; 32 mm Hg) to reduce CBV because dangerously low regional CBF and resultant cerebral ischemia can develop. The effect of hypocapnia is mediated by an increase in perivascular pH, which is attenuated over time, approximately 6 hours, as extracellular fluid bicarbonate levels fall to normalize interstitial pH. This decreases the longer-term efficacy of such intervention.

Arterial Oxygen Tension and Content

Classic teaching is that CBF is unchanged until arterial oxygen tension (Pa_{O_2}) falls below about 7 kPa (53 mm Hg) (Fig. 3-2) but rises sharply with further reductions. However, recent transcranial Doppler data suggest cerebral thresholds for vasodilation as high as 8.5 kPa (about 89% to 90% oxygen saturation). This nonlinear behaviour is due to arterial oxygen content (Ca_{O_2}) governing CBF. Ca_{O_2} is related primarily to haemoglobin oxygen carriage (and thus oxygen saturation) rather than Pa_{O_2}. Because of the shape of the hemoglobin-oxygen dissociation curve, Ca_{O_2} is relatively constant over this range of Pa_{O_2}. Below about 7 kPa, CBF exhibits an inverse linear relationship with Ca_{O_2}. Hypoxemia-induced vasodilation shows little adaptation with time but may be substantially modulated by Pa_{CO_2} levels.

Kety and Schmidt showed that Pa_{O_2} greater than 15 kPa (112 mm Hg) reduces CBF by 13% and increases CVR by 1.7 to 2.2 resistance units in healthy volunteers, indicative of cerebral vasoconstriction. This has been confirmed by other techniques. This vasoconstrictor response is impaired in cerebral ischemia. The physiologic benefit of hyperoxic vasoconstriction is unclear, but it may be a mechanism by which the brain protects itself against high Pao_2 and the subsequent production of oxygen free radicals.

Other Influences

Other global factors affecting CBF include hematocrit; sympathetic tone, with β_1-adrenergic stimulation causing vasodilation and α_2-adrenergic stimulation causing vasoconstriction predominantly in the larger cerebral vessels; and elevated central venous pressure, which may elevate ICP and reduce CPP. Temperature changes CBF by about 5% per 1° C and also decreases both $CMRO_2$ and CBF, whereas autoregulation, flow-metabolism coupling, and carbon dioxide reactivity remain intact. Hyperthermia increases the utilization of oxygen and therefore CBF.

REGIONAL CONTROL OF CEREBRAL BLOOD FLOW

Metabolic Factors

Local metabolic factors affecting vascular tone are of primary importance in the regulation of regional CBF (Table 3-1). Increased metabolic activity causes increased levels of these factors, which increases perfusion, and subsequent washout of these factors then acts as a negative feedback mechanism.

Originally identified as endothelium-derived relaxant factor (EDRF), nitric oxide (NO) is synthesized from l-arginine by enzymes known as NO synthases. Under basal conditions, endothelial cells synthesize NO, which diffuses into the muscular layer and produces cyclic guanosine monophosphate (cGMP)-mediated vasodilation. NO is thought to exert a tonic dilatory influence on cerebral vessels. It mediates cerebrovascular responses to functional activation, excitatory amino acids, hypercapnia, ischemia, subarachnoid hemorrhage, and volatile anesthetic agents.

Neural Factors

Although sympathetic neural control appears to be weaker than in other vascular beds, neurogenic pathways do play a role in control of CBF, especially autoregulation. Acetylcholine, NO, and possibly 5-hydroxytryptamine (serotonin), dopamine, substance P, and neuropeptide Y are thought to be released by nerve fibers to act on cerebral vessels.

EFFECTS OF ANESTHETIC AGENTS ON CEREBRAL BLOOD FLOW

Intravenous Agents

Propofol, thiopental, and etomidate all cause global reductions in cerebral metabolism and CBF. Although autoregulation, flow-metabolism coupling, and CO_2 responsiveness remain intact even with high doses of propofol and thiopental, care should be exercised to avoid arterial hypotension, which may compromise CPP.

Inhalational Agents

Even though volatile anesthetic agents decrease $CMRO_2$, they all cause cerebral vasodilation with a resultant increase in CBF. Autoregulation is impaired in a dose-dependent fashion. Hypocapnia attenuates these effects.

Table 3-1 Factors Regulating Regional Cerebral Blood Flow

Vasoconstrictors	Vasodilators
α_2-Adrenergic stimulation	β_1-Adrenergic stimulation
Free Ca^{2+}	Nitric oxide (NO)
Thromboxane A_2 (from arachidonate)	Prostaglandins (PGE_2 and PGI_2) (increase in ECF and CSF during hypotension)
Endothelin (via endothelin A receptors in vascular smooth muscle)	Perivascular K^+ (increase in hypoxia and seizures)
	Adenosine (increase in hypotension and hypoxia)

CSF, cerebrospinal fluid; ECF, extracellular fluid.

Other Drugs

Low-dose opiates have little effect on $CMRO_2$, CBF, or ICP, with sparing of autoregulation and CO_2 responsiveness. Benzodiazepines reduce $CMRO_2$ and CBF, whereas ketamine increases $CMRO_2$, CBF, and ICP, unless concomitant hypnotics are used. Nondepolarizing neuromuscular blockers have little effect on metabolism or CBF, and the transient increases in ICP and CBF with succinylcholine are not usually clinically significant and do not preclude its use.

MEASUREMENT OF CEREBRAL BLOOD FLOW

Measurement of CBF is described in Chapter 46.

KEY POINTS

- The high metabolic rate of the brain warrants high blood flow.
- CBF may be regulated by global factors such as flow-metabolism coupling, autoregulation, $Paco_2$, Pao_2, hematocrit, and the autonomic nervous system.
- Metabolic and neural factors influence regional CBF.
- Most intravenous anesthetic agents reduce CBF.
- Inhalational anesthetic agents increase CBF through potent vasodilation.

FURTHER READING

Fitch W: Physiology of the cerebral circulation. Baillieres Clin Anaesthesiol 1999; 13:487-498.
Fox PT, Raichle ME, Mintun MA, et al: Nonoxidative glucose consumption during focal physiologic neural activity. Science 1988; 241:462-464.
Hutchinson PJ, Menon DK, Czosnyka M, et al: Monitoring cerebral blood flow and metabolism. In Reilly PL, Bullock MR (eds): Head Injury. London, Hodder Arnold, 2005, pp 215-245.
Larsen FS, Olsen KS, Hansen BA, et al: Transcranial Doppler is valid for determination of the lower limit of cerebral blood flow autoregulation. Stroke 1994; 25:1985-1988.
Lebrun-Grandie P, Baron JC, Soussaline F, et al: Coupling between regional blood flow and oxygen utilisation in the normal human brain. Arch Neurol 1983; 40:230-236.
Menon DK: The cerebral circulation. In Matta BF, Menon DK, Turner JM (eds):Textbook of Neuroanaesthesia and Critical Care, London, Greenwich, 2000, pp 17-33.
Menon DK: Cerebral circulation. In Priebe H-J, Skarvan K (eds): Cardiovascular Physiology. London, BMJ Publishing, 2000, pp 240-277.
Zauner A, Daugherty WP, Bullock MR, et al: Brain oxygenation and energy metabolism: Part I—biological function and pathophysiology. Neurosurgery 2002; 51:289-302.

Chapter 4

The Intracranial Compartment and Intracranial Pressure

Ivan Timofeev

Pressure-Volume Relationship	**Clinical Features of Raised Intracranial Pressure**
Pathophysiologic Mechanisms and Causes of Raised Intracranial Pressure	**Radiologic Signs of Intracranial Hypertension**

Intracranial pressure (ICP) is the pressure within the intracranial space relative to atmospheric pressure. At present, it can be measured only by direct invasive techniques. ICP reflects the dynamic relationship between increases or decreases in volume of the craniospinal axis and the ability of the latter to accommodate such changes. "Normal" ICP is generally less than 10 to 15 mm Hg; however, it is rarely constant and is normally subject to substantial individual variations and physiologic fluctuations, for example, with change in position, straining, and coughing. Estimation of ICP by direct measurement of cerebrospinal fluid (CSF) pressure was introduced into clinical practice by Quincke, who invented the lumbar puncture technique in 1891. In the 20th century, methodology progressed to direct ventricular catheterization, pioneered by Lundberg and colleagues, and more recently to intraparenchymal or subdural monitoring techniques.

In 1948, Kety and Schmidt demonstrated that a substantial increase in ICP may lead to a reduction in cerebral blood flow (CBF), and this finding triggered interest in estimation of cerebral perfusion pressure (CPP = mean arterial pressure [MAP] − ICP), which remains one of the cornerstones of current neurointensive care management. After the introduction of ICP monitoring into clinical practice, evidence indicating a negative association between raised ICP (>20 to 25 mm Hg) and poor outcome began to accumulate and influenced many modern neurointensive care management protocols driven by ICP and CPP targets.

PRESSURE-VOLUME RELATIONSHIP

The volume of intracranial contents is approximately 1700 mL and can be divided into three physiologic compartments:

- Brain parenchyma ≈ 1400 mL (80%, of which ≈10% is solid material and ≈70% is tissue water)
- Cerebral blood volume (CBV) ≈ 150 mL (10%)
- CSF ≈ 150 mL (10%)

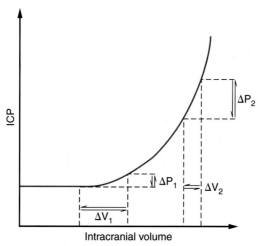

Figure 4-1 Intracranial pressure-volume relationship. Initially, additional intracranial volume is accommodated with minimal change in intracranial pressure (high compliance, $C_1 = \Delta V_1 / \Delta P_1$, "flat" part). Once this capacity is exhausted, further minimal increases in volume lead to a substantial rise in intracranial pressure (low compliance, $C_2 = \Delta V_2 / \Delta P_2$, "steep" part of the curve).

Monro and Kellie were among the first to describe the pressure-volume relationship between the intact adult skull and its contents by postulating that brain parenchyma is not compressible and therefore any flow of arterial blood into the cranium needs to be compensated by a matching outflow of venous blood if ICP is to remain constant. Later, their description was refined after recognizing the role of the CSF compartment, which can accommodate some increase in intracranial volume without a rise in pressure by altering the amount of intracranial CSF. The generalized Monro-Kellie doctrine states that *an increase in the volume of one intracranial compartment will lead to a rise in ICP unless it is matched by an equal reduction in the volume of another compartment.* Because brain parenchyma is predominantly represented by incompressible fluid, the vascular and CSF compartments play the key role in buffering additional intracranial volume by increasing venous outflow or reducing CBF and by displacing or reducing the amount of intracranial CSF. In infants, an open fontanelle provides an additional mechanism of volume compensation. Because the size of the CBV and CSF compartments is relatively small, many pathologic processes lead to increases in ICP by exceeding their compensatory capacity.

The dynamic relationship between changes in intracranial volume and pressure can be graphically presented as a "pressure-volume" curve (Fig. 4-1). It is evident from the shape of the curve that additional intracranial volume is initially accommodated with little or no change in ICP (flat part of the curve), but when craniospinal buffering capacity is exhausted (point of decompensation), further small increases in intracranial volume lead to substantial rises in ICP. Intracranial compliance can serve as measure of craniospinal compensatory reserve (position on the pressure-volume curve) and is described by the following equation, in which ΔV is change in volume and ΔP is change in pressure:

$$C = \Delta V / \Delta P$$

Cerebral compliance can be measured directly with invasive devices.

PHYSIOLOGY

PATHOPHYSIOLOGIC MECHANISMS AND CAUSES OF RAISED INTRACRANIAL PRESSURE

Progressive increases in volume of any intracranial compartment can lead to a rise in ICP. The most common mechanisms and causes of intracranial hypertension are presented in the following text. They are listed according to the involved compartment, but it should be noted that in the majority of clinical conditions characterized by high ICP, these causes and mechanisms are combined and jointly contribute to increases in ICP.

1. *Brain edema* leads to increased fluid content in brain parenchyma and has many causes. Commonly described types of brain edema are based on the underlying pathophysiologic mechanism and include the following:
   - Cytotoxic (intracellular swelling, usually caused by impaired cellular transport of ions and fluid as a result of injury or impaired energy metabolism)
   - Vasogenic (extracellular edema secondary to increased permeability of the blood-brain barrier)
   - Interstitial (tissue edema caused by osmotic or oncotic differences between plasma and cerebral tissue)
   - The predominant type of edema depends on the primary pathology, and commonly all three types are present.
2. *Increases in cerebral blood volume* are caused by a mismatch between inflow and outflow of blood, which can be due to pathologic or physiologic factors such as
   - Reduced venous outflow (mechanical obstruction of intracranial or extracranial venous structures, head-down position, obstructed ventilation, high positive end-expiratory pressure [PEEP], tight neck collar, etc.)
   - Increased CBF (loss of vascular autoregulation at low or high CPP, increase in $Paco_2$, hypoxia, acidosis, coupling to increased metabolism)
3. *Increases in intracranial CSF volume* not matched by CSF absorption usually lead to the development of hydrocephalus. The most common causes of increased CSF volume are
   - Decreased CSF absorption at the arachnoid villi—known as communicating hydrocephalus (subarachnoid hemorrhage, infection)
   - Obstruction to CSF circulation—obstructive hydrocephalus (neoplasm, traumatic and spontaneous hemorrhage, infection)
   - Increased production of CSF (meningitis, choroid plexus tumors)
4. *Intra- and extra-axial mass lesions* cause increases in ICP as a result of a direct contribution to intracranial volume. Their most common causes include
   - Neoplastic (intrinsic and extrinsic tumors)
   - Hemorrhagic
   - Traumatic (intracerebral, extradural, and subdural hematomas; contusions; CSF hygromas)
   - Infectious (abscess, subdural empyema, etc.)

Many current clinical strategies aimed at reducing ICP are based on the described pathophysiologic mechanisms, for example, correction of hypoxia and hypotension (prevention of cellular brain edema), osmotic agents (decrease in interstitial brain edema), head elevation (increase in venous outflow), moderate hyperventilation (reduction in CBF and therefore CBV via decreased $Paco_2$), sedation and muscle paralysis, hypothermia (reduction in metabolism with a coupled reduction in CBF/CBV), optimization of CPP (improvement in O_2 delivery without increasing vasogenic edema), ventriculostomy (CSF diversion), removal of mass lesions, and decompressive craniectomy (mechanical increase in intracranial volume).

28

CLINICAL FEATURES OF RAISED INTRACRANIAL PRESSURE

Common clinical symptoms of increased ICP include

- Headache caused by traction or distortion of cerebral blood vessels and dura mater. Headache is often exacerbated by recumbency, movement, and straining (lifting, coughing, sneezing). Classically, it is worse on waking up.
- Nausea and vomiting, which represent irritation of the vomiting center and vagus nucleus in the brainstem.
- Papilledema (optic disc swelling) caused by transmission of pressure through the optic nerve sheath, which is continuous with the subarachnoid space in the brain. It is a good clinical indicator of intracranial hypertension; however, it is not present in all cases of raised ICP and is often a feature of prolonged ICP elevation. Absence of papilledema does not rule out high ICP, but when present, its cause needs to be promptly investigated. Protracted papilledema may lead to visual deterioration.
- Cushing's ulcers—gastric, duodenal, or esophageal ulcers associated with elevated ICP.
- Neurologic deficits, which may point to a cause of increased ICP (e.g., mass lesion) or represent false localizing signs secondary to a generalized increase in pressure (e.g., abducens palsy caused by compression of the abducens against the base of the skull).

Progressive increases in ICP with associated brain tissue shifts may lead to

- Symptoms of brain herniation—a late feature of advanced intracranial hypertension. Transtentorial herniation is caused by a downward shift of the temporal lobe or lobes and diencephalon via the tentorial notch. With unilateral supratentorial mass lesions, compression of the oculomotor nerve nucleus and corticospinal tract in the cerebral peduncle by the temporal uncus (Kernohan's notch) is manifested as ipsilateral mydriasis and contra-lateral hemiplegia. Central or progressive unilateral transtentorial herniation leads to bilateral papillary dilation and absent light reflex, thereby preempting brainstem death. Pressure on the brainstem and cerebellum may lead to tonsillar herniation at the foramen magnum, usually manifested as respiratory or circulatory arrest.
- Cushing's triad, which is represented by increasing blood pressure, bradycardia, and widening pulse pressure. It is a sign of advanced intracranial hypertension and impending cerebral herniation but is not consistently seen.
- Respiratory problems, which may be manifested as frequent, irregular, Cheyne-Stokes breathing or apnea. Such symptoms commonly accompany high ICP and usually follow a depressed level of consciousness.

RADIOLOGIC SIGNS OF INTRACRANIAL HYPERTENSION

Computed tomography (CT) remains one of the main radiologic modalities in current neurocritical care. Despite the absence of reliable radiologic signs of elevated ICP, cranial CT helps reveal mass lesions and features of cerebral edema (Fig. 4-2). In the absence of a significant mass lesion, the following radiologic signs may point to acutely raised ICP:

- Effacement of cortical sulci and loss of gray-white matter differentiation (subtle signs of brain edema)
- Compression or complete obliteration of the cerebral ventricles or basal CSF cisterns, or both

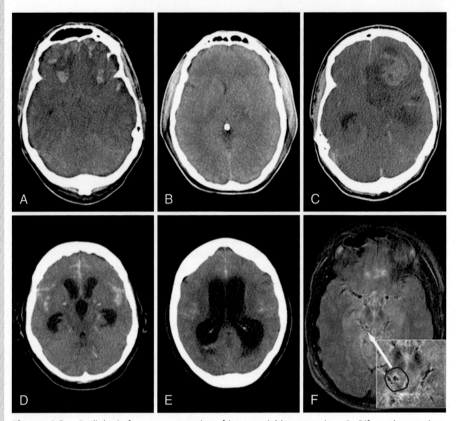

Figure 4-2 Radiologic features suggestive of intracranial hypertension. **A,** Bifrontal contusions and complete obliteration of the ambient cistern. **B,** Diffuse cerebral edema with a decrease in gray-white matter differentiation and effacement of the ventricles and sulci. **C,** Neoplastic mass lesion with surrounding edema and a mass effect causing compression of the ventricular system (note the dilated right temporal horn). **D** and **E,** Ventriculomegaly in acute hydrocephalus secondary to subarachnoid hemorrhage. **F,** Cerebral magnetic resonance imaging (MRI) may provide additional information on tissue injury. Brainstem injuries (*inset*) may be not detectable with computed tomography and could be better visualized with MRI.

- Displacement of intracranial contents (midline shift with predominantly unilateral pathology, signs of cerebral herniation)
- Presence of acute hydrocephalus (ventriculomegaly with periventricular "radiolucency," dilated temporal horns, evidence of obstruction)

Chronically raised ICP produces more subtle changes and is difficult to diagnose.

Magnetic resonance imaging provides superior spatial resolution and can therefore better delineate the pathologic changes in the brain; however, it has little advantage over CT in diagnosing raised ICP.

KEY POINTS

- ICP reflects the ability of the craniospinal axis to accommodate extra volume.
- Within a rigid skull any increase in one volume compartment needs to be matched by an equal decrease in another or ICP will rise (Monro-Kellie doctrine).
- The CSF and CBF compartments provide some buffering of increasing volume.

- Once compensatory capacity is exhausted, further small increases in volume lead to a large rise in ICP.
- The most common causes of raised ICP are mass lesions, brain edema, and increased cerebral blood or CSF volume.
- In patients with headache, altered consciousness, or papilledema, elevated ICP needs to be suspected.
- There are no pathognomonic radiologic signs of high ICP, although some features may suggest intracranial hypertension.

FURTHER READING

Cushing H: The blood-pressure reaction of acute cerebral compression, illustrated by cases of intracranial hemorrhage. Am J Med Sci 1903; 125:1017-1045.

Kellie G: An account of the appearances observed in the dissection of two of the three individuals presumed to have perished in the storm of the 3rd, and whose bodies were discovered in the vicinity of Leith on the morning of the 4th November 1821 with some reflections on the pathology of the brain. Trans Med Chir Sci 1824; 1:84-169.

Kety SS, Shenkin HA, Schmidt CF: The effects of increased intracranial pressure on cerebral circulatory functions in man. J Clin Invest 1948; 27:493-499.

Lundberg N, Troupp H, Lorin H: Continuous recording of the ventricular-fluid pressure in patients with severe acute traumatic brain injury. A preliminary report. J Neurosurg 1965; 22:581-590.

Monro A: Observations on the structure and function of the nervous system. Edinburgh, Creech & Johnson, 1823, p 5.

Marmarou A, Shulman K, LaMorgese J, Compartmental analysis of compliance and outflow resistance of the cerebrospinal fluid system. J Neurosurg 1975; 43:523-534.

Quincke H: Die Lumbalpunction des Hydrocephalus. Berl Kline Wochenschr 1891; 28:965-968. 929-923.

Rengachary SS, Ellenbogen RG (eds): Principles of Neurosurgery, 2nd ed. Edinburgh, Elsevier Mosby, 2005, p 880.

Unterberg AW, Stover J, Kress B, et al: Edema and brain trauma. Neuroscience 2004; 129:1021-1029.

4

Chapter 5

Cerebral Metabolism

Jonathan P. Coles

Mechanisms of Cerebral Metabolism
Glucose
Ketone Bodies, Organic Acids, and Amino Acids
Lactate

Flow-Metabolism Coupling

The human brain accounts for only 2% to 3% of total body weight but receives about 15% of resting cardiac output (750 mL/min) and consumes about 20% (150 μmol/100 g/min) of the oxygen and 25% (30 μmol/100 g/min) of the glucose required by the body at rest. This high energy expenditure results mainly from maintenance of transmembrane electrical and ionic gradients (≈60%), but also from maintenance of membrane structure and integrity and the synthesis and release of neurotransmitters (≈40%). Although the energy requirements of the brain are substantial, it has a very small reserve of metabolic substrates. Therefore, normal functioning of the central nervous system is highly dependent on adequate and continuous provision of energy substrates and removal of the waste products of metabolism.

MECHANISMS OF CELLULAR METABOLISM

Although the human brain has the capacity to metabolize ketones, lactate, fatty acids, glycerol, and a variety of amino acids, the conventional view is that glucose oxidation fuels the majority of the energy requirements. Indeed, the brain is the major consumer of glucose, and more than 90% of all glucose taken up by cerebral tissue is oxidized to CO_2 and water. The rest is metabolized through the pentose phosphate pathway to the reduced form of nicotinamide adenine dinucleotide phosphate (NADPH); to glycogen, galactose, and glycoprotein; or to lactate and pyruvate through glycolysis. The glycogen stores of the brain are very small and do not provide a useful reservoir of glucose. In fact, at the normal rate of adenosine triphosphate (ATP) production, the available stores of glycogen would be exhausted in less than 3 minutes.

Glucose

The body is well designed to ensure delivery of glucose to the brain and prevent falls in blood glucose levels. At rest the brain extracts about 10% of the glucose delivered within blood, but this can be increased if blood flow is decreased. In response to a decrease in blood sugar below 4 mmol/L (72 mg/dL), a set of regulatory mechanisms (glycogenolysis and gluconeogenesis) are initiated that act to restore blood glucose levels and prompt the subject to eat. However, if these initial mechanisms fail and plasma glucose levels fall below 3 mmol/L, brain function will deteriorate.

The rate-limiting step in glucose metabolism is transport of glucose into the cell. Glucose is transported via facilitated diffusion from the blood to the brain by membrane-based carrier systems. Once within the cell, glucose is metabolized through the processes of glycolysis, the citric acid cycle, and the electron transport chain. *Glycolysis* is the term given to a series of chemical reactions that occur in the cell cytoplasm and convert glucose into two molecules of pyruvic acid. This reaction results in a net gain of two molecules of ATP. In the absence of oxygen, pyruvic acid is reduced to lactic acid, which may remain within the cell for metabolism at a later date or be transported back into the bloodstream. Under aerobic conditions, pyruvic acid enters the mitochondria, where it passes through a cyclic series of reactions and is oxidized to form carbon dioxide and water. This is called the citric acid (Krebs) cycle and results in the generation of reduced coenzymes (NADH and flavin adenine dinucleotide), which contain stored energy, and guanosine triphosphate. The reduced coenzymes are oxidized by the transfer of electrons within the electron transport chain, and this generates 34 molecules of ATP. Therefore, 38 molecules of ATP can be generated from the aerobic metabolism of each molecule of glucose:

$$C_6H_{12}O_6 + 6O_2 + 38ADP + 38Pi \rightarrow 6CO_2 + 6H_2O + 38ATP$$

This is in contrast to the two molecules of ATP that can be generated under anaerobic conditions. It is clear from this summary that the energy requirements of the brain cannot be met from anaerobic metabolism alone. The brain has a high metabolic requirement for oxygen (40 to 70 mL O_2/min) that must be met by delivery within blood, which depends on the oxygen content of the blood (typically, 20 mL per 100 mL blood) and blood flow (typically, 50 mL per 100 g brain per minute). Therefore, under normal circumstances, delivery (150 mL/min) is much greater than demand (40 to 70 mL/min), and around 40% of the oxygen delivered in blood is extracted. This so-called oxygen extraction ratio (OER) or oxygen extraction fraction (OEF) can be increased for short periods when either delivery is reduced or demand is increased (see Fig. 5-1). However, if the supply of oxygen remains insufficient, the energy-requiring processes that sustain normal cellular function and integrity will fail.

Ketone Bodies, Organic Acids, and Amino Acids

Evidence of reduced responsiveness to hypoglycemia and better preservation of cerebral function after prolonged fasting suggest that the brain can use alternative substrates for metabolism, particularly after a period of adaptation. In states of prolonged starvation and in the developing brain, ketone bodies (acetoacetate and β-hydroxybutyrate) can become important metabolic substrates within the brain. In addition, some amino and organic acids can be taken up and metabolized within the brain. Overall, these are minor energy substrates except during periods of metabolic stress, such as during acute hypoglycemia and ischemia.

Lactate

The brain can consume lactate as a substrate, particularly during periods of hypoglycemia or elevated blood lactate. In fact, recent theories have suggested that lactate is produced by astrocytes and is then transferred and used by active neurons. This astrocyte-neuron lactate shuttle hypothesis (ANLSH) was proposed by Pellerin and Magistretti in 1994 and suggests a major metabolic role for brain-derived lactate as a

5

substrate for neuronal energy metabolism. This hypothesis has recently been critically debated and is currently the subject of further scientific review. Thus, although there is evidence that neurons can use lactate under certain conditions, the conventional view is that glucose is the major fuel for oxidative metabolism within active neurons.

FLOW-METABOLISM COUPLING

The brain possesses an intrinsic mechanism by which its blood supply is varied locally to match functional activity. Indeed, close matching of flow to metabolism normally results in remarkably little variation in OEF across the brain despite wide regional variations in cerebral blood flow (CBF) and oxygen metabolism ($CMRO_2$) (Fig. 5-1).

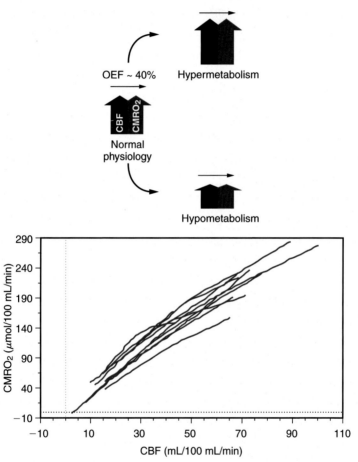

Figure 5-1 Flow-metabolism coupling. **Top,** In health, cerebral blood flow (CBF) and the cerebral metabolic rate of oxygen ($CMRO_2$) are tightly coupled such that the amount of oxygen extracted from blood is similar across the brain despite differing levels of regional metabolism. This local matching of flow to metabolic demand results in a normal oxygen extraction fraction (OEF) of approximately 40%. **Bottom,** Summary data from a group of 10 healthy controls who underwent physiologic imaging of CBF and $CMRO_2$ via [15]O positron emission tomography. The data demonstrate the close coupling between CBF and $CMRO_2$ across the healthy human brain. (Unpublished data obtained by the author within the Wolfson Brain Imaging Centre, Department of Clinical Neurosciences, University of Cambridge, UK.)

When cerebral function is depressed after coma, energy requirements are reduced and CBF, $CMRO_2$, and glucose use are decreased. Conversely, epileptiform activity or hypermetabolism associated with excitotoxicity may increase energy requirements and necessitate an increase in CBF. Anesthesia and hypothermia suppress brain metabolism and lead to coupled reductions in blood flow.

KEY POINTS

- Normal brain function is dependent on continuous delivery of oxygenated blood and energy substrates.
- Oxidation of glucose fuels the majority of energy requirements.
- CBF varies regionally to match differing metabolic needs across the brain.

FURTHER READING

Chih C-P, Roberts EL: Energy substrates for neurons during neural activity: A critical review of the astrocyte-neuron lactate shuttle hypothesis. J Cereb Blood Flow Metab 2003; 23:1263-1281.

Dienel GA: Energy generation in the central nervous system. In: Edvinsson L, Krause DN (eds): Cerebral Blood Flow and Metabolism, Philadelphia, Lippincott Williams & Wilkins, 2002.

Fitch W: Brain metabolism. In: Cottrell JE, Smith DS (eds): Anesthesia and Neurosurgery. St Louis, CV Mosby, 2001.

5

Chapter 6

Cerebral Ischemia

Piyush M. Patel

Cerebral Blood Flow and Ischemia	Apoptosis
Pathophysiologic Mechanisms	Nitric Oxide
Excitotoxicity	Inflammation
Tissue Acidosis	**Summary**

A fundamental characteristic of the central nervous system (CNS) is that despite its relatively high metabolic rate, it does not have substantial reserves of oxygen and energy substrates. The CNS is therefore intolerant of a reduction in cerebral blood flow (CBF) for all but brief periods. The pathophysiology of cerebral ischemia is complex; a wide variety of cellular processes, initiated by ischemia, have been shown to be integral to neuronal injury. Emphasis will be placed on CBF thresholds that result in specific patterns of injury, and a brief summary of the processes thought to play a major role in CNS injury is provided.

CEREBRAL BLOOD FLOW AND ISCHEMIA

Under normal circumstances, CBF is maintained at a relatively constant rate of 50 mL/100 g/min. With a reduction in cerebral perfusion pressure, CBF declines gradually. Physiologic indices of ischemia are not apparent until CBF is reduced to about 20 to 25 mL/100 g/min; at that time, electroencephalographic (EEG) slowing is apparent (Fig. 6-1). Such slowing indicates that the brain has a substantial blood flow reserve. Below a CBF of 20, the electroencephalogram is suppressed and evoked potentials are absent. It is not until the CBF is less than 10 that energy failure occurs. Neuronal depolarization, which is characterized by efflux of K^+ and influx of Ca^{2+}, follows rapidly. Once depolarized, neurons undergo death within a short time unless CBF is restored.

Cerebral ischemia is generally categorized into global ischemia and focal ischemia. The former is characterized by a global reduction in CBF (e.g., cardiac arrest). Lack of oxygen and glucose leads to energy failure, and cellular adenosine triphosphate (ATP) levels decrease dramatically within a few minutes. Neuronal injury occurs rapidly, and resuscitation becomes increasingly more difficult as the duration of ischemia increases. Not all neurons in the brain have the same vulnerability to ischemia. Neurons in the hippocampus, layer 3 of the cerebral cortex, the striatum, and the Purkinje cells of the cerebellum are more vulnerable; these neurons are referred to as *selectively vulnerable*. Upon restoration of CBF, there is a transient increase in CBF above basal levels. In several models of ischemia, postischemic hypoperfusion has

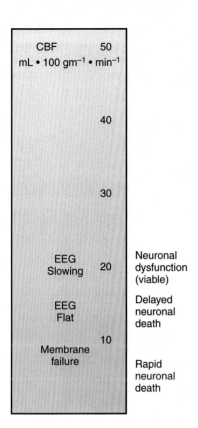

Figure 6-1 Flow thresholds for electrophysiologic dysfunction and cell death in the brain.

been described. Flow reductions of up to 50% of baseline flow, which persist for a variable period after reperfusion, contribute to neuronal injury.

Focal ischemia (e.g., stroke) is characterized by a reduction in flow of a major vessel in the brain. Within the ischemic territory, the region supplied by end arteries undergoes rapid death and is referred to as the *core*. Surrounding the core is a variable area of the brain called the penumbra. The penumbra is rendered sufficiently ischemic to be electrically silent but has not yet undergone ischemic depolarization. The penumbra is viable for several hours and can be salvaged by restoration of flow. If reperfusion is not established, the penumbra is gradually recruited into the core. A hallmark of focal ischemia is the development of brain infarction. Recent data have indicated that the size of this infarction is dynamic and a gradual increase can occur.

Cerebral edema is a frequent concomitant of ischemia. Within minutes of ischemia, flux of ions into neurons leads to uptake of water from the extracellular space. Neuronal swelling in the presence of an intact blood-brain barrier is referred to as *cytotoxic* edema. Depending on the severity of the injury, blood-brain barrier breakdown occurs about 2 to 3 days after injury. This permits the entry of plasma proteins into the brain substance, which further increases cerebral edema significantly and is called *vasogenic* edema. The development of postischemic edema can be significant enough to result in substantial increases in intracranial pressure.

The process of healing occurs over a period of weeks. Necrotic tissue is gradually resorbed and the resulting cystic cavity is lined by a glial scar. In the region surrounding the infarction, autoregulation and CO_2 reactivity are re-established in most situations in about 4 to 6 weeks.

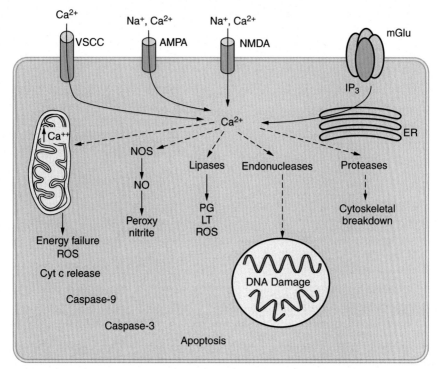

Figure 6-2 Excitotoxicity. Excessive release of glutamate leads to glutamate receptor activation, neuronal depolarization, influx of calcium, release of calcium from the endoplasmic reticulum, and unregulated enzyme activation. AMPA, α-amino-3-hydroxy-5-methyl-4-isoxazolepropionate; CBF, cerebral blood flow; Cyt c, cytochrome c; EEG, electroencephalogram; ER, endoplasmic reticulum; IP₃, inositol 1,4,5-triphosphate; LT, leukotriene; mGlu, metabotropic glutamate receptor; NMDA, N-methyl-D-aspartate; NO, nitric oxide; NOS, nitric oxide synthase; PG, prostaglandin; ROS, reactive oxygen species; VSCC, voltage-sensitive Ca^{2+} channels.

II

PATHOPHYSIOLOGIC MECHANISMS

Excitotoxicity

Energy failure is the central event in the pathophysiology of ischemia. Maintenance of normal ionic gradients across the cell membrane is an active process that requires ATP. When ATP levels reach critically low levels, ionic homeostasis is no longer maintained, and rapid influx of Na^+, efflux of K^+, and depolarization of the membrane take place (Fig. 6-2). Simultaneously, depolarization of presynaptic terminals leads to massive release of the excitatory neurotransmitter glutamate. Glutamate activates N-methyl-d-aspartate (NMDA) and α-amino-3-hydroxy-5-methyl-4-isoxazolepropionate (AMPA) glutamate receptors, the result being membrane depolarization and influx of Ca^{2+} and Na^+. Entry of Ca^{2+} via voltage-sensitive Ca^{2+} channels and release from endoplasmic reticulum via stimulation of metabotropic glutamate receptors result in an increase in intracellular Ca^{2+} to levels that are toxic to the cell. Excessive glutamate-mediated injury is referred to as *excitotoxicity*.

Calcium is a ubiquitous second messenger in cells and a cofactor required for the activation of a number of enzyme systems. A rapid, uncontrolled increase in cytosolic Ca^{2+} levels initiates the activation of a variety of cellular processes that contribute to injury.

Proteases cleave cytoskeletal proteins and other protein constituents of the neuron. Lipases attack cellular lipids and produce membrane damage. Free radicals, generated by lipid metabolism and mitochondrial injury, can lead to lipid peroxidation and membrane injury. Activation of platelets within cerebral microvessels, as well as the influx of white blood cells into damaged areas, aggravates ischemic injury by occluding the vasculature.

In neurons in which ATP production is severely compromised, death is rapid. This type of death, referred to as necrosis, is characterized by cellular swelling, nuclear pyknosis, and cell lysis. Necrosis is accompanied by a significant inflammatory response (see later).

Tissue Acidosis

In the absence of oxygen, anaerobic metabolism remains the only manner in which ATP synthesis can continue and results in the generation of lactate. The associated reduction in tissue pH can further compromise ischemic tissue. With hyperglycemia, a greater amount of substrate is available for anaerobic metabolism, and therefore the reduction in tissue pH is greater than might occur with normoglycemia. Indeed, hyperglycemia is associated with an exacerbation of ischemic cerebral injury.

Apoptosis

Programmed cell death is a cellular program in which the coordinated activation of a variety of proteases, called caspases, leads to the breakdown of key cellular constituents. Pathologically, a neuron undergoing apoptosis (or programmed cell death) manifests chromatin condensation, cell shrinkage, membrane blebbing, and apoptotic bodies. The neuron is fragmented in the later stages of the process and then resorbed. A fundamental difference between apoptosis and necrosis is that the former does not provoke inflammation whereas the latter does.

The consequences of excitotoxicity, increased intracellular concentration, acidosis, and the generation of free radicals all lead to mitochondrial injury. A key event that occurs in injured mitochondria is development of the mitochondrial permeability transition. With this transition, mitochondrial membranes undergo depolarization, and cytochrome c, an integral component of the electron transport system, is released from the space between the inner and outer mitochondrial membranes into the cytoplasm. Cytochrome c leads to the activation of caspases responsible for the proteolytic cleavage of a number of cellular constituents, thereby resulting in cell apoptosis. Inhibition of caspase 3 has been shown to be neuroprotective in a variety of experimental models of ischemia.

Apoptosis can occur relatively early during the evolution of ischemic injury. However, it can also contribute to ongoing neuronal loss for several weeks after the initial ischemia.

Nitric Oxide

A number of isoforms of nitric oxide synthase (NOS) produce NO in the setting of ischemia. Ischemia leads to the activation of neuronal NOS (nNOS) and the induction of inducible NOS (iNOS). The combination of NO and superoxide anion results in the production of peroxynitrite radical. This radical can damage cellular proteins and membranes and, importantly, DNA.

By contrast, the NO produced by endothelial NOS (eNOS) is a vasodilator. In addition, it has anti-inflammatory and antithrombotic effects. In the setting of ischemia, eNOS-produced NO maintains CBF and reduces neuronal injury. Therefore,

6

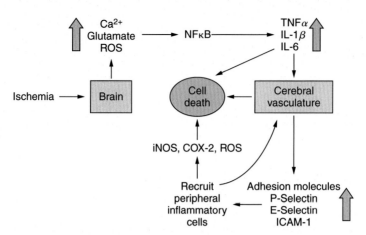

Figure 6-3 Ischemic brain inflammation. Activation of the nuclear transcription factor NFκB leads to the synthesis and subsequent release of inflammatory cytokines. Expression of adhesion molecules in cerebral vessels results in the recruitment of inflammatory cells into the brain. These inflammatory cells contribute to neuronal injury. COX-2, cyclooxygenase-2; ICAM-1, intercellular adhesion molecule-1; IL-1β, interleukin-1β; iNOS, inducible nitric oxide synthase; NFκB, nuclear factor κB; ROS, reactive oxygen species; TNF-α, tumor necrosis factor α.

NO has a dual role in the pathophysiology of cerebral ischemia: NO from nNOS and iNOS activity can enhance injury, whereas that from eNOS attenuates it. For the treatment of stroke, manipulation of specific isoforms of NOS is key.

Inflammation

Ischemia induces inflammation early in the process. Expression of adhesion molecules such as intercellular adhesion molecule (ICAM), vascular cell adhesion molecule (VCAM), and selectins on endothelial cells and the expression of integrins on leukocytes lead to the recruitment and adhesion of leukocytes in the microcirculation of the ischemic territory. In addition to occlusion of the microcirculation, leukocytes release proteolytic enzymes and free radicals, thereby augmenting injury. Efforts to block adhesion molecules reduce the influx of leukocytes into the brain and reduce injury.

Leukocytes, neurons, and glial cells also elaborate a variety of proinflammatory cytokines. These cytokines, which include interleukin-1 (IL-1), IL-6, and tumor necrosis factor α (TNF-α), mediate the inflammatory response and also serve to recruit more inflammatory cells. Cytokine receptor antagonists reduce cerebral infarction, at least in the acute phase. However, long-term suppression of these cytokines actually enhances injury. This suggests that proinflammatory cytokines, though deleterious in the *acute phase* of ischemia, are nonetheless necessary for *long-term* neuronal survival.

iNOS and cyclooxygenase-2 (COX-2), two enzymes that play a critical role in inflammation, are both activated by ischemia. The impact of iNOS activation was discussed earlier. Activation of COX-2 results in the production of injurious free radicals, as well as eicosanoids that enhance the inflammatory reaction. Inhibition of iNOS and COX-2 has been shown in experimental models to reduce injury (Fig. 6-3).

The role of microglia in CNS inflammation is gaining increasing interest. Activated microglia can elaborate proinflammatory cytokines and free radicals, both of which can increase injury. Inhibition of microglia by tetracycline has been shown

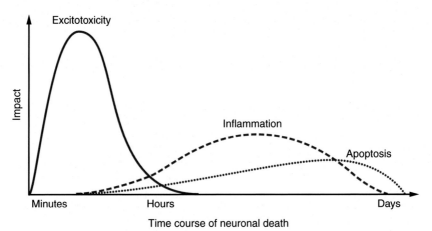

Figure 6-4 Time course of neuronal death after cerebral ischemia. Excitotoxicity rapidly leads to neuronal necrosis. Inflammation and neuronal apoptosis contribute to ongoing cell death for a period that extends from several days to weeks.

to reduce injury. Of importance is the observation that microglial activation can be observed as long as 6 months after ischemia (Fig. 6-4). This long-term inflammation in the brain has led some to characterize ischemic injury not as an acute process only but also as a chronic encephalopathic process.

SUMMARY

It is now clear that a multitude of processes contribute to neuronal injury after ischemia. Importantly, not all of these processes produce injury at the same time. Whereas necrosis occurs early in response to excitotoxicity, apoptosis and inflammation can produce ongoing neuronal loss well after the initial ischemic insult. It is therefore not surprising that attempts to reduce injury by interventions that target a single pathway have not met with success in humans. It is clear that combination therapies, each targeting a specific mechanism that is operative at specific times in the pathophysiology of stroke, are more likely to be effective. Finally, the demonstration of inflammation in the CNS as late as 6 to 8 months after ischemia in experimental models indicates that neuronal loss (and perhaps neuronal replacement through neurogenesis) is not limited to the acute phase of ischemia. As such, ischemic cerebral injury should be regarded as a chronic disease.

KEY POINTS

- Normal CBF is about 50 mL/100 g/min. EEG evidence of ischemia occurs at a CBF of 20 to 25. Below a CBF of 10, rapid neuronal death ensues.
- Focal cerebral ischemia (e.g., stroke) is characterized by a central area of severe ischemia, called the core, and a surrounding area of moderate ischemia called the penumbra. Brain infarction is a characteristic of focal ischemia.
- Global cerebral ischemia (e.g., cardiac arrest), produced by complete cessation of CBF, results in selective neuronal necrosis in the hippocampus, cortex, cerebellum, and striatum.

6

- Cytotoxic edema, a consequence of neuronal swelling, occurs early during ischemia. At later stages, breakdown of the blood-brain barrier results in the development of vasogenic edema.
- Excessive release of the excitatory neurotransmitter glutamate leads to the activation of postsynaptic glutamate receptors. The result is a massive increase in intracellular calcium concentration and unregulated activation of a number of processes that lead to neuronal death. This phenomenon is termed *excitotoxicity*.
- The development of tissue acidosis contributes to brain injury, which is of particular importance in hyperglycemic states.
- Neuronal injury is not restricted to the period of ischemia. Whereas neuronal necrosis occurs early in the pathophysiology of ischemia, delayed neuronal death occurs for a long period after ischemia. Apoptosis contributes to this delayed death.
- Influx of inflammatory cells such as leukocytes into the ischemic territory results in substantial collateral damage. Activation of astrocytes and microglia, together with the release of cytokines, augments the inflammation.
- Healing of the brain, together with restoration of cerebrovascular carbon dioxide reactivity and cerebral autoregulation, occurs over a period of 4 to 6 weeks.

FURTHER READING

Astrup J, Siesjo BK, Symon L: Thresholds in cerebral ischemia—the ischemic penumbra. Stroke 1981; 12:723-725.

Back T, Kohno K, Hossmann KA: Cortical negative DC deflections following middle cerebral artery occlusion and KCl-induced spreading depression: Effect on blood flow, tissue oxygenation, and electroencephalogram. J Cereb Blood Flow Metab 1994; 14:12-19.

Chen ST, Hsu CY, Hogan EL, et al: Thromboxane, prostacyclin, and leukotrienes in cerebral ischemia. Neurology 1986; 36:466-470.

Endres M, Laufs U, Liao JK, et al: Targeting eNOS for stroke protection. Trends Neurosci 2004; 90:281-289.

Hossmann KA: Ischemia-mediated neuronal injury. Resuscitation 1993; 26:225-235.

Polster BM, Fiskum G: Mitochondrial mechanisms of neural cell apoptosis. J Neurochem 2004; 90:1281-1289.

Rosenberg GA: Ischemic brain edema. Prog Cardiovasc Dis 1999; 42:209-216.

Siesjo BK: Pathophysiology and treatment of focal cerebral ischemia. Part I: Pathophysiology. J Neurosurg 1992; 77:169-184.

Zheng Z, Yenari MA: Post-ischemic inflammation: Molecular mechanisms and therapeutic implications. Neurol Res 2004; 26:884-892.

II

Chapter 7

Intraoperative Brain Protection

Piyush M. Patel

Influence of Anesthetics on an Ischemic Brain	Cerebral Ischemia—Influence of Physiologic Parameters
Barbiturates	Body Temperature
Volatile Anesthetics	Cerebral Perfusion Pressure
Propofol	Blood Glucose
Ketamine	Arterial Carbon Dioxide Tension
Etomidate	Seizure Prophylaxis
Summary	Summary

There is considerable risk for the occurrence of ischemic cerebral injury during neurosurgical, cardiac, and carotid artery surgery. Such risk has fostered a substantial amount of interest in identifying approaches that reduce the vulnerability of the brain to ischemia. In the present discussion, the available information about the neuroprotective efficacy of anesthetic agents and the physiologic management of a brain at risk are briefly reviewed.

INFLUENCE OF ANESTHETICS ON AN ISCHEMIC BRAIN

The approach to the problem of cerebral ischemia was initially focused on reducing the brain's requirement for energy. The rationale was that by reducing requirements for adenosine triphosphate (ATP), the brain would be able to tolerate ischemia for a longer time. Given that anesthetics suppress the cerebral metabolic rate (CMR) and, in some circumstances, increase cerebral blood flow (CBF), it is not surprising that they have been extensively investigated as potential neuroprotectant agents. Unfortunately, nearly all the evidence comes from animal studies, and very few human trials are available for guidance.

Barbiturates

Barbiturates can produce isoelectricity of the electroencephalogram, and they have been studied extensively. In the setting of *global* ischemia, barbiturates given in electroencephalographic (EEG) burst suppression doses do not reduce ischemia injury. By contrast, barbiturates can reduce the extent of *focal* cerebral injury. In humans, thiopental loading has been demonstrated in a single study to reduce post–cardiopulmonary bypass neurologic deficits. Although more recent studies in animals, in which brain temperature was rigidly controlled, have confirmed the protective efficacy of barbiturates, it should be noted that the magnitude of the protective effect is modest. In addition, high doses that produce burst suppression of the electroencephalogram may not be necessary to achieve protection; a dose of barbiturate that is approximately a third of that required to achieve EEG suppression can yield a reduction in injury that is of similar magnitude to that achieved with much larger doses. Note should be made of the fact that long-term neuro protection with barbiturates has not yet been demonstrated.

Volatile Anesthetics

A large number of animal investigations have shown that the volatile agents halothane, isoflurane, sevoflurane, and desflurane can reduce cerebral injury in the setting of focal ischemia. This protective efficacy of volatile agents is as large as that of barbiturates. However, there does not appear to be a substantial difference among the agents.

In most experimental studies of volatile anesthetic neuroprotection, injury was evaluated a few days after the ischemic insult. In a postischemic brain, neurons continue to die for a long period after the initial ischemic insult. Therefore, therapeutic strategies that are neuroprotective after short recovery periods may not produce long-lasting neuroprotection because of the continual loss of neurons in the postischemic period. Volatile anesthetics do produce neuroprotection for short periods. However, this protection is not sustained beyond 2 weeks with *moderate* and *severe* insults, which suggests that volatile anesthetics delay but do not prevent neuronal death. By contrast, in models of *very mild* focal ischemia, sustained neuroprotection with sevoflurane can be achieved. These data suggest that volatile agents can produce long-term neuroprotection *provided that the severity of injury is very mild*. Once even a small amount of neuronal injury occurs, infarct expansion will preclude long-term neuroprotection.

Propofol

Propofol shares a number of properties with barbiturates. In particular, propofol can also produce burst suppression of the electroencephalogram, thereby reducing $CMRO_2$ by up to 50%. Experimental studies have shown that propofol can substantially reduce the ischemic injury produced by stroke; its efficacy is similar to that of barbiturates and volatile anesthetics. Like volatile agents, propofol neuroprotection is not sustained with moderate to severe insults. With mild insults, sustained neuroprotection has been demonstrated.

Ketamine

Ketamine is a potent *N*-methyl-d-aspartate (NMDA) receptor antagonist. In models of focal ischemia, substantial neuroprotection has been demonstrated with the administration of ketamine. The adverse neuropsychiatric side effects of ketamine, however, have restricted its clinical use for neuroprotection.

Etomidate

Etomidate can reduce $CMRO_2$ by up to 50% by producing EEG burst suppression. Unlike barbiturates, etomidate is cleared rapidly and does not cause myocardial depression or hypotension. These properties make etomidate an ideal agent for purposes of neuroprotection. However, in human investigations of focal ischemia, administration of etomidate leads to a greater degree of tissue acidosis and hypoxia than noted with desflurane anesthesia. The detrimental effects of etomidate have been confirmed in experimental studies, which have shown that brain injury actually *increases* after the administration of etomidate. This injury-enhancing effect of etomidate has been attributed to its ability to reduce nitric oxide levels in ischemic brain tissue. Because nitric oxide is thought to be important in the maintenance of blood flow during ischemia, it is conceivable that etomidate might increase the severity of ischemia.

Summary

Collectively, the available data indicate that barbiturates can protect the brain and that doses required to achieve this protection may well be less than those that produce EEG burst suppression. Similarly, protection may also be achieved with clinically relevant concentrations of volatile anesthetics ($\approx$1 minimal alveolar concentration [MAC]) and with propofol. The available data indicate that it is the anesthetized state per se rather than the choice of specific anesthetics that reduces the vulnerability of the brain to ischemic injury.

CEREBRAL ISCHEMIA—INFLUENCE OF PHYSIOLOGIC PARAMETERS

Physiologic parameters such as mean arterial pressure (MAP), $Paco_2$, blood glucose, and body temperature have a significant influence on outcome after cerebral ischemia. In this section, information regarding the effect of these parameters on an ischemic brain is summarized. When possible, specific management recommendations have been suggested.

Body Temperature

Experimental studies have shown that a reduction in temperature of only a few degrees ($\approx$33° C to 34° C) can dramatically reduce the brain's vulnerability to ischemic injury. In light of these compelling experimental data, induction of mild hypothermia in the operating room has been advocated. Proponents of its use argue that hypothermia is readily achieved and is not accompanied by significant myocardial depression or arrhythmias. In addition, the patient can be readily rewarmed in the operating room after the risk of ischemia has subsided. However, in a multicenter trial mild hypothermia did not result in either short- or long-term improvement in neurologic outcome after cerebral aneurysm surgery. This finding is similar to that of another multicenter trial of hypothermia in head-injured patients that also did not show benefit. These important outcome studies have forced re-evaluation of the use of mild hypothermia in the operating room. Data do not favor the routine use of mild hypothermia for unruptured aneurysms and for grade I and II subarachnoid hemorrhage (SAH). However, for higher-grade SAH, the question of whether hypothermia should be applied remains to be answered.

In contrast, increases in brain temperature during and after ischemia aggravate injury. An increase of as little as 1° C can dramatically increase injury. Ischemia that normally results in scattered neuronal necrosis produces cerebral infarction when body temperature is elevated. It therefore seems prudent to avoid hyperthermia in patients who have suffered an ischemic insult or those who are risk for cerebral ischemia.

Cerebral Perfusion Pressure

CBF is normally autoregulated over a cerebral perfusion pressure (CPP) range of 60 to 150 mm Hg. In most patients, maintenance of CBF can be ensured with a CPP in excess of 60 mm Hg. The question is whether this CPP is adequate to maintain perfusion in a brain that has undergone ischemic injury. The ideal CPP in such patients has not been adequately studied. In head-injured patients, however, a higher than normal CPP is required to maintain normal CBF. Although optimal CPP should be tailored to the individual, a CPP of 60 to 70 mm Hg is adequate in head-injured patients (see Chapter 34). A CPP of 70 mm Hg is therefore a reasonable goal in patients who have undergone an ischemic insult, provided that the results of Chan and colleagues can be applied to such patients. In hypertensive patients, the lower limit of autoregulation is shifted to the right and higher CPP may be required. Maintenance of CPP that is close to the patient's normal baseline pressure is prudent.

By contrast, hypotension has been shown to be quite deleterious to an injured (ischemic or traumatic) brain. Hypotension can increase cerebral infarct volumes significantly and should be avoided in patients who have suffered a stroke. Similarly, hypotension has been demonstrated to be one of the most important contributors to a poor outcome in patients who have sustained head injury. Maintenance of adequate MAP and CPP is therefore critical. Elevation of MAP by α-agonists is reasonable.

Blood Glucose

In a normal brain that is adequately perfused, glucose is metabolized aerobically. When the brain is rendered ischemic, oxygen is no longer available and aerobic metabolism of glucose is inhibited. Glucose is then metabolized anaerobically through glycolysis. The end products of this pathway are lactic acid and ATP. The lactic acid produced contributes to the acidosis that occurs in many ischemic tissues.

Because the brain does not have glucose stores, the extent of lactic acidosis is limited. However, during hyperglycemia, the supply of glucose to the brain is increased. In this situation the amount of lactic acid produced is considerable and cerebral pH decreases. This acidosis contributes significantly to neuronal necrosis. Preexisting hyperglycemia has been shown to be associated with increased neurologic injury. As a corollary, treatment of hyperglycemia with insulin has been shown to reduce neurologic injury. Consequently, it has been suggested that hyperglycemia be treated in patients at risk for cerebral ischemia and in those who have suffered an ischemic insult. What is not certain is the threshold level of glucose beyond which treatment is indicated. Based on the available data, treatment of a blood glucose level above 150 mg/dL is reasonable. Of equal importance is prevention of hypoglycemia; frequent measurement of blood glucose levels is essential.

Arterial Carbon Dioxide Tension

Manipulation of arterial carbon dioxide tension is a potent means of altering CBF and cerebral blood volume (CBV). Hypocapnia can reduce CBF, CBV, and intracranial pressure (ICP). Hence, hyperventilation is often used in patients with expanding mass lesions and intracranial hypertension and in the operating room to produce brain relaxation. The advantages of short-term temporary use of hyperventilation are readily apparent.

A significant concern about hypocapnia in patients with ischemic or traumatic central nervous system injury is whether a reduction in blood flow can enhance injury. Prophylactic hyperventilation has not been shown to be of any benefit in patients with stroke. In fact, laboratory data have shown that hypocapnia can significantly decrease CBF in an ischemic brain; the net result is an increase in the amount of brain tissue in which the reduction in flow is severe (and within what is considered to be ischemia). In the setting of head injury, the application of prophylactic hyperventilation is associated with a worse outcome 3 and 6 months after injury. In such patients, the regions of the brain that are ischemic increase dramatically with hypocapnia. Based on these data, the Brain Trauma Foundation has recommended that prophylactic hyperventilation be avoided during the early stages after head injury.

Hyperventilation is not entirely innocuous and should be treated like other therapeutic interventions. It should be applied with an understanding of its complications. In the setting of head injury and cerebral ischemia, it has the potential to enhance injury. If applied, hyperventilation should be terminated when the intended goal has been achieved or is no longer necessary.

Seizure Prophylaxis

Seizures commonly occur in patients with intracranial pathology. Seizure activity is associated with increased neuronal activity, increased CBF and CBV (and consequently increased ICP), and cerebral acidosis. Untreated seizures can actually produce neuronal necrosis even with normal cerebral perfusion. Prevention plus rapid treatment of seizures is therefore an important goal (see Chapter 38).

Summary

At present, our ability to pharmacologically protect the brain and make it less vulnerable to ischemic injury is limited. In the operating room, our capacity to exacerbate brain injury, by contrast, is almost unlimited. Therefore, emphasis should be placed on maintenance of physiologic homeostasis rather than on pharmacologic interventions for purposes of brain protection.

KEY POINTS

- An anesthetized brain is less vulnerable to ischemic injury. There do not appear to be any differences among anesthetic agents with respect to their neuroprotective efficacy.
- Barbiturates, propofol, and ketamine have been shown to have neuroprotective efficacy. With regard to barbiturates, doses less than those that produce burst suppression of the electroencephalogram achieve the same degree of protection as higher doses do.
- All volatile anesthetics reduce the vulnerability of the brain to ischemic injury. There are no differences among the volatile anesthetics with respect to their neuroprotective efficacy.
- Maintenance of CPP within the normal range for a patient who is at risk for cerebral ischemic injury is essential. Modest increases in blood pressure (5% to 10%) may be of benefit to those who have suffered from an ischemic insult. Hypotension is deleterious.
- Arterial P_{CO_2} should be maintained in the normal range unless hyperventilation is used for short-term brain relaxation. Prophylactic hyperventilation should be avoided.
- Hyperglycemia exacerbates ischemic injury and should be treated with insulin. A reasonable threshold for treatment is 150 mg/dL. If insulin treatment is initiated, blood glucose should be closely monitored and hypoglycemia prevented.
- The routine induction of mild hypothermia for low-grade aneurysm clipping and for head injury may not be of benefit. In high-grade patients, the utility of mild hypothermia for purposes of brain protection remains to be defined. Hyperthermia should be treated.

PHYSIOLOGY

- Seizures can augment cerebral injury and should be treated with anticonvulsants.
- Our ability to protect the brain is limited. By contrast, our capacity to exacerbate ischemic brain damage is limitless. Emphasis should be placed on maintenance of physiologic homeostasis rather than on reliance on pharmacologic agents to protect the brain.

FURTHER READING

Bruno A, Levine SR, Frankel MR, et al: Admission glucose level and clinical outcomes in the NINDS rt-PA Stroke Trial. Neurology 2002; 59:669-674.

Chan KH, Dearden NM, Miller JD, et al: Multimodality monitoring as a guide to treatment of intracranial hypertension after severe brain injury. Neurosurgery 1993; 32:547-552.

Clifton GL, Miller ET, Choi SC, et al: Lack of effect of induction of hypothermia after acute brain injury. N Engl J Med 2001; 344:556-563.

Kawaguchi M, Furuya H, Patel PM: Neuroprotective effects of anesthetic agents. J Anesth 2005; 19:150-156.

Marzan AS, Hungerbuhler HJ, Studer A, et al: Feasibility and safety of norepinephrine-induced arterial hypertension in acute ischemic stroke. Neurology 2004; 62:1193-1195.

Todd MM, Hindman BJ, Clarke WR, et al: Mild intraoperative hypothermia during surgery for intracranial aneurysm. N Engl J Med 2005; 352:135-145.

The Brain Trauma Foundation: The American Association of Neurological Surgeons. The Joint Section on Neurotrauma and Critical Care. Hyperventilation. J Neurotrauma 2000; 17:513-520.

Warner DS, Takaoka S, Wu B, et al: Electroencephalographic burst suppression is not required to elicit maximal neuroprotection from pentobarbital in a rat model of focal cerebral ischemia. Anesthesiology 1996; 84:1475-1484.

Section III
Pharmacology

Chapter 8

Intravenous Anesthetic Agents

Anthony Absalom • Tamsin Poole

Propofol	Ketamine
Thiopental	Benzodiazepines
Etomidate	Total Intravenous Anesthesia

The mechanism of action of all anesthetic agents is currently under intense investigation. With the exception of ketamine, which acts via antagonism of the excitatory receptor N-methyl-D-aspartate (NMDA), most intravenous anesthetic agents (such as propofol, thiopental, and etomidate) probably act by an agonist effect at the γ-aminobutyric acid A ($GABA_A$) receptor that causes an increase in the duration of opening of $GABA_A$-dependent chloride channels. The increased channel-opening time permits increased passage of chloride ions, which causes membrane hyperpolarization and therefore inhibition of neuronal transmission. It is likely that each agent binds to a separate site on the $GABA_A$ receptor and that the different effects of each drug (such as amnesia, sedation, and hypnosis) are mediated by distinct subunits of the receptor. Although current evidence favors involvement of the $GABA_A$ receptor, it is likely that intravenous anesthetic agents also have significant effects on other receptors and ion channels.

Benzodiazepines have sedative rather than hypnotic effects. They also act at the $GABA_A$ receptor by binding to the α subunit of the activated receptor. Two subtypes of benzodiazepine receptors have thus far been identified. BZ_1 is responsible for anxiolysis, and the receptors are located mainly in the cerebellum and spinal cord. BZ_2 receptors facilitate the anticonvulsant and sedative effects of benzodiazepines. They are located in the cerebral cortex, hippocampus, and spinal cord.

Functional imaging studies using techniques such positron emission tomography and functional magnetic resonance imaging show that although intravenous anesthetic agents can have similar clinical effects, they cause distinct (and very different) effects on *regional* blood flow and metabolism. Nonetheless, as will be seen later, with the exception of ketamine they all cause *global* reductions in cerebral blood flow (CBF) and metabolism.

Although intravenous anesthetic agents cause slowing of the surface electroencephalogram, the only exception being ketamine, there are agent-specific differences that are discernible to an expert or expert system. In general, the agents other than ketamine cause a dose-dependent progressive shift of power from the higher to the lower frequencies. At deep levels of anesthesia, a burst suppression pattern occurs. With increasing levels of suppression, fewer bursts occur, and finally at excessively deep levels of anesthesia or overdose, an isoelectric pattern will be found.

8

An "ideal" intravenous anesthetic agent for use in neuroanesthesia and neurocritical care should possess certain properties. Such an agent would

- Allow rapid recovery of consciousness to permit early assessment of neurologic status
- Be easily and rapidly titratable
- Have minimal effects on other organ systems
- Provide analgesia
- Be nonepileptogenic (or even have antiepileptic properties)
- Have advantageous effects on cerebral hemodynamics, in particular,
  Maintenance of cerebrovascular autoregulation
  Maintenance of vasoreactivity to CO_2
  Prevention of increases in cerebral blood volume (CBV)
  Reduction of the cerebral metabolic rate (CMR) coupled with a decrease in CBF
  No increase in intracranial pressure (ICP) or even a reduction in ICP

No agent currently available fulfills all of these criteria. The agents most commonly used for induction of anesthesia for neurosurgery are propofol, thiopental, and etomidate. Although all three agents can induce anesthesia, they have distinct advantages and disadvantages, particularly during neurosurgery.

PROPOFOL

Propofol is now the most widely used agent for intravenous induction and maintenance of anesthesia during neurosurgical procedures. It has also recently been used successfully for providing conscious sedation during awake craniotomy.

Propofol provides smooth induction of anesthesia with minimal excitatory effects and rapid, clear-headed recovery. Although there have been case reports of convulsions, most are believed to be "pseudoseizures" because they have not been found to be associated with abnormal electroencephalographic (EEG) activity. Propofol is generally regarded as having anticonvulsive effects and is sometimes used to treat refractory status epilepticus. It causes a dose-dependent reduction in arterial blood pressure, which may in turn compromise cerebral perfusion pressure (CPP).

With regard to neuroanesthesia, propofol

- Produces a progressive reduction in CBF coupled to a reduction in $CMRO_2$
- Produces a reduction in ICP, particularly in patients with elevated baseline ICP
- Maintains cerebral autoregulation
- Maintains the responsiveness of the cerebral circulation to CO_2
- Provides protection against focal ischemia in animals
- Has free radical–scavenging properties (greater than thiopental)
- Has calcium channel–blocking and glutamate antagonist properties (in vitro)

THIOPENTAL

Thiopental is the only barbiturate that remains in widespread clinical use. It is still an important agent in the neurocritical care setting for its role in reducing ICP in head-injured patients and those whose intracranial hypertension is refractory to other treatments. This effect is achieved by reduction of $CMRO_2$ to minimal levels in conjunction with an isoelectric electroencephalogram. However, when thiopental is given by prolonged infusion, hepatic enzyme saturation changes its metabolism from a first-order to a zero-order process, which together with a very large volume of distribution, causes accumulation. Accumulation of thiopental may result in extended elimination times and very delayed recovery.

Thiopental

- Produces a reduction in CBF coupled to a decrease in $CMRO_2$
- Causes a decrease in CBV
- Causes a decrease in ICP
- Provides protection against focal ischemia in animals
- Possesses free radical–scavenging properties
- Reduces calcium influx
- Probably also causes blockade of sodium channels
- Provides treatment of status epilepticus

ETOMIDATE

Etomidate remains a drug of interest because of its cardiovascular stability on induction of anesthesia, which may be relevant when maintenance of CPP is vital. It has similar effects on CBF, $CMRO_2$, and autoregulation as thiopental and propofol. However, it is a potent suppressant of corticosteroid synthesis, an effect that may occur after a single dose, particularly in critically ill patients. For this reason the widespread use of etomidate has declined.

In susceptible patients, seizures may be elicited with low-dose etomidate (6 to 10 mg). It has therefore been used to unmask seizure foci during operative EEG mapping for epilepsy surgery.

KETAMINE

Ketamine is an antagonist at NMDA receptors. The use of ketamine in neuroanesthesia has been limited because of the perception that it raises ICP. Additionally, its side effects include nightmares and hallucinations.

Ketamine causes

- Increased CBF (but not when used with other sedatives or in a brain-injured patient)
- Increased ICP (but not when used with other sedatives or in a brain-injured patient)
- Specific increases in regional CMR and CBF in limbic structures
- Cerebral protection via NMDA antagonism in animals

BENZODIAZEPINES

The use of benzodiazepines may be associated with prolonged sedation, which limits their use as induction agents for neuroanesthesia. However, at lower doses, benzodiazepines may be of use for premedication before induction of anesthesia. They are also useful agents for sedation in the intensive care unit, particularly in head-injured patients in whom hypothermia is being used and when propofol administration is inadvisable (e.g., hypothermia causes impaired propofol metabolism and lipid accumulation).

53

Benzodiazepines

- Cause a modest reduction in CBF
- Cause a modest reduction in $CMRO_2$
- Cause a modest reduction in ICP
- Preserve vasoreactivity to CO_2
- Preserve cerebral autoregulation
- Increase the seizure threshold

However, a plateau effect occurs whereby increasing doses do not produce greater reductions in these variables. All effects are reversed by flumazenil, a competitive benzodiazepine. The use of flumazenil may precipitate seizures.

TOTAL INTRAVENOUS ANESTHESIA

The use of intravenous induction agents for maintenance of anesthesia is becoming increasingly popular. Propofol is the agent most suited to prolonged infusion because its context-sensitive half-time does not increase appreciably with time. Therefore, after prolonged infusion, there is relatively rapid return of consciousness, which facilitates assessment of neurologic status.

Remifentanil is a pure μ-receptor agonist. It possesses ester linkages that are degraded by nonspecific tissue and plasma esterases. It has a constant context-sensitive half-time, thus making it ideal for use in addition to propofol for maintenance of anesthesia, allowing good analgesia and muscle relaxation during the surgery, but minimizing the postoperative sedation, nausea, and vomiting that may occur with longer-acting opiates. Provision of alternative adequate postoperative analgesia (e.g., morphine, 0.05 to 0.1 mg/kg, or fentanyl, 1 to 1.5 μg/kg) is essential in situations in which pain is likely.

Both propofol and remifentanil can be used by simple infusion for maintenance of anesthesia. Usual dose ranges are 3 to 12 mg/kg/hr for propofol and 0.05 to 0.5 μg/kg/min for remifentanil. With the development of commercially available microprocessor-controlled infusion pumps, propofol and remifentanil can now be given by target-controlled infusion (TCI) for both induction and maintenance of anesthesia. The pumps require that the patient's weight and age be entered and then calculate the appropriate infusion rate according to an estimated plasma concentration from internal algorithms based on a three-compartment model. Usual target propofol levels are 4 to 6 μg/mL for induction and 2 to 4 μg/mL for maintenance. The use of TCI systems has been shown to result in improved hemodynamic stability, particularly during induction of anesthesia, and this is particularly beneficial in neurosurgical procedures.

KEY POINTS

- Propofol, thiopental, and etomidate have similar effects on overall cerebral hemodynamics and metabolism.
- All three agents reduce $CMRO_2$ and maintain responsiveness to CO_2 and autoregulation.
- Ketamine may be associated with an increase in CBF and ICP in the absence of other sedatives.
- Benzodiazepines have a small effect on blood flow and metabolism.
- Propofol and remifentanil are ideal agents for continuous infusion for maintenance of anesthesia. They allow rapid return of consciousness and assessment of neurologic status despite prolonged infusion.

FURTHER READING

Absalom AR, Pledger DR, Kong A: A single dose of etomidate may be associated with adrenal suppression for 24 hours in the critically ill. Anaesthesia 1999; 54:861-867.

Absalom AR, Struys MR: An Overview of TCI and TIVA, Belgium, Gent, Academic Press, 2005.

Hemmings HC Jr, Akabas MH, Goldstein PA, et al: Emerging molecular mechanisms of general anesthetic action, Trends Pharmacol Sci 2005; 26:503-510.

Marik PE, Varon J: The management of status epilepticus. Chest 2004; 126:582-591.

Petersen KD, Landsfeldt U, Cold GE, et al: Intracranial pressure and cerebral hemodynamic in patients with cerebral tumors: A randomized prospective study of patients subjected to craniotomy in propofol-fentanyl, isoflurane-fentanyl, or sevoflurane-fentanyl anesthesia. Anesthesiology 2003; 98:329-336.

Ravussin P, Guiard JP, Ralley F, Thorin D: Effect of propofol on cerebrospinal fluid pressure and cerebral perfusion pressure in patients undergoing craniotomy. Anaesthesia 1988; 43(Suppl):37-41.

Ravussin P, Tempelhoff R, Modica PA, et al: Propofol vs thiopental-isoflurane for neurosurgical anesthesia: Comparison of hemodynamics, CSF pressure, and recovery. J Neurosurg Anesthesiol 1991; 3:85-95.

Sneyd JR: Propofol and epilepsy. Br J Anaesth 1999; 82:168-169.

8

Chapter 9

Volatile Anesthetic Agents

Olga Afonin • Adrian W. Gelb

Common Effects of Inhaled Anesthetic Agents
Nitrous Oxide
Isoflurane
Desflurane
Sevoflurane

Volatile anesthetics are frequently an integral part of anesthesia for complex neuro-surgical procedures. They can have profound effects on neurophysiologic processes, both desirable and adverse, and knowing these effects allows tailoring of the optimal anesthetic regimen for the patient and neurosurgical needs.

COMMON EFFECTS OF INHALED ANESTHETIC AGENTS

Volatile anesthetics affect cerebral vascular tone by both a reduction in the cerebral metabolic rate (CMR) and a direct vasodilatory effect. All cause a dose-dependent decrease in oxygen consumption ($CRMO_2$) as a result of the reduction in cerebral activity, and this decrease is approximately the same for all the currently used agents. This metabolic depression leads to a reduced need for substrate and therefore an associated vasoconstriction, which initially balances the direct vasodilator effect. However, as the concentration increases above 0.6 minimal alveolar concentration (MAC), direct vasodilating effects start to predominate over vasoconstriction. At 1 MAC, desflurane produces the greatest vasodilation, then isoflurane, and sevo-flurane exhibits the least. The dilation results in an increase in cerebral blood flow (CBF). This increase in blood flow in the face of a reduction in metabolism is frequently referred to "uncoupling." However, experimental data indicate that although flow has been reset to a higher level, it will still track metabolic changes appropriately (i.e., it is a resetting rather than an uncoupling).

Normally, cerebral autoregulation preserves CBF at a relatively constant rate despite changes in perfusion pressure. This is mediated through vascular responses to local metabolic, neurogenic, stretch, and endothelial mechanisms. Inhaled anes-thetic agents progressively impair autoregulation at greater than 0.5 MAC, with the exception of sevoflurane. At 1 to 1.5 MAC sevoflurane cerebrovascular autoregula-tion is still intact, although the fast dynamic component is slightly impaired. When autoregulation is abolished, blood flow passively follows blood pressure, thus making ischemia or luxury perfusion with edema or hemorrhage more likely.

Vascular changes in response to Pa_{CO_2} are preserved, and hypocapnia may (partially) overcome the drug-induced vasodilation. The reduced blood flow with hyperventilation has been associated with increased O_2 extraction, evidence of (potential) ischemia, and a worse outcome in head trauma. Common clinical practice is to apply a $PaCO_2$ of 32 to 35 mmHg, when a vapor is being used.

Vasodilation also increases cerebral blood volume, which increases intracranial volume and can increase intracranial pressure (ICP). This is particularly concerning in patients with a space-occupying intracranial lesion or cerebral edema. Isoflurane, desflurane, and sevoflurane all increase ICP, with sevoflurane having the least effect. All also reduce mean arterial pressure (MAP) and therefore cerebral perfusion pressure in a dose-dependent manner.

All inhaled anesthetics cause a progressive, dose-dependent slowing of the electrocardiogram (EEG) and eventually isoelectricity. They also cause a progressive increase in latency and a decrease in the amplitude of motor evoked potential (MEP), somatosensory evoked potential (SSEP), brainstem auditory evoked potential (BAEP), and visual evoked potential (VEP) responses in a dose-dependent manner. MEP and VEP are the most sensitive and BAEP the least.

Most anesthetic agents exhibit neuroprotective properties in rodents, but there are no human studies to support their use for such an indication in clinical practice.

Nitrous Oxide

Nitrous oxide (N_2O), when given on its own, has stimulatory effects that result in an increase in $CMRO_2$ and CBF. The vasodilation can be partially or completely attenuated by hypocapnia or combination with an anesthetic that also reduces CBF, such as propofol, barbiturate, or midazolam. There is synergism between N_2O and other volatile anesthetics in the increase in CBF, and as such this combination should not be used in patients with critically increased ICP. Autoregulation is not altered by N_2O.

N_2O expands air-filled spaces, can cause worsening of pneumocephalus, and should therefore be avoided in any situation in which a closed intracranial gas space may exist.

Isoflurane

In low doses, isoflurane decreases $CRMO_2$ and has minimal effect on CBF at less than 0.6 MAC, but it increases CBF by about 20% at 1.1 MAC. Autoregulation is impaired by 1.0 MAC. A dose-dependent vasodilation thus occurs that can increase ICP. By 2 MAC the EEG is isoelectric.

Desflurane

Desflurane has effects on CBF, $CRMO_2$, and autoregulation similar to those of isoflurane (i.e., metabolic suppression with dose-dependent increasing vasodilation). Autoregulation is lost at greater than 1 MAC. Experimentally, it is the only commonly used vapor that alters cerebrospinal fluid (CSF) dynamics in that it increases CSF production. This effect may be of consequence with a closed cranium, but with a craniotomy it is probably of minimal importance. The vasodilation, perhaps together with the altered CSF production, increases ICP.

An advantage over isoflurane is its low blood/gas partition coefficient, which enables one to more rapidly titrate desflurane to the patient's needs, level of surgical stimulation, or neuromonitoring requirements. In addition, the desflurane-associated sympathetic stimulation may be helpful in maintaining blood pressure and cerebral perfusion pressure.

Sevoflurane

Sevoflurane is less vasoactive than the other inhaled anesthetics. Although the initial animal studies found that sevoflurane was similar to isoflurane in its effects on CBF, the experience in patients is that it causes less intrinsic vasodilation and does not increase CBF until greater than 1 MAC. ICP does not increase until greater than 1 to 1.5 MAC, and autoregulation remains intact at these concentrations.

Spiking or seizure-like changes on the EEG have been seen in adults and children, especially those taking anticonvulsive medications, patients with a history of febrile convulsion, or during inhalational induction with high concentrations of sevoflurane. No enduring sequelae are currently evident. Sevoflurane anesthesia is thought to be safe in seizure-prone patients as long as hyperventilation is avoided and the sevoflurane dose is less than 1.5 MAC.

Decreased pungency and lesser effects on ICP in comparison to other inhaled anesthetics make sevoflurane the best agent for inhalational induction in pediatric patients or adults. A low blood/gas partition coefficient allows more rapid changes in depth of anesthesia than is the case with isoflurane.

Up to 40% of preschool children experience emergence agitation after sevoflurane anesthesia. Agitation could potentially increase $CRMO_2$, MAP, CBF, and ICP. It can be prevented by small doses of clonidine, dexmedetomidine, or propofol or by switching to another vapor for surgical closure.

KEY POINTS

- All inhaled vapors decrease cerebral metabolism.
- All inhaled vapors are cerebral vasodilators, but at differing concentrations.
- Desflurane and isoflurane produce more vasodilation than sevoflurane does.
- The vasodilation is associated with increases in CBF, blood volume, and ICP.
- The vasodilation progressively impairs autoregulation.
- Hypocapnia (partially) prevents the vasodilation.
- There are no human outcome data to substantiate neuroprotection by vapors.

FURTHER READING

Constant I, Seeman R, Murat I: Sevoflurane and epileptiform EEG changes. Pediatr Anesth 2005; 15:266-274.

Engelhard K, Werner C: Inhalational or intravenous anesthetics for craniotomies? Pro inhalational. Curr Opin Anaesthesiol 2006; 19:504-508.

Holmstrom A, Akeson J: Sevoflurane induces less cerebral vasodilation than isoflurane at the same A-line autoregressive index level. Acta Anaesthesiol Scand 2005; 49:16-22.

Kaisti KK, Langsjo JW, Aalto S, et al: Effects of sevoflurane, propofol, and adjunct nitrous oxide on regional cerebral blood flow, oxygen consumption, and blood volume in humans. Anesthesiology 2003; 99:603-613.

Petersen KD, Landsfeldt U, Cold GE, et al: Intracranial pressure and cerebral hemodynamic in patients with cerebral tumors: A randomized prospective study of patients subjected to craniotomy in propofol-fentanyl, isoflurane-fentanyl, or sevoflurane-fentanyl anesthesia. Anesthesiology 2003; 98:329-336.

Sponheim S, Skraastad O, Helseth E, et al: Effects of 0.5 and 1.0 MAC isoflurane, sevoflurane and desflurane on intracranial and cerebral perfusion pressures in children. Acta Anaesthesiol Scand 2003; 47:932-938.

Strebel S, Lam AM, Matta B, et al: Dynamic and static cerebral autoregulation during isoflurane, desflurane, and propofol anesthesia. Anesthesiology 1995; 83:66-76.

Summors AC, Gupta AK, Matta BF: Dynamic cerebral autoregulation during sevoflurane anesthesia: A comparison with isoflurane. Anesth Analg 1999; 88:341-345.

Chapter 10

Opioids and Adjuvant Drugs

Balachandra Maiya • Anthony Absalom

Opioids	**Neuromuscular Blocking Agents**
Cardiovascular Effects	**Antihypertensives**
Respiratory Effects	Direct-Acting Vasodilators
Cerebral Hemodynamics	Adrenoreceptor Antagonists
Electrical Activity	Calcium Channel Blockers
Analgesia	
Other Effects	**Miscellaneous Agents**
Naloxone	Glucocorticoids
	Osmotic Agents
α₂-Adrenergic Agonists	

OPIOIDS

Opioid analgesics are an important adjunct to the sedative and hypnotic anesthetic agents. In addition to providing analgesia, the opioids have a hypnotic-sparing effect that can result in improved intraoperative hemodynamic stability and more rapid emergence. The opioid analgesics commonly used in neuroanesthesia include morphine, fentanyl, sufentanil, remifentanil, and alfentanil. Sufentanil is a highly selective opioid agonist used in North America and Europe, but not in the United Kingdom. It is 10 to 15 times more potent than fentanyl and has a shorter elimination half-life. Remifentanil has distinct advantages over other opioids in that its unique pharmacokinetic characteristics result in more rapid onset and offset of action than is the case with the other agents. As a result of ester linkages, remifentanil is susceptible to the nonspecific esterases widely present in blood and tissues, and it has a context-insensitive duration of action after an infusion (i.e., its duration of effect is independent of the duration of administration).

Cardiovascular Effects

Opioids reduce sympathetic tone and increase parasympathetic tone. Thus, in large doses all opioids are associated with bradycardia. Hypotension secondary to bradycardia usually responds to a small dose of atropine or glycopyrrolate. It is important to remember that opioids also profoundly potentiate hypnotic agents. Even moderate blood concentrations of remifentanil, for example, more than halve the propofol concentration required to ablate the response to noxious stimuli. Opioids also potentiate the cardiovascular effects of hypnotics, so when moderate or large doses of opioid agents are used, hypotension will occur if the dose of hypnotic agent is not reduced accordingly.

Respiratory Effects

There is profound synergism between the depressant respiratory effects of opioids and hypnotics. Moderately large doses of opioids markedly attenuate the airway reflexes, including coughing in response to the presence of an endotracheal tube. Thus, the pharmacokinetics of remifentanil makes it an ideal agent for use in combination with a hypnotic during operations in which limited or no paralysis is required but coughing or movement is undesirable. Examples are skull base surgery, such as excision of acoustic neuromas, in which facial nerve monitoring is necessary, and scoliosis surgery, in which recording of motor evoked potentials may be required.

Cerebral Hemodynamics

High opioid doses may cause modest reductions in cerebral blood flow and cerebral oxygen metabolism if normocapnia is maintained. The effects are probably minimal with clinically used doses. Some studies have shown an increase in intracranial pressure (ICP) after the administration of opioids, which may be secondary to autoregulatory vasodilation after a reduction in mean arterial (and cerebral perfusion) pressure. Werner and colleagues showed that opioids have no effect on ICP when mean arterial pressure was maintained with vasopressors. Opioids are useful for attenuating the adverse effects of stimulating procedures on cerebral hemodynamics, such as intubation, endotracheal tube suctioning, and application of skull pins for stabilizing the head for surgery.

Electrical Activity

Electroencephalographic (EEG) changes depend on the dose. Fentanyl and sufentanil in small doses produce minimal EEG changes. There may be a ceiling effect for the EEG changes produced during sufentanil infusion, but very high doses of fentanyl, 30 to 70 μg/kg, can result in delta wave activity (high voltage, slow waves).

Even though higher-dose opioids may alter the latency and amplitude of sensory evoked potentials, this effect does not preclude their use for monitoring spinal cord function. Opioids generally have minimal effects on auditory evoked potentials.

Analgesia

Although craniotomy was believed to produce minimal postoperative pain, it is now clear that the pain can be quite significant. Opioids have been underused in the perioperative period for fear of sedation, pupillary changes, nausea, and suppression of cough reflexes despite studies showing that the use of morphine does not significantly increase the incidence of these adverse effects. Codeine is the most common opioid analgesic used in the United Kingdom for postcraniotomy analgesia. Codeine itself possesses little analgesic efficacy and must first be metabolized to morphine before it can be clinically effective. The main metabolic pathway is glucuronidation mediated by the genetically polymorphic enzyme CYP2D6, which is absent or defective in a significant proportion of the population (so-called poor metabolizers, in whom codeine will be largely ineffective).

Other Effects

Opiates have the potential to cause nausea and vomiting by stimulation of serotonin (5-HT$_3$) and dopamine receptors in the chemoreceptor trigger zone, and prolonged infusions or repeated doses of longer-acting agents can cause impaired gastric emptying, ileus, constipation, pupillary constriction, pruritus, and blurred vision. Nausea and vomiting are rare after propofol/remifentanil anesthesia, possibly because of the antiemetic effect of propofol, combined with the rapid clearance of remifentanil. Large intraoperative doses of all strong opioids (other than remifentanil) may result in delayed emergence from anesthesia.

NALOXONE

Naloxone has high affinity for the μ opioid receptor, where it acts as a competitive antagonist. It also acts as a weaker competitive antagonist at the κ and δ opioid receptors. Naloxone on its own has minimal effects on cerebral blood flow and oxygen metabolism. Although it can be used to reverse opioid-induced sedation and respiratory depression, it should be used with caution because it also antagonizes the analgesic effects. Abrupt opioid reversal with naloxone can thus result in pain, hypertension, arrhythmias, myocardial ischemia, and intracranial hemorrhage. Naloxone should be avoided altogether if possible and should be used cautiously in doses of approximately 1.5 μg/kg titrated to clinical effect. It should be remembered that the effects of a bolus of naloxone last only 20 to 30 minutes and thus the patient may return to a narcotized state if a longer-acting opioid has been used.

α_2-ADRENERGIC AGONISTS

This class of drugs produces sedation, analgesia, and anxiolysis. Clonidine and dexmedetomidine are the two commonly used drugs. Dexmedetomidine is more selective, with 1600-fold greater sensitivity toward α_2 than α_1 receptors. They produce their sedative effects by action on α_2 receptors in the locus ceruleus, where they reduce neural activity in projections to the hypothalamus. Dexmedetomidine reduces cerebral blood flow without affecting oxygen metabolism, but it does not produce cerebral ischemia. The reduction in cerebral blood flow is secondary to cerebral vasoconstriction via postsynaptic α_2 receptors. Dexmedetomidine may be used as an adjuvant for general anesthesia or for sedated (awake) procedures in countries in which it is commercially available.

10

NEUROMUSCULAR BLOCKING AGENTS

Coughing, straining, and intolerance of the endotracheal tube cause increases in ICP, which can be avoided by the administration of neuromuscular blocking agents, provided that patients receive adequate hypnosis and analgesia. Although succinylcholine has the potential to increase ICP, the rise is minimal and transient. The clinical significance of the increase in ICP is unknown, which should not preclude its use in situations in which rapid control of the airway is required. The rise in ICP can be minimized by pretreatment with nondepolarizing neuromuscular blockers. Nondepolarizing neuromuscular blocking agents do not have significant effects on cerebral hemodynamics. Laudanosine, one of the metabolites of atracurium, crosses the blood-brain barrier and can induce seizures. This was seen only when large doses were used in animals and has no clinical significance in humans.

Chronic phenytoin or carbamazepine use accelerates recovery from muscle relaxants, possibly because of a combination of central and peripheral effects. Carbamazepine almost doubles the clearance of vecuronium.

ANTIHYPERTENSIVES

In patients with disturbed cerebral autoregulation, sudden hypertensive episodes result in increased ICP and the potential for intracranial hemorrhage. These episodes may occur during laryngoscopy, at incision, or during extubation and can be treated with either direct-acting vasodilators or adrenoreceptor antagonists.

Direct-Acting Vasodilators

Direct-acting vasodilators reduce blood pressure by relaxing vascular smooth muscle and decreasing vascular resistance. They must be used with caution because the vasodilation can result in increased cerebral blood volume and ICP with a reduction in cerebral perfusion. Moreover, if the blood vessels in the abnormal regions of the brain are selectively sensitive to vasodilators, a steal-phenomenon and worsening of ischemic injury could result.

The common agents include sodium nitroprusside (SNP), glyceryl trinitrate, and hydralazine. SNP is a nonselective organic nitrate vasodilator that reacts with the sulfhydryl groups on endothelium to release nitric oxide (NO), a smooth muscle relaxant. NO produces vasodilation through the cyclic guanosine monophosphate pathway within vascular smooth muscle. It acts on both resistance and capacitance vessels and hence can increase ICP and reduce cerebral perfusion pressure. Moreover, in patients with reduced cerebral compliance, SNP can make the cerebral vasculature less responsive to the vasoconstrictive effects of hypocapnia. Glyceryl trinitrate is another vasodilator acting via NO, but unlike SNP, it acts predominantly on capacitance vessels. It increases ICP, possibly because of dilation of cerebral veins, and can reduce cerebral blood flow in patients with increased ICP. Hydralazine causes direct relaxation of smooth muscle tissue in vascular resistance vessels, predominantly in the arterioles. The cellular mechanism of action responsible for this effect are not fully understood, but may involve formation of NO and activation of guanylate cyclase. It may also affect intracellular Ca^{2+} mobilization and phosphorylation processes. Like all other drugs in this group it may elevate ICP.

In addition to exercising caution with the use of these drugs, they must be withdrawn cautiously to reduce the risk of rebound hypertension.

Adrenoreceptor Antagonists

Labetalol is one of the more commonly used adrenoreceptor blockers. It has α- and noncardioselective β-adrenergic blocking action. The ratio of β-to-α blocking effects is 7:1. Unlike direct-acting vasodilators, it reduces mean arterial pressure without a concomitant increase in ICP. In postoperative neurosurgical patients with refractory hypertension, labetalol improved cerebral perfusion pressure when compared with SNP. Esmolol is an ultrashort-acting β receptor antagonist commonly used to control perioperative surges in blood pressure. It has the advantage of rapid onset and offset. The short half-life results from rapid biotransformation by esterases.

Calcium Channel Blockers

These agents are of little use in hypertensive emergencies because of their long duration of action and potential to cause cerebral vasodilation. Several calcium channel antagonists are used for long-term control of hypertension, and the use of nimodipine in patients with subarachnoid hemorrhage is discussed elsewhere (see Chapter 17).

MISCELLANEOUS AGENTS

Glucocorticoids

Glucocorticoids stabilize the blood-brain barrier and increase absorption of cerebrospinal fluid. They are beneficial in reducing edema in primary and metastatic brain tumors. Their use in brain tumors improves generalized symptoms (such as headache and altered mental status) more than focal ones. In traumatic brain injury, glucocorticoids have been associated with an increased risk of death. The use of steroids in acute spinal cord injury has not been shown to improve long-term motor function.

Osmotic Agents

Mannitol and hypertonic saline are commonly used to treat acute increases in ICP. Mannitol is an osmotic agent and a free radical scavenger. It acts by drawing fluid out of tissue into the vascular compartment. It also reduces blood viscosity and hence increases cerebral blood flow, which results in an autoregulatory vasoconstriction that may reduce ICP. It is administered as an intermittent bolus of 0.25 to 0.5 g/kg but should not be used if serum osmolality exceeds 320 mOsm/kg. Mannitol can accumulate in injured tissues and can thus lead to rebound effects. Hypertonic saline is increasingly being used to control ICP in traumatic brain injury. Studies have shown better control of ICP with hypertonic saline than with mannitol, but no difference in mortality or neurologic outcome.

KEY POINTS

- Opioids have minimal effect on cerebral blood flow, metabolism, and intracranial pressure, provided that normocapnia and normotension are maintained.
- Pain after craniotomy can be significant.
- Perioperative use of modest doses of morphine does not increase the incidence of sedation, nausea, and depression of airway reflexes.
- Naloxone is best avoided in neurosurgical patients because abrupt opioid reversal has several detrimental effects.
- Succinylcholine causes a mild, temporary elevation in ICP and is not contraindicated when rapid airway control is required.
- For control of intraoperative or postoperative hypertension, adrenoceptor antagonists such as labetalol are preferred over vasodilators because they reduce blood pressure without increasing cerebral blood volume and ICP.

10

FURTHER READING

Cohen J, Royston D: Remifentanil. Curr Opin Crit Care 2001; 7:227-231.

Crabb I, Thornton C, Konieczko KM, et al: Remifentanil reduces auditory and somatosensory evoked responses during isoflurane anaesthesia in a dose-dependent manner. Br J Anaesth 1996; 76:795-801.

Fagerlund TH, Braaten O: No pain relief from codeine… ? An introduction to pharmacogenomics. Acta Anaesthesiol Scand 2001; 45:140-149.

Roberts I, Yates D, Sandercock P, et al: Effect of intravenous corticosteroids on death within 14 days in 10008 adults with clinically significant head injury (MRC CRASH trial): Randomised placebo-controlled trial. Lancet 2004; 364:1321-1328.

Stoneham MD, Cooper R, Quiney NF, Walters FJ: Pain following craniotomy: A preliminary study comparing PCA morphine with intramuscular codeine phosphate. Anaesthesia 1996; 51:1176-1178.

Talke PO, Gelb AW: Post craniotomy pain remains a real headache! Eur J Anaesthesiol 2005; 22:325-327.

Tietjen CS, Hurn PD, Ulatowski JA, Kirsch JR: Treatment modalities for hypertensive patients with intracranial pathology: Options and risks. Crit Care Med 1996; 24:311-322.

Werner C, Kochs E, Bause H, et al: Effects of sufentanil on cerebral hemodynamics and intracranial pressure in patients with brain injury. Anesthesiology 1995; 83:721-726.

Chapter 11

Anticonvulsants

Peter M.C. Wright

Chronic Anticonvulsant Administration

Acute Anticonvulsant Administration

Summary

Commonly used anticonvulsant drugs are phenytoin, carbamazepine, valproic acid, and ethosuximide. The formerly commonly used drugs phenobarbital and its prodrug primidone are used less frequently now because of prominent sedative side effects (see Table 19-3 for indications and side effects). There are also a number of newer agents available whose place in therapy has not yet been fully established.

Phenytoin has been in use for more than 50 years and still has a very prominent role in the management of "grand mal" epilepsy. It is a potent inducer of cytochrome P-450 enzymes, and because of its highly nonlinear kinetics combined with a narrow therapeutic range, it is difficult to dose. Phenytoin can be given intravenously, but this route of administration carries the risk of hypotension or severe dysrhythmia—a risk that can be diminished by using the prodrug fosphenytoin instead. Carbamazepine is also commonly used for epilepsy syndromes, trigeminal neuralgia, and other chronic pain syndromes. It is similar to the tricyclic antidepressants in structure and has a similar profile of side effects. Like phenytoin, it is an inducer of liver enzymes. It can lead to electrolyte disturbances such as hyponatremia. Valproic acid is used in epilepsy syndromes, as well as for migraine and bipolar depression. Like many other anticonvulsant drugs it has nonlinear pharmacokinetics, and it is occasionally associated with thrombocytopenia. Ethosuximide is most commonly used in the treatment of "petit mal" epilepsy in children.

For a variety of reasons, anticonvulsants are encountered more frequently in patients undergoing neurosurgical operations than in the general surgical population. Patients being treated neurosurgically for epilepsy are the obvious case, but in such patients anticonvulsant drugs are usually titrated down and stopped before surgery so that the anticonvulsants do not interfere with the electroencephalographic signals recorded during the operation. The more common experience is a patient undergoing management of a space-occupying lesion who is receiving anticonvulsant drugs for control of seizures that occur as a result of the primary pathology. Practitioners of anesthesia for neurosurgery are therefore frequently called on to manage the implications of interactions between anticonvulsant drugs and the requirements of neurosurgery. This requirement is dominated by the fact that anticonvulsant drugs interact strongly with the actions of other drugs. Any drug that is metabolized by the liver is predisposed to reduced action in a patient taking an anticonvulsant drug.

Although there is no good evidence that these drugs reduce the effect of fentanyl and morphine in such patients, clinical observations would indicate that any such effect is not marked. The dose of inhalational anesthetics does not seem to be altered, and the response to propofol does not appear to be markedly altered. The hepatic toxicity of halothane may be enhanced in patients taking anticonvulsants.

The anticonvulsant drugs as a class have profound effects on the activity of neuromuscular blocking drugs. Given that the different anticonvulsant drugs are not similar chemically, it remains unknown why they should interact with neuromuscular blocking drugs so profoundly as a class. Experience is greatest with the anticonvulsant drugs phenytoin and carbamazepine. Patients taking these two drugs have a profoundly altered response to neuromuscular blocking drugs in comparison to patients not receiving anticonvulsant therapy. Valproic acid and ethosuximide likewise seem to have this effect, and it is probably wise to assume that the newer anticonvulsant agents also do until there is evidence one way or the other.

CHRONIC ANTICONVULSANT ADMINISTRATION

Patients taking anticonvulsants for more than a few days are resistant to the effects of neuromuscular blocking drugs. The magnitude of the interaction varies depending on the exact drugs involved. Steroid-based neuromuscular blocking drugs seem to be the most affected by the interaction, and for these drugs a recent study estimated a fivefold increase in vecuronium requirement in patients taking phenytoin. There are a variety of possible mechanisms for this profound interaction. Anticonvulsants induce hepatic enzymes, and it is therefore likely that metabolism and elimination of the muscle relaxant are increased; increased clearance of muscle relaxants has been demonstrated after chronic phenytoin use. Phenytoin also has effects that might alter the apparent sensitivity of the neuromuscular junction to muscle relaxants. For instance, phenytoin itself has mild blocking action at the neuromuscular junction, which may lead to up-regulation of the acetylcholine receptor. It might also alter the protein binding of muscle relaxants or have effects at presynaptic acetylcholine receptors. The relative contribution of these various possible mechanisms to this interaction is not known, but the extent to which pharmacokinetic and pharmacodynamic mechanisms contribute can be determined. In the study cited earlier the authors estimated that the kinetic and dynamic mechanisms were equally important.

Both steroidal and benzylisoquinoline neuromuscular blocking drugs have been observed to have reduced effect in patients taking anticonvulsant drugs. For steroidal neuromuscular blocking drugs this interaction has been observed with phenytoin, carbamazepine, and other anticonvulsant drugs. For the benzylisoquinoline neuromuscular blocking drugs the evidence is less clear, with some studies reporting an effect and others not. These differences might be explained by the typical metabolism of these drugs. For steroidal neuromuscular blocking drugs liver metabolism is an important route of drug elimination. Many anticonvulsant drugs are potent inducers of liver enzymes. Thus, a possible explanation for the reduced effect of steroid neuromuscular blocking drugs is that they are eliminated more rapidly because of liver enzyme induction. More rapid elimination of the neuromuscular blocking drug has been demonstrated for vecuronium, pancuronium, and rocuronium in patients taking phenytoin. In contrast, benzylisoquinoline neuromuscular blocking drugs are typically not dependent on liver metabolism or excretion. Yet patients taking anticonvulsant drugs are also resistant to their effects, though to a lesser extent than with the steroidal drugs, presumably because these effects are mediated through a pharmacodynamic mechanism.

11

The clinical implication of profound resistance to neuromuscular blocking drugs in a patient undergoing neurosurgery is that it alters the strategies used to ensure that the patient does not strain or cough on the endotracheal tube at times when this would disrupt the surgery or place the patient at risk for harm. The anesthesiologist needs to be aware that the duration of action of normal doses of neuromuscular blocking drugs may be surprisingly short (or similarly, an infusion may have surprisingly little effect). Thus, if the anesthesiologist is to rely on neuromuscular blocking drugs to prevent straining, unusually high doses must be administered. The actual dose required is variable and may be surprisingly large. Neuromuscular monitoring is therefore highly advisable. An alternative strategy would involve the use of a high dose of an opioid drug to reduce the patient's likelihood of movement or straining.

ACUTE ANTICONVULSANT ADMINISTRATION

In contrast to the interaction seen with chronic phenytoin treatment, acute treatment produces a weak neuromuscular block and enhances the action of nondepolarizing neuromuscular blocking drugs. A wide range of anticonvulsant drugs also have similar effects. These observations provide a further putative mechanism for resistance to the action of neuromuscular blocking drugs seen with chronic anticonvulsant administration. The weak neuromuscular blocking properties of anticonvulsant drugs results in postjunctional acetylcholine receptor up-regulation. Thus, the enhancement of the action of nondepolarizing neuromuscular blocking drugs that occurs with the acute administration of phenytoin gives way to resistance after a few days of treatment. This would be consistent with the observation that acute phenytoin administration reduces the effect of suxamethonium (in contrast to its acute interaction with nondepolarizing neuromuscular blocking drugs). Other possible explanations for resistance to vecuronium that do not involve changes in vecuronium's disposition include alterations in the protein binding of vecuronium or a presynaptic effect of phenytoin. For instance, phenytoin increases α_1-acid glycoprotein concentrations, which might alter the free fraction of neuromuscular blocking drug. However, a study that examined this proposal concluded that altered protein binding does not cause resistance to vecuronium.

SUMMARY

Anticonvulsant drugs are commonly encountered in the neurosurgical population. Frequently, the anticonvulsant has been introduced within the preceding days or weeks. The response of these patients to anesthesia differs from that in patients not taking anticonvulsant drugs, mainly in the response to neuromuscular blocking drugs. There is resistance to nondepolarizing neuromuscular blocking drugs in patients taking anticonvulsant drugs for more than a few days. Evidence of this interaction is stronger for drugs with liver-based metabolism, such as vecuronium or rocuronium, but is also present for drugs that are eliminated independently of liver function. The dose requirements of neuromuscular blocking drugs are therefore increased in patients taking phenytoin, carbamazepine, and to a lesser extent other anticonvulsant drugs, and this effect may be greater for steroid-based neuromuscular blocking drugs than others. In a typical case the expected dose of vecuronium needed to maintain a given degree of block will be increased fourfold to fivefold in patients taking phenytoin chronically.

KEY POINTS

- Anticonvulsants are commonly encountered in patients undergoing neurosurgery.
- Abrupt withdrawal of anticonvulsants should be avoided.
- There is a marked interaction between many anticonvulsants and many neuro-muscular blocking drugs.
- Patients taking phenytoin and carbamazepine have a greatly increased dose requirement for nondepolarizing neuromuscular blocking drugs.

FURTHER READING

Gage PW, Lonergan M, Torda TA: Presynaptic and postsynaptic depressant effects of phenytoin sodium at the neuromuscular junction. Br J Pharmacol 1980; 69:119-121.

Gray HS, Slater RM, Pollard BJ: The effect of acutely administered phenytoin on vecuronium-induced neuromuscular blockade. Anaesthesia1989; 44:379-381.

Gandhi IC, Jindal MN, Patel VK: Mechanism of neuromuscular blockade with some antiepileptic drugs. Arzneimittelforschung 1976; 26:258-261.

Hans P, Brichant JF, Pieron F, et al: Elevated plasma alpha 1-acid glycoprotein levels: Lack of connection to resistance to vecuronium blockade induced by anticonvulsant therapy. J Neurosurg Anesthesiol 1997; 9:3-7.

Martyn JA, White DA, Gronert GA, et al: Up-and-down regulation of skeletal muscle acetylcholine receptors. Effects on neuromuscular blockers. Anesthesiology 1992; 76:822-843.

Melton AT, Antognini JF, Gronert GA: Prolonged duration of succinylcholine in patients receiving anticonvulsants: Evidence for mild up-regulation of acetylcholine receptors? Can J Anaesth1993; 40:939-942.

Norris FH, Colella J, McFarlin D: Effect of diphenylhydantoin on neuromuscular synapse. Neurology 1964; 14:869-876.

Wright PM, McCarthy G, Szenohradszky J, et al: Influence of chronic phenytoin administration on the pharmacokinetics and pharmacodynamics of vecuronium. Anesthesiology 2004; 100:626-633.

11

Section IV
Neuroanesthesia

Chapter 12

Preoperative Assessment

Rowan Burnstein • James Stimpson

Preoperative assessment is the cornerstone of safe neuroanesthetic practice. The important elements are identification of specific problems that may be associated with the procedure, as well as those related to any comorbid conditions, and formulation of a plan for care in the early postoperative period. As in all areas of anesthesia, preoperative assessment also allows the patient to better understand the role of the anesthetist and provides time for delivering information to the patient and addressing any patient concerns. Neurologic deficits should be documented and comorbid conditions and opportunities for preoperative optimization identified. Preoperative assessment should also document current medications and recommend any necessary premedication as it relates to these medications or the specific needs of the procedure. Requirements of the surgical position, intraoperative monitoring, and postoperative care requirements should all be borne in mind. A significant proportion of neurosurgical patients will be referred from the critical care unit and are likely to require management in a critical care or high-dependency facility postoperatively. However, rarely is any patient such an emergency that no assessment can be made.

WHY IS THE PATIENT HAVING THIS PROCEDURE NOW?

The timing and urgency of any neurosurgical procedure are crucial. Certain procedures result in a worse neurologic outcome if undertaken either too early or too late. For example, pretreatment of patients who have significant peritumor edema with steroids may significantly improve preoperative neurologic status, whereas delaying surgery because of rapidly expanding extradural hematomas will have an adverse effect on outcome. Any decision to delay surgery on the basis of anesthetic risk must take into account the neurosurgical benefits of the procedure. Communication with the surgical team is paramount. Frequently, suboptimally prepared patients need their procedures even if hazardous from an anesthetic perspective. This has implications for perioperative strategy and postoperative care.

Certain procedures such as craniotomy are generic terms and do not describe the extent of surgery or the actual procedure. The extent of the procedure (biopsy, resection, debulking, clipping, etc.) and the approach (frontal, temporal, occipital, supine, lateral, prone, burr hole versus craniotomy) should be ascertained because they directly affect positioning, monitoring, size and location of intravenous access, and provision of cross-matched blood.

OBTAINING INFORMATION FROM THE PATIENT AND OTHER SOURCES

Neurosurgical patients vary in their ability to communicate, so information will need to be gathered from multiple sources, including the patients themselves, family members, hospital notes, referral letters, and hospital information systems.

Confirmation of the patient's identity is important in a population with neurologic disease. In a specialty in which the laterality of signs, symptoms, and pathology differs and the sequelae of surgery on the wrong site can be so devastating, it is crucial to confirm that the correct operation is being performed at the correct site. The site of the symptoms and signs can be checked with the patient, and scans will confirm the site of pathology. Any confusion or disagreement must be clarified before proceeding to surgery.

History

A routine general anesthetic assessment should be undertaken. However, specific features should be embellished in neuroanesthetic patients.

The size and location of lesions should be identified and their progression appreciated. In most patients computed tomography (CT) or magnetic resonance imaging (MRI) will be performed to assist in this matter. Surgery in critical brain regions is well known to be associated with typical postoperative sequelae, such as swallowing difficulties and other cranial nerve palsies in posterior fossa and brainstem surgery and seizures after temporal lobe surgery. Any treatment up to this point, such as steroids, mannitol, anticonvulsants, chemotherapy, radiotherapy, neurovascular ablation, biopsy, or formal surgery, should be noted.

Many neurosurgical patients have had multiple similar previous operations and anesthetics, so old anesthetic charts are a source of very useful information. Current comorbidity helps assess overall fitness and suitability for anesthesia and provides areas for optimization if appropriate. A high index of suspicion is needed for establishing comorbidity. Patients may have disease states directly associated with their neurosurgical pathology (Table 12-1).

Any identified disease associations need to be evaluated in terms of their severity, duration, progression, treatment, and complications. Occasionally, specialists may need to be contacted to appropriately guide perioperative care, such as patients with pituitary lesions, who are likely to require long-term endocrinology management.

Current and previous medications should be reviewed and documented, any allergies documented along with the reaction, and any specific investigations performed. Therapeutic drug levels (e.g., for anticonvulsants) should be ascertained when appropriate. Smoking history should be quantified in terms of daily amount, overall duration, and any associated reduction in respiratory function or underlying infection. A significant smoking history may indicate a high probability of coughing and wheezing at induction and extubation. Likewise, alcohol consumption has implications for disease causality, nutritional status, hepatic enzyme induction, and

Table 12-1	Disease States Directly Associated with Patients' Neurosurgical Pathology
Intracranial aneurysm	Hypertension
	Adult polycystic disease
	Marfan's syndrome
	Amphetamine abuse
Arteriovenous malformations	Sturge-Weber syndrome
	Osler-Weber-Rendu syndrome
Carotid endarterectomy	Diffuse atherosclerosis
	Hypertension
	Chronic obstructive pulmonary disease
Pituitary lesions	Hypopituitarism or hyperpituitarism
Acoustic neuroma	Multiple neurofibromatosis
Kyphoscoliosis	Restrictive lung disease
Cervical arthritis	Rheumatoid arthritis

withdrawal phenomena. Recreational drug use and drug addiction may have significant implications for perioperative care, and thus a high index of suspicion is necessary.

Finally, a systems review may identify other areas for concern, such as unidentified comorbidity that requires further investigation.

Examination

Examination of a neurosurgical patient aims to verify any neurologic signs, assess the airway, and establish baseline cardiorespiratory status.

This population of patients usually has symptoms and signs of their neuropathology. An accurate baseline neurologic status is invaluable to guide the expected level of recovery in the immediate postoperative period and also to anticipate any complications that may occur. After surgery, any changes in neurologic status may be entirely appropriate to the location and extent of the procedure, but they may also represent incomplete surgery, extension of the pathologic insult, localized edema, or surgical or anesthetic mishap. Ideally, there will be a complete and carefully documented preoperative neurologic assessment by a neurologist or neurosurgeon in the patient's notes. It is reasonable to confirm these findings with the patient. However, occasionally there is a discrepancy, so repeat examination can clarify the situation. In the acute situation it is critical at the very least to establish the level of consciousness (preferably quantified within a repeatable scoring system such as the Glasgow Coma Scale), reactivity of the pupils, and limb strength and movement to guide the likelihood of successful extubation and appropriate postoperative placement.

Assessment of the airway is important to allow appropriate planning of induction of anesthesia to facilitate smooth induction with minimal delay, trauma, or hemodynamic consequence. A proportion of these patients will satisfy the requirements for fiberoptic intubation (potentially awake) (see Chapter 25). A standardized approach to the airway consisting of a history, inspection, palpation, and further investigation is necessary.

Any significant history may have already been noted, but specific details should be disclosed, including problems with previous airway management; previous prolonged intubation or tracheotomy care; comorbid conditions influencing the airway, such as head or neck carcinoma, goiter, cervical spine pathology, or rheumatoid arthritis; symptoms or signs suggesting obstructive sleep apnea; smoking history; and aspiration risk. Rigid collars or halo traction obviously predicts limitations in airway access. This latter group does not necessarily consist of only those undergoing cervical surgery (e.g., trauma patients with supratentorial lesions).

For cervical spine surgery, patients should have imaging available that details the laryngeal and thoracic inlet anatomy. In other individual cases it may be helpful to request such imaging. The degree of stability of the cervical spine is also important. Cervical spine pathology may limit neck flexion or head extension, or both; again, fiberoptic intubation is invaluable in these patients. In the acute situation, all patients who are to undergo neurosurgery and have a history of trauma, whether they are conscious or unconscious, should be considered to have an unstable cervical spine until formal radiologic clearance has been obtained. In an unconscious patient it is not always possible to clear the spine, even on the basis of plain cervical imaging and reconstituted cervical images or MRI. A decision regarding awake versus asleep intubation may need to be based on the mechanism of injury, a high index of suspicion, and discussion with the surgeon.

Assessment of the cardiorespiratory system allows prediction of cardiovascular instability, airway irritability and coughing, laryngospasm, bronchospasm, breath-holding, approximation of $Etco_2$ to $Paco_2$, and alveolar-to-arterial gradients and may suggest either areas for optimization or the need for postoperative ventilation. Patients with cranial nerve palsies or a depressed level of consciousness preoperatively are at high risk for perioperative aspiration pneumonia. Specific note should be made of the ease of peripheral venous and arterial access, blood pressure, oxygen saturation on room air, heart rate, presence or absence of murmurs and their character, and the clarity of breath sounds in all lung regions. When possible, walking a patient through the ward or clinic while discussing the anticipated care provides insight into any functional impairment that may not be apparent from a bedside discussion.

Investigations

A complete blood count, clotting profile, and electrolyte assay should be performed before any neurosurgical procedure. Blood should be drawn for cross-matching as appropriate to the particular lesion and anticipated blood loss. If seizures have been a symptom, assessment of magnesium and calcium levels, as well as serum levels of anticonvulsant drugs, is appropriate. When endocrine abnormalities are anticipated, baseline investigation of the adrenocortical axis should be established. Other blood investigations are guided by comorbidity.

The electrocardiogram may highlight hypertensive heart disease, rhythm abnormality, or occult ischemia, thus adding to the perioperative management strategy. Preoperative chest radiographs are necessary only when specifically indicated.

All neurosurgical patients will have additional imaging of the surgical field, either CT, contrast-enhanced CT, CT angiography, MRI, or formal angiography. These studies should be reviewed, the pathology identified, the site confirmed, and further features noted such as the degree of tissue edema, size of the ventricles, degree of midline shift, amount of space around the basal cisterns and posterior fossa, and in the case of trauma, the presence of coexisting injuries such as maxillofacial trauma, depressed skull fractures, and cervical spine disruption. These findings have a direct influence on patient handling, the induction technique, the approach to intubation, instigation of invasive monitoring, the use of mannitol, and anticipation of delayed postoperative recovery.

Additional Information

Specific questions need to be addressed to complete the assessment of the patient. Having established the exact procedure, it is important to ascertain the position required, whether head pins or frames are being used, and whether any additional procedures are to be performed, such as rescanning under general anesthesia, bone graft from the iliac wing, plastic surgery input for closure, or insertion of an extraventricular drain or intracranial pressure–monitoring device.

DELIVERING INFORMATION TO THE PATIENT

Communication with a neurosurgical patient can be awkward and difficult to achieve. Patients may be aphasic, dysphasic, or dysarthric, and the dysphasia may be expressive or receptive. The patient's level of consciousness may be depressed. Patients may be agitated or combative or may have total neglect on one side. Hearing and visual abnormalities are not uncommon.

Assumptions regarding the mental capacity of a patient to comprehend should not be made. However awkward it may feel, a full explanation about the anesthesia and its risks and benefits in the perioperative period should be undertaken.

Consent becomes a difficult issue for patients who have diminished capacity to understand. There are now special consent forms for patients who are already unconscious or in whom there is no doubt about reduced capacity. If there is any uncertainty, a pragmatic approach is to ensure that the procedure is explained in the clearest way possible to the patient and verbal assent obtained. This discussion should ideally take place with relatives or other guardian present and any questions answered fully. For a patient with diminished capacity, the consent of relatives is not mandatory if two clinicians are in agreement that the procedure is essential and in the patient's best interests.

PREOPERATIVE OPTIMIZATION OF NEUROSURGICAL PATIENTS

For elective surgery any requirement for optimization may mean rescheduling of the procedure. The problems identified by preoperative assessment need to be balanced against the risks associated with delaying surgery while taking into consideration that the majority of neurosurgical pathology is progressive, although the time scale of such progression varies according to the condition. Hazards are always relative, and weighing of the risk-benefit ratio should be undertaken in consultation with neurosurgical staff.

Electrolyte disturbances are common and are often a consequence of either the neurosurgical pathology or medications, such as diuretics, anticonvulsants, steroids, or antihypertensives.

PREMEDICATION BEFORE NEUROSURGICAL PROCEDURES

Premedication with sedative drugs needs to be cautiously implemented in neurosurgical patients. In particular, patients with space-occupying intracranial lesions may be well compensated, but the introduction of a sedative agent with the potential to depress ventilation or precipitate airway obstruction may be enough to increase intracranial pressure and result in neurologic decompensation. Patients will, however, be naturally anxious about their impending surgery, and therefore reassurance and an explanation are important. Although a short-acting benzodiazepine is sometimes used for anxiolysis in patients with uncompromised neurology, sedative premedication should never be given to patients with an already reduced level of consciousness.

12

PLANNING FOR POSTOPERATIVE MANAGEMENT

The preoperative assessment should be used to plan for postoperative care of the neurosurgical patient. A high proportion of neurosurgical patients will require elective admission to a critical care or high-dependency area by virtue of the procedure that has been undertaken and the probable or potential complications of surgery. This does, however, vary between centers and is to some extent influenced by the recovery facilities available. Such issues should be discussed with the patient and family before the procedure, as should the presence of any invasive monitoring techniques (invasive arterial monitoring, central venous pressure monitoring, transcranial Doppler ultrasound, intracranial pressure monitoring, etc.) that might be required in the postoperative period.

KEY POINTS

- Preoperative assessment is the cornerstone of safe neuroanesthetic practice.
- An accurate baseline of neurologic status is invaluable as a recovery tool, not only to guide the expected level of recovery in the immediate postoperative period but also to anticipate complications that may occur at this time.
- Any patient with a space-occupying lesion should be considered to have raised intracranial pressure, even if well compensated.
- Preoperative assessment of neurosurgical patients should also take into account the extent of surgery and positioning for surgery, as well as anticipation of postoperative sequelae as a result of the location of surgery or disruption of the neuroendocrine axis.

FURTHER READING

Fischer SP.<http://www.ncbi.nlm.nih.gov/sites/entrez?Db=pubmed&Cmd=ShowDetailView&TermToSearch=8956062&ordinalpos=8&itool=EntrezSystem2.PEntrez.Pubmed.Pubmed_ResultsPanel.Pubmed_RVDocSum> Preoperative evaluation of the adult neurosurgical patient. Int Anesthesiol Clin. 1996 Fall; 34(4):21-32. Review.

Fleisher LA, et al: ACC/AHA 2007 guidelines on perioperative cardiovascular evaluation and care for non cardiac surgery. J Am Coll Cardiol 2007; 50(17):161-241.

Lefevre F, Woolger JM: Surgery in the patient with neurologic disease. Med Clin North Am. 2003 Jan; 87(1):257-271. Review.

IV

Chapter 13

Basic Concepts of Neuroimaging

Daniel Scoffings • Jonathan H. Gillard

Magnetic Resonance Imaging Sequences	**Subarachnoid Hemorrhage**
Spinal Trauma	**Raised Intracranial Pressure**
Intracranial Appearances in Trauma	**Intracranial Tumors**

Imaging of patients who have not undergone neurologic surgery is usually performed for cases of trauma and subarachnoid hemorrhage. The primary objectives of imaging focus on clearing the cervical spine and defining the extent and prognosis of any intracranial injury with the use of plain films, computed tomography (CT) and magnetic resonance imaging (MRI). Imaging of patients for elective neurosurgery is performed primarily to assess the position and character of a lesion, mass effect, cerebral edema, and postoperative hemorrhage.

MAGNETIC RESONANCE IMAGING SEQUENCES

A number of different MRI sequences are in common use for imaging the brain and spine. The sequence used depends on which tissue needs imaging most usefully.

T1-weighted images show white matter with a higher signal intensity than gray matter, and cerebrospinal fluid (CSF) is also of low signal. On *T2-weighted* images, white matter is of lower signal than gray matter and CSF, which have high signal intensity. The fluid-attenuated inversion recovery (FLAIR) sequence suppresses CSF signal so that it is of low intensity. For this reason, at first glance FLAIR images can be confused with T1-weighted images; however, FLAIR images have T2 weighting, so white matter is of lower signal than gray matter, which is the opposite of a T1-weighted image.

Diffusion-weighted images are sensitized to the movement of water protons. When diffusion is restricted, such as in acute infarcts and within cerebral abscesses, diffusion-weighted images show high signal. These images also contain an element of T2 weighting, which means that high signal on a diffusion-weighted image may also be caused by conditions that cause high signal on T2-weighted images ("T2 shine through").

Perfusion-weighted imaging can be obtained with CT or MRI. Both techniques require rapid imaging before and during the injection of a bolus of contrast medium. The whole brain can be studied with MR perfusion, whereas coverage with CT is usually limited to two slices. Postprocessing of the images allows the production of maps of cerebral blood flow, cerebral blood volume, mean transit time, and time to peak enhancement. Perfusion-weighted imaging is most often used for the assessment of acute ischemic stroke and may be of benefit in assessing vasospasm after subarachnoid hemorrhage.

13

Table 13-1 Assessing the Cervical Spine Radiograph

Lateral Projection	Frontal Projection
Alignment of the anterior margins of vertebral bodies	Orientation of the spinous processes
Alignment of the posterior margins of vertebral bodies	The distance between spinous processes should be equal
Facet joint alignment	Orientation of the facet joints
Alignment of the bases of the spinous processes (spinolaminar line)	The lateral margins of C1 should be in alignment with those of C2
Alignment of the tips of the spinous processes	
Prevertebral soft tissue swelling (does not exclude a significant injury)	
C7/T1 included	
Vertebral body height equal from C2 to C7	
Intervertebral disc spaces should be equal	

SPINAL TRAUMA

There is a high incidence of cervical spine injury associated with multiple trauma. A lateral cervical spine radiograph is invariably obtained in the emergency department on admission. Further views involve an anteroposterior projection of the whole cervical spine, as well as an open-mouth anteroposterior projection to demonstrate the C1/C2 articulation. Tracing curves connecting the anatomic landmarks outlined in Table 13-1 is a simple and essential part of interpretation (Fig. 13-1). The presence of a step in one of these lines or soft tissue swelling suggests a fracture or dislocation. It is important to ensure that the C7/T1 junction is imaged; a swimmer's projection may sometimes be necessary. Adequate radiographs are obtained in only 80% of multiply injured patients; multislice CT with multiplanar reconstruction is now being used increasingly in this scenario.

Normal prevertebral soft tissue should measure less than 6 mm at C3 and less than 20 mm at C6, although these figures are unreliable in intubated patients. Prevertebral soft tissue swelling secondary to hematoma may be the only sign of a fracture.

In cases of suspected ligamentous injury, flexion and extension radiographs should be considered. Alternatively, MRI has a role in evaluating ligamentous injury. It should be remembered that cervical trauma might also lead to intracranial consequences as a result of dissection of the carotid or vertebral arteries.

The traditional approach to clearing the thoracolumbar spine has been with radiographs. However, multiplanar reconstruction of CT scans of the chest and abdomen, obtained in cases of visceral injury, is an adequate substitute.

INTRACRANIAL APPEARANCES IN TRAUMA

The main aims of CT in head injury are to define the type and site of hemorrhage, evaluate depressed skull fractures, and recognize complications such as cerebral edema and brain herniation. Conventional CT is relatively insensitive in demonstrating nondepressed skull fractures, particularly when they are parallel to the plane of the CT slice. Sensitivity for skull fractures is increased with the use of multiplanar reconstruction of thin-section, multislice CT data. Indications for urgent CT are listed in Table 13-2. Traumatic intracranial hemorrhage can be parenchymal, such

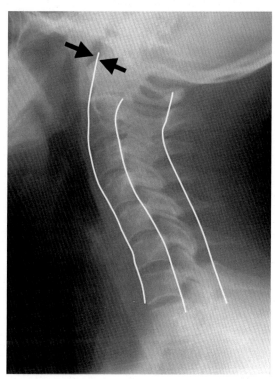

Figure 13-1 Lines connecting the anterior and posterior margins of the vertebral bodies, as well as the bases of the spinous processes. A further smooth curve can be traced between the tips of the spinous processes. The space between the odontoid peg and C1 should measure 3 mm or less in an adult (*arrows*).

Table 13-2	**Indications for Urgent Computed Tomography in Acute Head Injury**

Within 1 Hour

GCS score <13 at any point since the injury
GCS score equal to 13 or 14 at 2 hours after the injury
Suspected open or depressed skull fracture
Any sign of basal skull fracture
Post-traumatic seizure
Focal neurologic deficit
More than one episode of vomiting in patients older than 12 years
Age >65 years with loss of consciousness, amnesia, or coagulopathy

Within 8 Hours

Dangerous mechanism of injury
Amnesia of events before impact for longer than 30 minutes

GCS, Glasgow Coma Scale.
From National Institute of Clinical Excellence: Head Injury. Triage, Assessment, Investigation and Early Management of Head Injury in Infants, Children and Adults. 2003. Available online at http://www.nice.org.uk/CG56

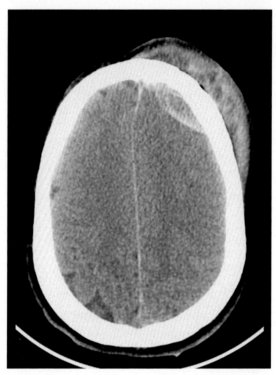

Figure 13-2   Axial computed tomography in a patient after head trauma showing an acute left frontal extradural hematoma. The presence of low attenuation within the collection implies active hemorrhage. Note the marked extracranial soft tissue swelling.

as contusions (including contrecoup injuries) or extra-axial, including subdural or extradural hematomas and subarachnoid hemorrhage.

Extradural hematomas classically have a biconvex configuration (Fig. 13-2) and are typically limited by the cranial sutures. They are associated with an adjacent skull fracture in up to 90% of cases (Fig. 13-3). Sixty percent of extradural hematomas have a concomitant tear in the middle meningeal artery; the remaining 40% are due to trauma to venous structures. Areas of low density within an extradural hematoma (the "swirl sign") suggest the presence of active hemorrhage. A lucid interval after injury is a frequent occurrence, possibly as a result of slow blood loss or initial hypotension.

Subdural hematomas are associated with significant head injury, and up to 30% of patients with severe head injury will have a subdural collection. They are much more common than extradural hematomas and result from shearing of bridging veins. Collections are concave medially and can cross suture lines (Fig. 13-4). Although in the acute stage blood is dense on CT, untreated collections become isodense to normal brain before becoming hypodense in the chronic stage. This situation can lead to diagnostic confusion. The most common site for subdural collections is over the frontal convexities, but they can also occur in the tentorium and posterior and middle cranial fossae. MRI is more sensitive in delineating these collections.

Diffuse axonal injury is associated with shearing of axons and disruption of white matter tracts. Certain sites are associated with axonal injury, including the body and splenium of the corpus callosum, the brainstem in the region of the superior cerebellar peduncle, and the internal capsule. Severe hyperextension injuries may

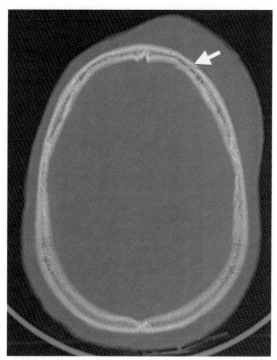

Figure 13-3   Bone algorithm reconstruction of Figure 13-2 showing a left frontal bone fracture (*arrow*).

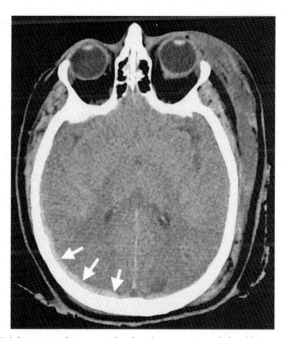

Figure 13-4   Axial computed tomography showing an acute subdural hematoma (*arrows*) with a typical concave medial margin.

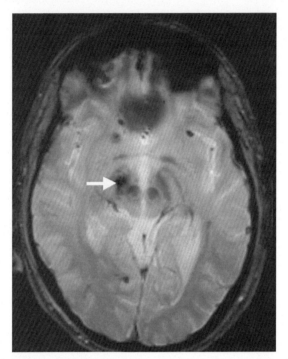

Figure 13-5 Axial T2*-weighted gradient-echo magnetic resonance imaging showing the typical features of diffuse axonal injury with multiple low–signal intensity foci of hemorrhage at the gray-white junction and in the right cerebral peduncle (*arrow*).

result in axonal damage to the cerebral peduncles and at the pontomedullary junction. MRI is more sensitive in identifying diffuse axonal injury, particularly gradient-echo sequences (Fig. 13-5).

SUBARACHNOID HEMORRHAGE

Spontaneous subarachnoid hemorrhage is most often caused by rupture of an aneurysm or arteriovenous malformation. It is less frequently associated with dural arteriovenous fistulas, hemorrhagic tumor, or bleeding diatheses. The initial diagnosis is invariably made by CT, on which hyperdense blood products are usually readily identifiable (Fig. 13-6). The sensitivity of CT is 98% within 24 hours of bleeding but falls to 50% by 7 days. In the setting of a good history for subarachnoid hemorrhage, negative CT findings without signs of impending brain herniation should lead to lumbar puncture. The extent and location of blood on the CT scan may indicate the probable source of hemorrhage. Although digital subtraction angiography (DSA) remains the "gold standard," CT angiography (CTA) is now frequently the first-line investigation for detection of aneurysms and has equivalent diagnostic accuracy (Fig. 13-7). In many cases CTA can be used to plan treatment, either by surgical clipping or by endovascular embolization with detachable coils. If CTA is negative, DSA should be performed. DSA is negative in up to 20% of cases. Repeat angiography approximately 5 to 7 days later may identify an occult aneurysm that may have been tamponaded by local hemorrhage. A negative repeat conventional angiogram suggests nonaneurysmal subarachnoid hemorrhage (occurring in up to

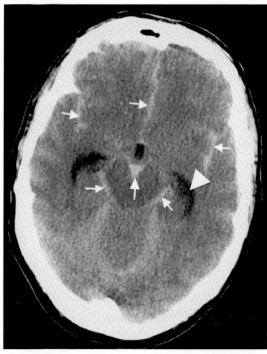

Figure 13-6   Axial computed tomography showing extensive acute subarachnoid hemorrhage in the basal cisterns, anterior interhemispheric fissure, and sylvian fissures (arrows). Note dilatation of temporal horn of lateral ventricle, indicating hydrocephalus (arrowhead).

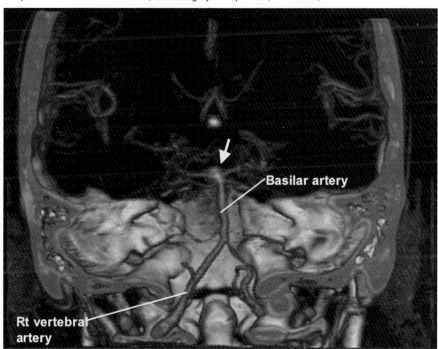

Figure 13-7   Volume-rendered image of a computed tomography angiogram of the patient in Figure 13-6. An aneurysm is located at the tip of the basilar artery (*arrow*).

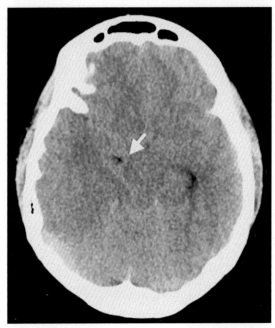

Figure 13-8 Axial computed tomography in a patient with raised intracranial pressure. Right uncal herniation with medial displacement of the temporal horn of the right lateral ventricle (*arrow*) and generalized effacement of the basal cistern are apparent.

15% of cases), which is frequently perimesencephalic. Such hemorrhage is possibly venous in origin and carries a good prognosis. Aneurysms are multiple in up to 20% of patients, and in such cases the presence of an irregular "nipple" on one of them suggests recent rupture.

RAISED INTRACRANIAL PRESSURE

Herniation of brain can take a number of forms: tonsillar or cerebellar herniation through the foramen magnum, superior vermian herniation, temporal lobe (uncal) herniation (Fig. 13-8), subfalcine herniation, and transtentorial herniation. A mass effect can lead to associated hydrocephalus (e.g., effacement of the fourth ventricle causing dilation of the third and lateral ventricles, as well as uncal herniation causing contralateral temporal horn dilation). Raised intracranial pressure itself causes effacement of the ventricles and extra-axial CSF spaces (Fig. 13-9). The diagnosis of raised intracranial pressure can be difficult to make in young people because the lateral and third ventricles could be small in normal individuals.

INTRACRANIAL TUMORS

A full account of the imaging appearances of intracranial tumors is beyond the scope of this chapter, but a few generalizations can be made.

Low-grade infiltrating gliomas typically appear as nonenhancing areas of increased signal intensity in the white matter and cortex on T2-weighted and FLAIR images.

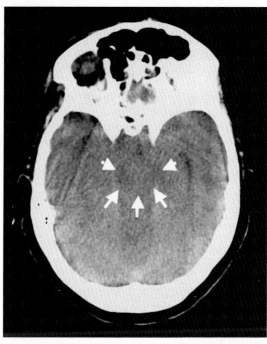

Figure 13-9   Axial computed tomography in a patient with raised intracranial pressure showing complete effacement of the perimesencephalic and quadrigeminal cisterns (*arrows*).

A mass effect results in effacement of the cortical sulci and expansion of the gyri. Though apparently well circumscribed, the tumor extends beyond the abnormality shown by imaging.

Glioblastoma multiforme is characterized by an irregular rind of peripheral enhancement around a central region of nonenhancing necrosis that is of low attenuation on CT, low signal on T1-weighted images, and high signal on T2-weighted images. Variable amounts of high T2 signal surround the enhancing part of the lesion and extend into the hemispheric white matter. Though often described as vasogenic edema, this peritumoral signal change represents a combination of edema and tumor cells.

Metastases tend to occur at the gray-white matter junction and are solitary in up to 50% of cases. Enhancement, which may be homogeneous or ring shaped, is a characteristic feature, and peritumoral vasogenic edema is often disproportionately extensive for the size of the lesions.

Primary cerebral lymphoma tends to occur in locations that abut the ependyma, leptomeninges, or both. In immunocompetent patients it appears as well-defined masses of relatively low T2 signal that enhance homogeneously after the administration of intravenous gadolinium. In the setting of acquired immunodeficiency syndrome, cerebral lymphoma tends to show more heterogeneous ring enhancement.

The extra-axial location of a meningioma is often shown by a thin rim of CSF signal between the tumor and the brain or by a broad dural base. Homogeneous enhancement is typical, calcification occurs in 20%, and vasogenic edema in the adjacent brain is not unusual. Meningiomas induce hyperostotic change in the adjacent skull in 20% of cases.

13

KEY POINTS

- Cervical spine radiographs are inadequate in 20% of multiply injured patients.
- Reconstructions of chest/abdomen CT scans are adequate to clear the thoracolumbar spine.
- Low density in an extradural hematoma suggests active bleeding.
- Subdural hematomas can cross cranial sutures.
- MRI is more sensitive than CT for diffuse axonal injury.
- CT angiography is the first-line investigation for patients with proven subarachnoid hemorrhage.
- Normal CT findings do not exclude raised intracranial pressure.

FURTHER READING

Agid R, Lee SK, Willinsky RA, et al: Acute subarachnoid haemorrhage: Using 64-slice multidetector CT angiography to "triage" patients' treatment. Neuroradiology 2006; 48:787-794.

Blackmore CC, Linnau KF: Controversies in clearing the spine. In Schwartz ED, Sanders AE (eds): Spinal Trauma: Imaging, Diagnosis and Management. Philadelphia, Lippincott Williams & Wilkins, 2007, pp 63-72.

National Institute of Clinical Excellence: Head Injury. Triage, Assessment, Investigation and Early Management of Head Injury in Infants, Children and Adults, 2003. Available online at http://www.nice.org.uk/CG56.

Osborn AG (ed): Diagnostic Cerebral Angiography. Philadelphia, Lippincott Williams & Wilkins, 1999.

Zulaga A, Núñez DB Jr: Plain film radiography and computed tomography of the cervical spine: Part 1. Normal anatomy and spinal injury identification. In Schwartz ED, Sanders AE (eds): Spinal Trauma: Imaging, Diagnosis and Management. Philadelphia, Lippincott Williams & Wilkins, 2007, pp 73-92.

IV

Chapter 14

Neurosurgical Operative Approaches

Rose Du • Michael W. McDermott

General Principles

Unilateral Frontotemporal Approaches

Bifrontal and Extended Bifrontal
Approaches

Interhemispheric Approach

Transsphenoidal Approach

Petrosal Approach (Retrolabyrinthine–
Middle Fossa Approach)

Midline Suboccipital Approach

Retrosigmoid Suboccipital Approach

Far Lateral Suboccipital Approach

GENERAL PRINCIPLES

The choice of surgical approach depends largely on the location of the lesion, the surrounding anatomy, the characteristics of the tumor, other comorbid conditions of the patient, and the experience of the surgeon. We discuss some of the major and common neurosurgical approaches that are used. Although the specialized approaches described in this chapter are used mainly for skull base and vascular lesions, the same principles apply to convexity lesions.

The main goal of any approach is to be able to reach the lesion with minimal brain retraction, thereby limiting any potential for brain injury. In many instances this means more bone removal to minimize brain retraction. The amount of exposure that can be gained with each approach is therefore variable and depends on the amount of bone removed, as well as the extent of arachnoid dissection, which will allow separation of lobes from one another (e.g., frontal from temporal lobe along the sylvian fissure), and the presence of vessels from the surface of the brain or surrounding nerves. The head should be elevated above the heart to avoid venous congestion. The use of a lumbar subarachnoid or external ventricular drain should also be considered to reduce the volume of the intracranial cavity and thereby the force of retraction necessary for a given exposure. In craniotomies around the venous sinuses, injury to the sinus can usually be controlled with direct pressure and the use of hemostatic agents, but there is a potential for large amounts of blood loss and air emboli. In general, management of intraoperative complications can best be facilitated by preoperative discussions between the attending surgeon and anesthesiologist about position, approach, expected blood loss, and common occurrences (such as bradycardia with coagulation of the tentorium) and by regular intraoperative discussions across the sterile drapes about what is happening and what to expect next. What follows here is the description of common neurosurgical approaches that can be used for a variety of pathologies (Table 14-1).

14

Table 14-1   Neurosurgical Approaches by Intracranial Compartment

Approaches	Compartment	Typical Pathology
Pterional	ACF, MCF	Tumor: glioma, meningioma,
Subfrontal	ACF	schwannoma, craniopha-
Bifrontal	ACF	ryngioma, giant pituitary
Extended frontal	ACF	adenoma
Orbitozygomatic	ACF, MCF	Vascular: aneurysm, AVM,
Extended middle fossa	MCF, PCF	AV fistula
Interhemispheric	Supratentorial, lateral, and third ventricle	Tumor: glioma, meningioma, intraventricular tumors Vascular: AVM, ACA aneurysm
Transnasal transsphenoidal	Sphenoid, ethmoid sinuses, sella, clivus, ACF	Tumor: pituitary adenoma, craniopharyngioma, chor- doma, esthesioneuroblas- toma, meningioma
Petrosal	MCF, PCF, CPA, clivus	Tumors meningioma, schwannoma, chordoma Vascular: AVM, basilar trunk aneurysm
Midline suboccipital	PCF, pineal region, fourth ventricle, FM	Tumor: glioma, choroid plexus papilloma, ependy- moma, medulloblastoma, pineal Vascular: AVM, rare distal PICA aneurysms
Retrosigmoid	PCF, CPA, FM	Tumor: schwannoma, meningioma, glioma, epidermoid cyst
Far lateral suboccipital	PCF, CPA, FM, cervico- medullary junction	Tumor: meningiomas Vascular: PICA aneurysm, medullary CVM

ACA, anterior cerebral artery; ACF, anterior cranial fossa; AV, arteriovenous; AVM arteriovenous malformation; CPA, cerebellopontine angle; CVM, cerebral venous malformation; FM, foramen mag- num; MCF, middle cranial fossa; PCF, posterior cranial fossa; PICA, posterior inferior cerebral artery.

IV

UNILATERAL FRONTOTEMPORAL APPROACHES

The unilateral frontotemporal approaches (Fig. 14-1) are used for unilateral tumors and vascular lesions. Some examples of lesions that can be treated with a unilateral frontotemporal approach include small olfactory groove meningiomas, small tuber- culum sella meningiomas, anterior circulation aneurysms, and basilar apex aneu- rysms. Variations of the frontotemporal approach include (1) the medial subfrontal approach, in which the bone flap is extended to the midline; this approach can be modified to include the orbital rim as a secondary osteotomy bone piece and is called a cranio-orbital approach; (2) the lateral frontotemporal approach, the so-called pterional approach, in which the bone flap extends in a curvilinear manner toward the supraorbital rim just above the superior temporal line, then parallel to the supra- orbital rim to the frontozygomatic process, then below this and posteriorly cross- ing the sphenoid wing, down into the squamous portion of the sphenoid bone, and then back up toward the superior temporal line posteriorly; (3) the orbitozygomatic approach (commonly referred to as the O-Z approach) (Fig. 14-2), which includes a bone flap as for the pterional approach and then removal of the supraorbital rim,

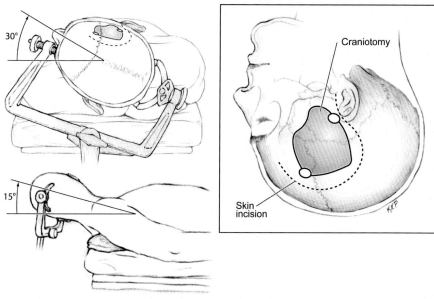

Figure 14-1   Unilateral frontotemporal (pterional) approach showing positioning, skin incision, and bone flap.

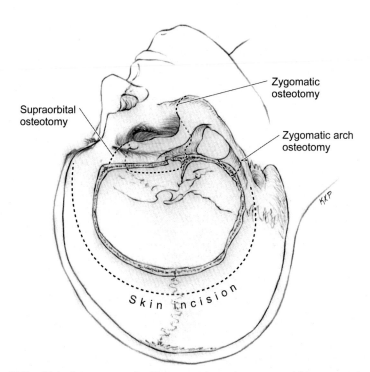

14

Figure 14-2   Right frontotemporal orbitozygomatic craniotomy. In addition to craniotomy for the pterional approach, osteotomies can be performed through the medial supraorbital margin, body of the zygoma, and zygomatic arch above the temporomandibular joint.

frontozygomatic process, posterior half of the body of the zygoma, and the arch of the zygoma in a second osteotomy all in one piece and; and (4) the extended middle fossa approach, which consists of removal of the petrous apex between the foramen ovale anteriorly, the arcuate eminence of the cochlea posteriorly, and the greater superficial petrosal nerve laterally (Kawase approach).

For the medial subfrontal approach the patient is placed supine, the neck flexed on the chest, and the head extended on the neck without rotation. For the pterional and O-Z approaches the patient is placed supine on the operating table with ipsilateral shoulder elevation and the head rotated 30 degrees. A frontotemporal craniotomy is usually accompanied by varying degrees of bone removal from the sphenoid ridge, posterior orbital roof, and anterior clinoid and may be extended by removal of the orbital rim with or without the zygoma (cranio-orbital and orbitozygomatic approaches). Removal of the orbital rim requires dissection of the periorbita from the orbital roof. During the orbital dissection, the trigemino-ocular reflex may be provoked, which consists of bradycardia, hypotension, apnea, and gastric hypermotility. Lesions are often accessed by splitting the sylvian fissure. Structures that can potentially be injured include the internal carotid artery, anterior cerebral artery, middle cerebral artery, posterior communicating artery, olfactory nerve, optic nerve, optic chiasm, oculomotor nerve, and pituitary stalk.

BIFRONTAL AND EXTENDED BIFRONTAL APPROACHES

The bifrontal approach (Fig. 14-3) is used for midline tumors. Lesions that are treated via the bifrontal approach include large olfactory groove meningiomas, large planum sphenoidale meningiomas, tuberculum sellae meningiomas, and some large

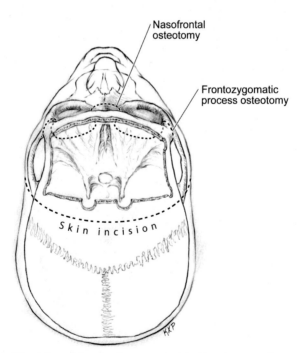

Nasofrontal osteotomy

Frontozygomatic process osteotomy

Skin incision

Figure 14-3 Bifrontal craniotomy using a coronal incision from ear to ear. For skull base approaches, bilateral supraorbital osteotomy can be done by removing the supraorbital bar in one piece (extended bifrontal craniotomy).

craniopharyngiomas. A lumbar subarachnoid drain may be placed for large tumors before positioning to help with relaxation of the brain. The patient is placed supine on the operating table with the neck flexed on the chest and the head extended at the neck with no rotation. A bicoronal incision is made from zygomatic arch to zygomatic arch. The scalp is reflected to the point where the supraorbital nerves are seen. Laterally, the temporalis muscle is reflected inferiorly and posteriorly while preserving the frontalis branch of the facial nerve. A bifrontal bone flap is elevated while taking care to not violate the superior sagittal sinus.

For large tumors that extend superiorly, an extended bifrontal approach may be necessary. In this approach, dissection is carried out around the orbit so that the orbital bar can be removed. During orbital dissection the trigemino-ocular reflex may be provoked. Other structures that can potentially be injured include the superior sagittal sinus, olfactory nerves, optic nerves and chiasm, and anterior cerebral arteries. Recent experience indicates that despite the extensive bone removal, the incidence of complications is acceptably low and infections are uncommon.

INTERHEMISPHERIC APPROACH

The interhemispheric approach (Fig. 14-4) is used for lesions at or close to the midline, including distal anterior cerebral artery aneurysms, falcine meningiomas, lesions of the corpus callosum, and lateral and third ventricular lesions. A lumbar subarachnoid drain may be placed for large tumors before positioning to help with relaxation of the brain. The patient is placed supine on the operating room table with the head slightly flexed. In a variation of this approach, the patient is placed semilateral with the head turned 90 degrees to the table and bent laterally up at a 45-degree angle.

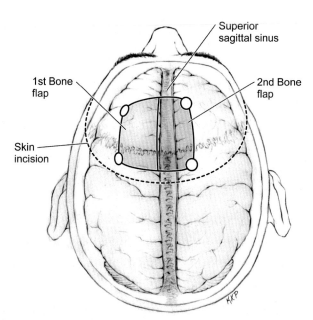

Figure 14-4   Bipartite bone flap crossing the midline for an interhemispheric approach. The first portion of the bone flap is lateral to the midline to avoid the risk of injury to the venous lakes and superior sagittal sinus. Under direct vision the midline dura can then be dissected to the opposite side and a second bone piece created.

For both positions, the craniotomy involves crossing the superior sagittal sinus. Injury to the sinus may result in air embolism or large amounts of blood loss, which is usually easily controlled with direct pressure. Other structures that can potentially be injured include the distal anterior cerebral artery and sensory and motor cortex. If a transcallosal transventricular approach is used, there is potential for injury to the thalamus and the deep venous drainage system, as well as for intraventricular hemorrhage.

TRANSSPHENOIDAL APPROACH

The transsphenoidal approach (Fig. 14-5) is used for sellar lesions with or without suprasellar extension or for clival lesions. The patient is placed supine on the operating room table with the body flexed and the head in a sniffing position. A lumbar subarachnoid drain may be placed for lesions with suprasellar extension. Saline is infused into the lumbar drain to help push the tumor inferiorly so that it can be reached easily. Maintaining normal or elevated Pa_{CO_2} is also helpful. The drain is sometimes left in place postoperatively for management or prevention of cerebrospinal fluid leakage. Structures that can potentially be injured during the exposure include the cavernous sinus, internal carotid artery, optic chiasm, and pituitary stalk. Injury to the cavernous sinus can easily be controlled with hemostatic agents. Injury to the internal carotid artery may result in massive blood loss requiring endovascular treatment.

Currently, sublabial, transnasal, and endonasal transsphenoidal approaches are practiced. For the sublabial approach the labial mucosa just past the gingival crease above the upper central incisors is opened and the nasal cavity accessed via

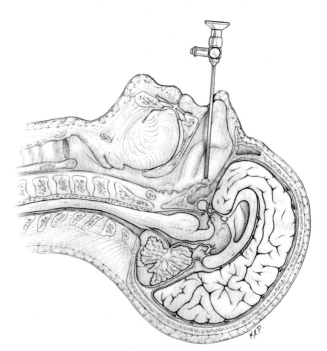

Figure 14-5   Transnasal transsphenoidal approach using an endoscope. The same approach can be taken with a nasal speculum and microscope (transnasal transsphenoidal microsurgical approach) without need for any sublabial or external incisions.

submucosal dissection. The mucosa is tripped all the way back to the rostrum of the sphenoid and the sphenoid sinus entered with a rongeur. Most experienced surgeons have now moved to the transnasal microsurgical approach, in which a smaller speculum introduced through a single nostril provides all the visibility and access necessary. The opening can be extended anteriorly up the front wall of the sella to include the tuberculum and planum, whereby larger suprasellar tumors can be removed, the so-called extended transsphenoidal approach. The endonasal endoscopic approach is the current minimally invasive technique coming to the fore; it uses nothing but the endoscope for visualization and working instruments up both nostrils.

PETROSAL APPROACH (RETROLABYRINTHINE–MIDDLE FOSSA APPROACH)

There are a number of approaches in which part of the petrous bone is removed. Here, we describe the retrolabyrinthine–middle fossa approach (Fig. 14-6), which is used for lesions that arise on the upper two thirds of the clivus, such as petro-clival meningiomas and chordomas. Neurophysiologic monitoring of the trigeminal, abducens, facial, and vestibulocochlear nerves is typical practice. A lumbar subarachnoid drain is often inserted. The patient is placed supine on the operating room table with a bolster underneath one shoulder and the head turned 60 degrees. A small temporoparietal craniotomy is performed, followed by a mastoidectomy/posterior fossa craniectomy, exposure of the sigmoid sinus, and retro-labyrinthine exposure of the presigmoid dura of the posterior fossa and toward the petrous apex below the superior petrosal sinus. The temporal dura and presigmoid dura are opened and the cuts connected with sectioning of the superior petrosal sinus and tentorium. Structures that can potentially be injured include the sigmoid sinus and jugular bulb; the hearing apparatus; cranial nerves IV, V, VI, VII, and

14

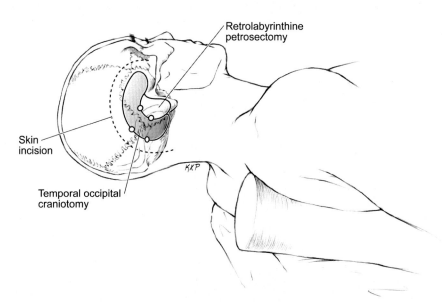

Retrolabyrinthine petrosectomy

Skin incision

Temporal occipital craniotomy

Figure 14-6 Petrosal approach for tumors involving the posterior and middle cranial fossa. A temporal craniotomy is combined with presigmoid, retrolabyrinthine bone removal. The dura is opened anterior to the sigmoid sinus along the floor of the middle fossa and the tentorium incised.

VIII; the brainstem; and the vein of Labbé. For larger tumors in this region such as meningiomas, the incidence of new neurologic deficits can be greater than 50% in published reports.

MIDLINE SUBOCCIPITAL APPROACH

The midline suboccipital approach (Fig. 14-7) is used for lesions in the cerebellar hemispheres, as well as for lesions near the midline in the dorsal medulla and pons. For tumors in the pineal region, this opening provides access to the superior cerebellar surface for the infratentorial supracerebellar approach. A lumbar drain is not needed here because the cisterna magna is easily accessible for release of cerebrospinal fluid. The patient is placed prone on the operating room table with the head flexed and chin tucked. Patients who are obese, large breasted, or of large size present problems with elevated venous and airway pressure in the prone position that may compromise conditions such that a sitting position may be required. In such a case in which the risk for air embolism is higher, a bubble echocardiogram is required to rule out a right-to-left shunt. Whether prone or sitting, a midline incision is made a few centimeters above the inion and extended down to C3-C4. The craniotomy is carried out superior to the transverse sinus and inferior to or through the foramen magnum. A C1 laminectomy may also be required for tumors that extend from the fourth ventricle into the upper cervical spine (e.g., ependymoma). The potential danger with this approach is injury to the transverse sinus, posterior inferior cerebellar artery, and brainstem. For large tumors around the confluence of the sinuses (torcular Herophili), a larger craniotomy may be required, including removal of bone over both occipital lobes and the cerebellum.

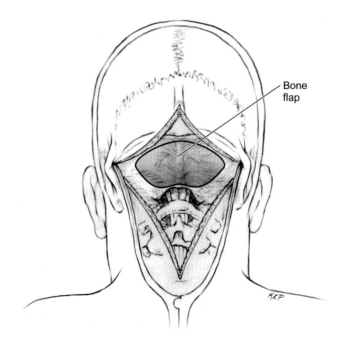

Bone flap

Figure 14-7   Midline suboccipital approach involving a craniotomy below the transverse sinuses and down to or including the lip of the foramen magnum.

RETROSIGMOID SUBOCCIPITAL APPROACH

The retrosigmoid suboccipital approach (Fig. 14-8) is used mainly for lesions in the middle third of the clivus, such as cerebellopontine angle tumors, microvascular decompression, anterolateral pontine lesions, and anterior inferior cerebellar artery aneurysms. A lumbar subarachnoid drain is sometimes inserted preoperatively. The patient is placed semilateral on the operating room table with a bolster underneath one shoulder. The head is turned 90 degrees with respect to the floor. The margins of the transverse and sigmoid sinuses are exposed with the craniotomy, often under image guidance. Bleeding from the transverse and sigmoid sinuses can occur during

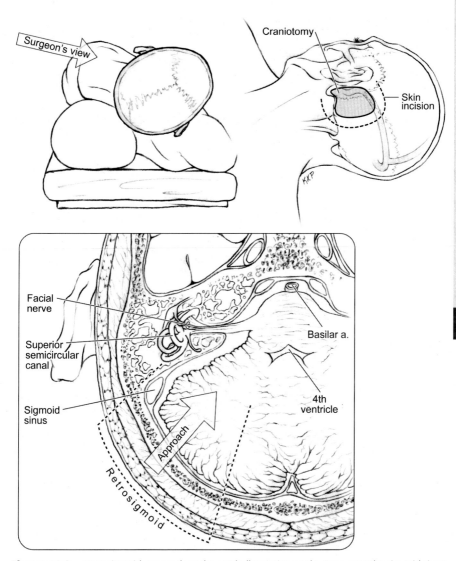

Figure 14-8 Retrosigmoid approach to the cerebellopontine angle. Bone over the sigmoid sinus is drilled off with a diamond bur to avoid injury. This is a common approach for meningiomas, acoustic neuromas, trigeminal neuralgia, and hemifacial spasm.

the craniotomy but can usually be controlled with pressure. With opening of the dura, the cerebellum is generally bulging, which necessitates release of cerebrospinal fluid from the cisterna magna or the cerebellopontine angle cistern for decompression. Retraction of the cerebellum allows exposure of the brainstem and cranial nerves. Depending on the lesion, neurophysiologic monitoring of the cranial nerves may be done. Structures that can potentially be injured include the pons and cranial nerves, mainly the trigeminal, abducens, facial, and vestibulocochlear nerves. For lesions that are lower, the vagus nerve can also be injured.

FAR LATERAL SUBOCCIPITAL APPROACH

The far lateral approach (Fig. 14-9) is used for lesions in the lateral and anterolateral region of the foramen magnum and the lower third of the clivus, such as foramen magnum meningiomas, posterior inferior cerebellar artery aneurysms, and medullary cavernous malformations. A lumbar subarachnoid drain is not necessary because the cisterna magna is easily accessible for release of cerebrospinal fluid. The patient is placed in a three-quarter prone park bench position with the head flexed toward the neck, rotated 120 degrees from vertical, and laterally flexed 20 degrees. The contralateral arm is secured in a sling over the edge of the top of the table. A suboccipital craniotomy is performed from midline to the sigmoid sinus laterally. The occipital condyle can be drilled down to the hypoglossal canal. A C1 cervical laminectomy is also performed. Structures that can potentially be injured include the vertebral artery, posterior inferior cerebellar artery, jugular bulb, lower brainstem, and lower cranial nerves.

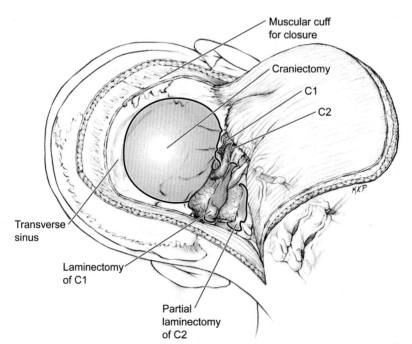

Figure 14-9 Far lateral suboccipital approach. A suboccipital craniotomy was extended into the posterior third of the occipital condyle combined with C1 (occasionally C2) hemilaminectomy,

KEY POINTS

- The frontotemporal approach and its modifications are the most common neurosurgical approaches for pathology in the anterior and middle cranial fossa.
- A bifrontal craniotomy can be used for pathology in the anterior skull base, those that extend into the nasal cavity, and those that extend back to the suprasellar region.
- Transsphenoidal approaches can be performed sublabially, transnasally, or completely endoscopically.
- Posterior fossa approaches can be complicated by transient trigeminal or vagal reflexes that cause profound bradycardia.
- Before sitting/semisitting procedures, a bubble echocardiogram should be obtained to exclude a right-to-left shunt.

FURTHER READING

Chi JH, McDermott, MW: Tuberculum sellae meningiomas. Neurosurg Focus 2003; 14(6): Article 6.

Chi JH, Parsa AT, Berger MS, et al: Extended bifrontal craniotomy for midline anterior fossa meningiomas: Minimization of retraction-related edema and surgical outcomes. Neurosurgery 2006; 59(4 Suppl 2):ONS426-ONS434.

McDermott MW, Durity FA, Rootman J, Woodhurst WB: Combined frontotemporal-orbitozygomatic approach for tumors of the sphenoid wing and orbit. Neurosurgery 1990; 26:107-116.

McDermott MW, Parsa AT: Surgical management of olfactory groove meningiomas. In Badie B (ed): Neurosurgical Operative Atlas. Neuro-oncology, 2nd ed, New York; Thieme 2007.

Quinones-Hinojosa A, Chang EF, Khan SA, et al: Renal cell carcinoma metastatic to the choroid plexus mimicking intraventricular meningioma. Can J Neurol Sci 2004; 31:115-120.

Quinones-Hinojosa A, Chang EF, McDermott MW: Falcotentorial meningiomas: Clinical, neuroimaging, and surgical features in six patients. Neurosurg Focus 2003; 14(6): Article 11.

14

Chapter 15

Surgical Positioning

Rose Du • Chanhung Z. Lee

Positioning of patients is critical in neurosurgical procedures. Proper positioning allows the most optimal exposure of the lesion with minimal injury to the brain while ensuring that the position is physiologically and physically safe for the anesthetized patient. Thus, in addition to exposure considerations, one must also be cognizant of positions that can result in immediate adverse effects on the operation or the patient, such as increased intracranial pressure and airway compromise, as well as those that can result in neurologic deficits or skin breakdown from prolonged compression or stretching of certain regions. Although patient positioning has been extensively discussed in standard anesthesia textbooks, this chapter discusses the most common positions for neurologic surgery and the related anesthesia complications.

GENERAL PRINCIPLES

Intraoperative problems can occur as a result of increased intracranial pressure, venous congestion, and airway compromise. Increased intracranial pressure can be due to increased abdominal pressure, venous congestion from kinking of the internal jugular vein, and positioning of the head below the level of the heart. Venous congestion itself can exacerbate brain swelling and lead to excessive venous bleeding, which can hinder the operation. Such congestion can result from prone positioning with insufficient abdominal bolstering, increased positive end-expiratory pressure (PEEP), or venous obstruction from hyper-rotation or hyperflexion of the neck. Hyperflexion of the neck can also result in airway compromise from kinking of the endotracheal tube. Kinking of the endotracheal tube can often be avoided by using armored tubes. As a general rule, a distance

IV

of one or two fingerbreadths should be maintained between the chin and chest during neck flexion.

Postoperative complications can result from prolonged pressure on presure points, which can cause skin breakdown or compression of periperal nerves. Common pressure points are the elbows (ulnar nerve), heels, iliac crests, breasts, and male genitalia. Other peripheral nerve injuries can occur as a result of stretching of nerves, particularly the brachial plexus. In general, the patient should be positioned in a way that would be comfortable for an awake patient over a prolonged period. The American Society of Anesthesiologists has published a practice advisory for the prevention of perioperative peripheral neuropathies. Corneal abrasions should be avoided in all cases by sealing the eyes shut. In prolonged cases, sealing should be augmented with ophthalmic ointment.

In the following sections, specific positioning considerations for common neurosurgical approaches are discussed.

SUPINE POSITION (FRONTOTEMPORAL, BIFRONTAL SUBFRONTAL, AND INTERHEMISPHERIC APPROACHES)

The bifrontal, subfrontal, and interhemispheric approaches and other frontotemporal approaches that involve only mild turning of the neck are performed by positioning the patient supine on the operating room table. This is the least involved of the operative positions. The influence of gravity on the circulation is minimal in the horizontal supine position. The head may be flexed slightly for interhemispheric approaches to the lateral or third ventricles or extended slightly in the subfrontal approaches. Neck flexion or extension in these approaches is generally mild. Extreme neck flexion can lead to kinking of the endotracheal tube. When extreme neck flexion is accompanied by placing the patient in the reverse Trendelenburg position, the patient may be at increased risk for air embolism, particularly with bifrontal craniotomies in which the superior sagittal sinus is traversed and at risk for injury.

Attention must also be paid to the extremities. The upper extremities are usually positioned at the patient's sides, in which case the shoulders should not be abducted more than 90 degrees to prevent injury to the brachial plexus. When the arm is tucked or held in a bent position across the body, foam padding should be applied to the elbow and wrist to avoid injury to the ulnar and median nerves. The knees should be elevated to decrease tension on the lower part of the back. The heels should also be padded to avoid skin breakdown.

15

SEMILATERAL POSITION OR SUPINE POSITION WITH A BOLSTER (PETROSAL, RETROSIGMOID, AND UNILATERAL FRONTOTEMPORAL APPROACHES)

The petrosal and retrosigmoid approaches, as well as any unilateral approach that requires moderate rotation of the neck, are performed by placing the patient in a supine position with the ipsilateral shoulder elevated (Fig. 15-1). The use of a shoulder bolster is particularly important in elderly patients with less flexible necks and to avoid kinking of the internal jugular vein with neck rotation. In the petrosal and retrosigmoid approaches, the elevated shoulder is often pulled down inferiorly with tape to minimize obstruction of the surgical view. Excessive traction on the shoulder can result in stretch injury to the brachial plexus. Other considerations are similar to those for the supine position.

Semilateral or supine position (petrosal, retrosigmoid, and unilateral frontotemporal approaches)

① Bolster
② Padding arm board
③ Padding between knees and ankles
④ Padding under heels
⑤ Adequate distance between chin and clavicle

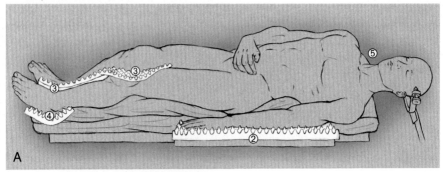

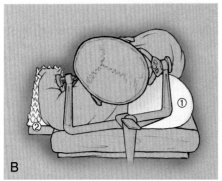

Figure 15-1   Semilateral position (**A**) or supine position with a bolster (**B**). There should not be any excessive traction on the brachial plexus or obstruction of venous drainage in the neck.

SITTING POSITION (SUPRACEREBELLAR INFRATENTORIAL APPROACH)

The sitting position is sometimes used for approaches to the posterior fossa such as the supracerebellar infratentorial approach. Major complications with this position include the risk of air embolism, which occurs in 9% to 43% of patients undergoing neurosurgery in the sitting position, hypotension, and postoperative tension pneumocephalus. Given the high risk of air embolism, all patients undergoing craniotomy in the sitting position should be preoperatively imaged with a echocardiogram to rule out a patent foramen ovale. Monitors such as precordial Doppler ultrasonography, capnography, and a right heart catheter are useful for detecting air embolism and should be placed immediately preoperatively. Nitrous oxide should be avoided if venous air embolism is a concern.

When the sitting position is used for the supracerebellar infratentorial approach, the extreme neck flexion may lead to kinking of the endotracheal tube, and it has also been associated with cervical cord ischemia.

Lateral position (posterior parietal or occipital craniotomies)

① Axillary roll
② Back and abdomen support
③ Bottom knee bent
④ Padding between legs
⑤ Padding under knee and ankle
⑥ Ipsilateral shoulder pulled inferiorly
⑦ Head in neutral position

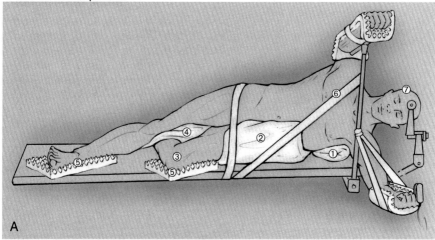

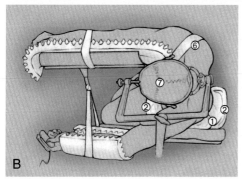

15

Figure 15-2 A and **B,** Lateral position. A variation is to place and tape the upper part of the arm along the length of the torso. The lower part of the arm can be folded across the chest with the hand in proximity to the upper part of the shoulder. Note that the axillary roll is placed under the chest to prevent pressure on and injury to the axillary structures.

LATERAL POSITION (POSTERIOR PARIETAL OR OCCIPITAL CRANIOTOMY)

The lateral position is often used for posterior parietal or occipital craniotomy (Fig. 15-2). The key feature of lateral positioning is the use of axillary rolls. The purpose of an axillary roll is to prevent brachial plexus compression or pressure on the dependent shoulder when the patient is in the lateral decubitus position. Complications can occur from the axillary rolls themselves, such as brachial plexus injury, and can be prevented by proper placement of the "axillary" roll under the upper part of the chest rather than the axilla.

101

To maintain the lateral position, a means of support should be placed along the patient's back and abdomen. The knees should be flexed with padding between the knees to avoid pressure over the fibular head and peroneal nerve.

PARK BENCH OR THREE-QUARTER PRONE POSITION (FAR LATERAL APPROACH)

The park bench or three-quarter prone position is used in far lateral approaches (Fig. 15-3). It involves placing the patient sufficiently superiorly on the operating table such that the dependent arm is hanging over the edge of the table and secured with a sling. The dependent arm should be well supported and protected. Care must be taken to pad all the pressure points. An axillary roll should be placed under the dependent chest for the same reason as for the lateral position. The trunk is rotated 15 degrees from the lateral position into a semiprone position and supported with pillows/blankets. The ipsilateral shoulder is pulled inferiorly. Too much tension on the shoulder can result in stretching of the brachial plexus.

The head is flexed at the neck and then rotated to look toward the floor (i.e., 120 degrees from vertical and laterally flexed 20 degrees). This results in considerable rotation and flexion of the neck and can result in kinking of the endotracheal tube, as well as the internal jugular vein. An armored endotracheal tube may be preferred. The head also needs to be properly positioned to prevent obstruction of cerebral venous outflow. In addition, excessive flexion can press the mandible onto the clavicle.

PRONE POSITION (SUBOCCIPITAL APPROACH)

The prone position is used for the suboccipital approach and posterior spinal surgery (Fig. 15-4). The potential for complications is very high. Turning the patient to a prone position could also cause hemodynamic changes, impairment of ventilation, and spinal cord injury. In this approach the patient is placed on two bolsters or a support device with arms to the side of the body. To ensure that abdominal and femoral venous return is not unduly compromised, as well as to allow adequate diaphragmatic excursion, the bolsters should be sufficiently far apart and large enough to not cause pressure on the abdomen. Breasts and male genitalia should be checked to minimize any pressure on them. Arms and knees should be padded. The ankles should be elevated so that the toes are hanging freely. The chin is tucked in the suboccipital approach, which may cause kinking of the endotracheal tube, so an armored tube may be preferred. Facial and airway edema occurs with longer procedures and may necessitate postoperative intubation. Though a rare occurrence, blindness has been reported after surgery in the prone position, particularly in procedures with a prolonged duration, significant blood loss, and hypotension.

KEY POINTS

- Increased intracranial pressure can result from increased abdominal pressure, venous congestion, and positioning of the head below the level of the heart.
- Venous congestion can result from venous outflow obstruction caused by hyperrotation or hyperflexion of the neck.
- Increased PEEP and airway compromise can result from kinking of the endotracheal tube caused by neck flexion.

Park bench or three-quarter prone position (far lateral approach)

① Dependent arm hangs off table
② Axillary roll
③ Back and abdomen support
④ Bottom knee bent
⑤ Padding between and under legs
⑥ Ipsilateral shoulder pulled inferiorly

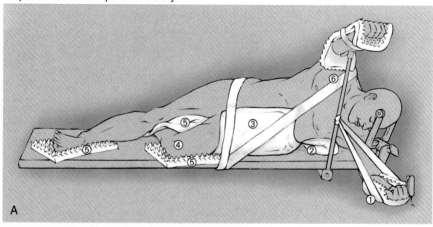

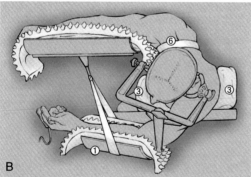

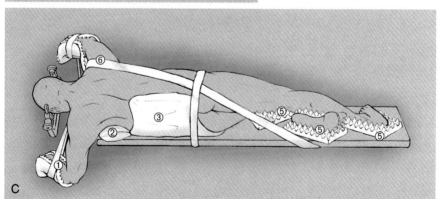

Figure 15-3 **A** to **C,** Park bench or three-quarter prone position. A variation is to place and tape the upper part of the arm along the length of the torso. The lower part of the arm can be folded across the chest with the hand in proximity to the upper part of the shoulder. Inappropriate flexion and rotation can obstruct venous drainage and ventilation.

Prone position-A (suboccipital approach)
Head in Mayfield clamp

① Bolster
② Arms down side
③ Avoid pressure on abdomen
④ Avoid pressure on male genitals and breasts
⑤ Arm and knee padding
⑥ Chin tucked
⑦ Mayfield head clamp

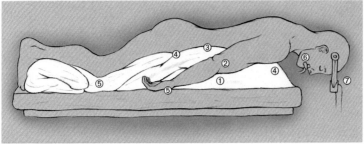

Prone position-B (suboccipital approach)
Head on face pillow

① Bolsters
② Arms alongside the head
③ Avoid pressure on abdomen
④ Avoid pressure on male genitals and breasts
⑤ Arm and knee padding
⑥ Face pillow with eyes and nose free of compression

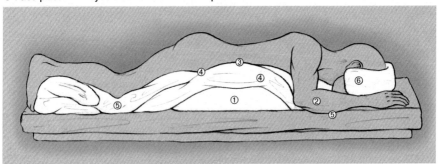

Figure 15-4   Prone position. **A,** Fixation of the head and cervical spine is needed for suboccipital and upper spine procedures. **B,** For lower spinal procedures the head is supported in a foam or other device. Care should be taken to ensure that no pressure is placed on the eyes and nose.

- Given the high risk for air embolism, all patients undergoing craniotomy in the sitting position should have an echocardiogram performed preoperatively to rule out a patent foramen ovale.
  - In the prone position, bolsters should be adequately placed to minimize pressure on the abdomen and thorax.

FURTHER READING

Benumof JL, Mazzei W, Roth S, et al: Multifactorial etiology of postoperative vision loss. Anesthesiology 2002; 96:1531-1532.

Engelhardt M, Folkers W, Brenke C, et al: Neurosurgical operations with the patient in sitting position: Analysis of risk factors using transcranial Doppler sonography. Br J Anaesth 2006; 96:467-472.

IV

Faust RJ, Cucchiara RF, Beehtle PS: Patient positioning. In Miller RD (ed): Miller's Anesthesia, 6th ed. New York, Churchill Livingstone, 2005, pp 1151-1167.

Furnas H, Canales F, Buncke GM, et al: Complications with the use of an axillary roll. Ann Plast Surg 1990; 25:208-209.

Leslie K, Hui R, Kaye AH: Venous air embolism and the sitting position: A case series. J Clin Neurosci 2006; 13:419-422.

McDermott MW, Wilson CW: Meningiomas. In Youmans JR (ed): Neurological Surgery. Philadelphia, WB Saunders, 1996, pp 2782-2825.

Practice advisory for the prevention of perioperative peripheral neuropathies: A report by the American Society of Anesthesiologists Task Force on Prevention of Perioperative Peripheral Neuropathies. Anesthesiology 2000; 92:1168-1182.

Warner MA, Matin JT: Patient positioning. In Barash PG, Cullen BF, Stoelting RK (eds): Clinical Anesthesia, 4th ed. Philadelphia, Lippincott Williams & Wilkins, 2001, pp 639-666.

15

Chapter 16

Anesthesia for Supratentorial Surgery

Rowan Burnstein • Arnab Banerjee

Anesthetic goals for supratentorial surgery include the following:

- Appreciation of the type, severity, and location of the lesion
- Swift, smooth anesthetic induction and emergence from general anesthesia
- Adequate cerebral perfusion pressure (CPP) throughout surgery and into the postoperative period
- Immobility, control of vital signs, and brain relaxation throughout surgery
- Adequate analgesia in the postoperative period

IV

THE LESIONS

Approximately 60% of supratentorial neoplasms are primary brain tumors, of which gliomas are the most common. These neoplasms range from relatively benign pilocytic and well-differentiated astrocytomas to aggressive anaplastic astrocytomas and glioblastoma multiforme. Other common benign tumors include meningiomas and pituitary adenomas. Brain abscesses can also be manifested as space-occupying lesions.

Glial tumors disrupt the blood-brain barrier and show a significant amount of contrast enhancement on computed tomography (CT) and magnetic resonance imaging (MRI). Although tumor blood flow varies, autoregulation is usually impaired within the tumor and induced hypertension can lead to an increase in tumor blood flow, which can worsen edema and cause bleeding. These tumors are frequently surrounded by large areas of edema, particularly prominent around fast-growing tumors, usually responds to corticosteroids. This edema can persist or even rebound after surgical excision of the tumor. The brain tissue surrounding a tumor may be relatively ischemic, perhaps as a result of compression. Meningiomas, which account for 15% of primary brain tumors, are slow growing and very vascular and can be difficult to dissect. They may require multiple attempts at resection and this may be preceeded by embolisation of the tumor.

Approximately 35% of supratentorial tumors are secondary neoplasms arising predominantly from the lung (50%) and breast (10%). The incidence of secondary tumors rises with increasing age. Excision of solitary lesions is justified in patients in whom the underlying disease is well controlled.

Other supratentorial lesions include brain abscesses, which may arise as a result of local spread from sinuses or ear infections and are especially common in immunocompromised and diabetic patients, those with right-to-left cardiac shunts, and intravenous drug abusers.

Most brain neoplasms tend to grow slowly and allow adaptive mechanisms to be established so that the tumors may become very large before becoming symptomatic. Patients commonly present with symptoms of raised intracranial pressure (ICP), seizures, or a focal neurologic deficit that may respond initially to steroids.

Patients with supratentorial tumors may present for surgical diagnosis (biopsy) or for curative resection/debulking of the lesion.

SURGICAL APPROACHES

Biopsy of supratentorial lesions is usually undertaken via a stereotactic approach or a mini-craniotomy. Debulking procedures are usually undertaken through either a pterional or a frontal craniotomy (see Chapter 14). The former accesses the temporal and parietal lobes and necessitates that the patient's head be turned away from the site of the lesion in the supine position, whereas the latter approach includes bifrontal craniotomy for bilateral or midline lesions. When intraoperative brain swelling is significant, the bone flap may not be replaced at the time of surgery but some months later instead (cranioplasty).

PREOPERATIVE MANAGEMENT

Specific preoperative assessment should include an accurate evaluation of the lesion, as well as lesion site and size, positioning of the patient, ease of surgical access, and information regarding blood loss and changes in ICP; such patients are likely to have raised ICP even if it is not evident clinically or seen on computed tomography/magnetic resonance imaging. Accurate clinical assessment of the patient's neurologic state should be undertaken, including any specific focal neurologic signs and preoperative Glasgow Coma Scale (GCS) score, as well as evaluation of concurrent disease.

Premedication should be given only if the patient is particularly anxious and there is no evidence of significantly raised ICP. A short-acting benzodiazepine is usually adequate. Medications such as anticonvulsants and steroids are continued in the perioperative period.

Based on the preoperative assessment, a plan should be made for postoperative management, including whether the patient is likely to require management in a high-dependency or critical care setting.

16

INTRAOPERATIVE MANAGEMENT

The aims of general anesthesia are

- Smooth induction
- Hemodynamic stability (hypotension can lead to ischemia in areas of impaired autoregulation; hypertension increases the risk for hemorrhage and vasogenic edema)

- Relaxed brain (for optimal surgical access and to reduce the risk for retractor damage)
- Rapid and smooth emergence from anesthesia to allow early neurologic assessment

Induction

Induction of anesthesia should be achieved with an intravenous anesthetic agent of choice, usually propofol or thiopental, combined with an opiate and a nondepolarizing muscle relaxant. Normotension should be maintained by anticipating hemodynamic responses. The hypertensive response to laryngoscopy can be obtunded by an additional bolus of induction agent, a short-acting opioid or β-blocker, or intravenous lidocaine.

After induction of anesthesia, standard routine monitoring should be instituted, including a nasopharyngeal temperature probe, urinary catheter, and a central venous line (if indicated, e.g., significant fluid/blood loss anticipated, cardiopulmonary disease). Continuous intra-arterial blood pressure monitoring is used for major craniotomies. Other neuromonitoring, such as electroencephalography, somatosensory evoked potentials, depth-of-anesthesia monitor, transcranial Doppler ultrasound, and jugular bulb catheterization, may be used in specific circumstances.

Once all monitoring is established, skull pins are generally applied. This is a potent stimulus and the hypertensive response can be obtunded in a fashion similar to the response to laryngoscopy. Scalp infiltration with local anesthetic at the pin site is also effective.

Positioning the Patient

A neutral head position, elevated to 15 to 30 degrees, is recommended to decrease ICP by improving venous drainage. Flexing or turning of the head may obstruct cerebral venous outflow and lead to dramatic elevation of ICP, which resolves on resumption of neutral head position. However, a skilled surgeon should be able to position and turn the head for surgical access without obstructing venous return. Lowering of the head impairs cerebral venous drainage and results in an increase in ICP. Application of positive end-expiratory pressure (PEEP) can increase ICP. PEEP should be applied cautiously with appropriate monitoring to minimize decreases in cardiac output and increases in ICP. PEEP levels of 10 cm H_2O or less have been used without a significant increase in ICP or decrease in CPP.

Maintenance of Anesthesia

The choice of anesthetic agents is largely at the discretion of the anesthetist, and either a total intravenous technique with propofol or an inhalational agent (sevoflurane, desflurane, isoflurane) in combination with a short-acting opioid and muscle relaxant may be used. The technique used should not increase ICP or decrease CPP and should allow rapid emergence at the end of surgery.

Unless there is a need to monitor cranial nerve function or motor responses, continuous muscle relaxation should be used and monitored with a nerve stimulator. The patient's ventilation should be controlled to maintain normocapnia, and body temperature should be maintained at normothermia, although most anesthesiologists will tolerate a fall in body temperature to 35° C to 36° C during surgical resection while ensuring that the patient is normothermic before starting to wake up.

IV

Table 16-1	Management of Intraoperative Cerebral Edema

Optimize oxygenation
Maximize venous drainage: ensure an adequate head-up position (15- to 30-degree tilt)
Reduce oxygen metabolism: deepen anesthesia, bolus intravenous anesthetic agents, or lidocaine
Reduction in brain extracellular fluid volume with mannitol or hypertonic saline; furosemide may be used as an adjunct
Cerebrospinal fluid drainage
Consider hypocapnia
Consider hypothermia (not proven)
Consider anticonvulsants

Fluid Management

Maintenance and resuscitation fluids in routine neurosurgical patients are provided with glucose-free iso-osmolar crystalloid and colloid solutions to prevent increases in brain water content from hypo-osmolality. Glucose-containing solutions are avoided in all neurosurgical patients with normal glucose metabolism; these solutions can potentially exacerbate ischemic damage and cerebral edema. Both hypoglycemia and hyperglycemia must be avoided because both have been demonstrated to potentiate cellular damage. However, there is currently no evidence to support "tight" glycemic control.

Intraoperative Complications

Severe complications include hemorrhage, intraoperative cerebral edema, and air embolism. Management of air embolism is dealt with elsewhere.

Blood products should be readily available in the event of major bleeding, with a goal of resuscitation to a hematocrit of 0.3. Thromboplastin release causing disseminated intravascular coagulopathy may occur, and clotting factors should be given early.

Acute cerebral edema requires aggressive management. Its management is presented in Table 16-1.

POSTOPERATIVE MANAGEMENT

Patients whose preoperative level of consciousness was depressed should be managed in a critical care setting. These patients may be electively ventilated postoperatively, but the decision to do so will be based on preoperative and intraoperative factors and discussion with the neurosurgeon.

Patients with a preoperative GCS score of 13 to 15 are usually extubated once they open their eyes to command and have a gag reflex. The overall aim is to achieve smooth emergence with minimal coughing or straining, which may increase ICP. Hypertension in the postoperative period is often due to inadequate analgesia, but once this has been excluded, the hypertension can be treated with a short-acting β-blocker such as esmolol or labetalol. Direct-acting vasodilators should be avoided because they may increase ICP.

Numerous studies have demonstrated that these patients frequently receive inadequate postoperative analgesia. The sedative effects of strong opiates need to be balanced against their analgesic properties. Postoperatively, longer-acting agents such as morphine or codeine phosphate are necessary to provide adequate analgesia. Paracetamol or acetaminophen is often used as an adjunct in the postoperative period.

16

KEY POINTS

- Preoperative assessment aims to assess neurologic status, determine the presence of raised ICP, optimize underlying disease, and plan for management in the postoperative period.
- Aim for smooth induction and smooth rapid emergence postoperatively.
- Total intravenous anesthesia or inhalational agents with muscle relaxation should be used intraoperatively.
- Aim for normotension, normothermia, controlled ventilation with normocapnia, and a relaxed brain intraoperatively.
- Tailor analgesic agents to the patient.

FURTHER READING

Hirsch N: Advances in neuroanaesthesia. Anaesthesia 2003; 58:1162-1165.

Randell T, Niskanen M: Management of physiological variables in neuroanaesthesia: Maintaining homeostasis during intracranial surgery. Curr Opin Anaesthesiol 2006; 19:492-497.

Ravussin P, Wilder-Smith OHG: Supratentorial masses: Anaesthetic considerations. In Cottrell JE, Smith DS (eds): Anaesthesia and Neurosurgery, 4th ed. St Louis, CV Mosby, 2001, pp 297-318.

van Hemelrijck J: Anaesthetic considerations for specific neurosurgical procedures. In Van Aken H (ed): Neuroanaesthetic Practice. London, BMJ Publishing, 1995, pp 214-239.

Chapter 17

Anesthesia for Intracranial Vascular Lesions

Vinodkumar Patil • Derek T. Duane

SUBARACHNOID HEMORRHAGE

Epidemiology

The incidence of subarachnoid hemorrhage (SAH) secondary to rupture of a cerebral aneurysm is 10 to 16 cases per 100,000 population per year, and aneurysms account for 80% of nontraumatic cases of SAH. It is more common in people older than 40 years, the average age at initial evaluation is 55 years, and it has a female-to-male ratio of 3:2.

Death from SAH occurs in 15% of patients before they reach the hospital, and approximately 25% of inpatients die within the first 2 weeks. Death commonly results from (1) overwhelming neuronal injury after the initial bleeding; (2) rebleeding, which occurs in 4% of untreated patients in the first 24 hours and in 20% within 2 weeks; and (3) profound cerebral ischemic damage from vasospasm. The 30-day mortality rate is close to 50%, whereas the incidence of moderate to severe neurologic morbidity can reach 30%.

Pathophysiology of Cerebral Aneurysms

The most common cause of spontaneous SAH is rupture of a cerebral aneurysm. Aneurysms are described as either saccular (berry-like) or fusiform, and the majority are less than 12 mm in diameter and classified as "small." Giant aneurysms (>24 mm in diameter) are found in less than 2% of all cases. Degenerative changes in the cerebral arterial wall induced by turbulent blood flow at a vessel's branching point contribute to the formation of aneurysms. This susceptibility to hemodynamic stress may be related to structural abnormalities in these arteries. Predisposing factors include a family history of the disease, atherosclerosis, hypertension, coarctation of the aorta, polycystic kidney disease, fibromuscular dysplasia, and connective tissue disorders such as Ehlers-Danlos and Marfan's syndrome.

The most common locations for aneurysms are the anterior cerebral artery (40%), posterior communicating artery (25%), and middle cerebral artery (25%). Only 10% of aneurysms develop in the vertebrobasilar system, mostly on the basilar artery.

The pathophysiologic changes that occur when an aneurysm ruptures include

- A sudden large increase in intracranial pressure (ICP)
- A decrease in cerebral perfusion pressure (CPP)
- Spread of blood through the subarachnoid space causing inflammation and meningism
- Cerebral vasoconstriction
- A decrease in cerebral blood flow (CBF), which may help stop further bleeding
- Loss of cerebrovascular autoregulation

Direct neural destruction by the force of extravasated blood, cerebral ischemia, and sympathetically mediated cardiac dysfunction are primarily responsible for the morbidity and mortality. The likelihood of aneurysm rupture depends on its size (more likely if >6 mm), morphology, location, and any previous history of SAH. During the initial bleeding blood can spread through the subarachnoid space, but with rebleeding, intracranial hemorrhage is more common and can be intraparenchymal (20% to 40%), intraventricular (10% to 20%), or subdural (5%).

Diagnosis and Investigations

The clinical manifestations of SAH include sudden severe headache with vomiting, neck pain (meningismus), photophobia, seizures, cranial nerve signs, focal neurologic deficits, transient loss of consciousness, or prolonged coma. An urgent, non–contrast-enhanced, high-resolution computed tomography (CT) head scan will diagnose SAH in more than 95% of patients.

Digital subtraction angiography (DSA) is the "gold standard" investigation. Recently, contrast-enhanced CT angiography, which involves three-dimensional reconstruction of cerebrovascular images after intravenous injection of dye, can help supplement DSA or even replace it as the first-line investigation.

A negative DSA finding can occur when SAH results from trauma, arteriovenous malformations (AVMs), arterial dissection, dural sinus thrombosis, coagulation disorders, pituitary apoplexy, or cocaine abuse. Doubt about the presence of an aneurysm may require a repeat angiographic procedure after a suitable time interval.

Treatment of Cerebral Aneurysms

Surgical or endovascular treatment of a patient within 2 to 3 days of a ruptured aneurysm minimizes the risk of rebleeding. Grading systems help stratify the degree of clinical impairment, assess the likelihood of complications, and guide prognosis. A combination of the Hunt and Hess, World Federation of Neurological Surgeons, and the Fischer grading systems is used (Tables 17-1 to 17-3).

Patients who are Hunt and Hess grade I or II may undergo prompt treatment, whereas patients with a Glasgow Coma Scale score less than 8 often have their intervention delayed until neurologic improvement occurs. Some centers treat patients graded III to IV to allow aggressive management of vasospasm with induced hypertension. Surgical treatment of aneurysms involves craniotomy, microsurgical dissection, and the application of a clip across the aneurysm's neck. Some aneurysms may be able to be managed only by wrapping in muslin gauze, by trapping between clips, or by proximal occlusion of the common carotid artery.

IV

Table 17-1   Hunt and Hess Grading Scale

Grade 0	Unruptured aneurysm
Grade 1	Asymptomatic or minimal headache and slight nuchal rigidity
Grade 2	Moderate to severe headache, nuchal rigidity, no neurologic deficit other than cranial nerve palsy
Grade 3	Drowsiness, confusion, or mild focal deficit
Grade 4	Stupor, moderate to severe hemiparesis, possible early decerebrate rigidity, vegetative disturbances
Grade 5	Deep coma, decerebrate rigidity, moribund appearance

From J Neurosurg 1968; 28:14-20.

Table 17-2   World Federation of Neurological Surgeon Grading Scale

WFNS Grade	Glasgow Coma Scale Score	Motor Deficit
I	15	Absent
II	14-13	Absent
III	14-13	Present
IV	12-7	Present or absent
V	6-3	Present or absent

From J Neurosurg 1988; 68:985.

Table 17-3   Fisher Grading System

Fisher Group	Blood on Computed Tomography
1	No subarachnoid blood detected
2	Diffuse vertical layers <1 mm thick
3	Localized clot and/or vertical layer ≥1 mm thick
4	Intracerebral or intraventricular clot with diffuse or no subarachnoid hemorrhage

From Neurosurgery 1980; 6:1-9.

17

Up to 80% of aneurysms can now be treated by endovascular occlusion with platinum coils. Results from the International Subarachnoid Aneurysm Trial indicated that despite a greater incidence of rebleeding, there was a 25% reduction in poor outcome at 1 year in patients undergoing coil embolization versus surgical clipping. Benefits of coil embolization include a less invasive procedure, greater suitability for patients with significant comorbidity, and a better outcome for posterior circulation aneurysms. However, repeat procedures may be necessary to completely pack the aneurysm with coils because the incidence of incomplete obliteration or aneurysmal regrowth can be as high as 30%.

Preoperative Anesthetic Assessment

Patients need to be assessed for the presence and extent of all intracranial and extracranial complications of SAH. Intracranial complications include

- Rebleeding
- Vasospasm leading to cerebral ischemia/infarction
- Hydrocephalus
- Expanding intracerebral hematoma
- Seizures

Important extracranial complications include (1) myocardial ischemia/infarction, (2) cardiac dysrhythmias, (3) neurogenic pulmonary edema, and (4) gastric hemorrhage. These complications are discussed in more detail in Chapter 35. Patients who are grade I or II will have minimal disturbance in cerebral hemodynamics, whereas those with grades III and IV can show loss of CBF autoregulation and CO_2 response.

Preoperative assessment includes a complete history and physical examination, especially a neurologic evaluation. It is essential that pulmonary and cardiac function be optimized before induction of anesthesia. Such optimization may involve treatment of (1) dysrhythmias, (2) hypovolemia to minimize vasospasm, (3) hyponatremia secondary to the syndrome of inappropriate antidiuretic hormone secretion or cerebral-induced salt wasting, and (4) hypoxia resulting from neurogenic pulmonary edema. Medical therapy for coexisting conditions should be continued, and patients should be maintained on nimodipine throughout the perioperative period or according to local practice. Baseline investigations must include a complete blood count, electrolyte studies, coagulation profile, 12-lead electrocardiograph, and a chest radiograph. Premedication may be appropriate in good-grade patients but should be avoided in poorer-grade patients.

Anesthetic Management

The goals of anesthetic management, whether for surgery or endovascular coiling, involve (1) avoiding increases in aneurysmal transmural pressure gradients, which may cause rupture (transmural pressure is the difference between the pressure inside the aneurysm, which equals blood pressure, and the pressure outside, which equals local ICP); (2) maintaining adequate CPP and cerebral oxygenation; and (3) preventing the development of a "tight" brain from cerebral edema or vascular engorgement.

Anesthesia for endovascular coiling follows the same basic principles as for surgery (see Chapter 27).

Monitoring

In addition to routine cardiac, respiratory, urine output, and temperature monitoring, direct measurement of intra-arterial blood pressure is essential and for some patients is appropriate before induction. Monitoring of central venous pressure or pulmonary artery wedge pressure may help guide vascular filling, especially if myocardial dysfunction is suspected. More specialized intraoperative monitoring can be performed, including jugular bulb or cerebral oximetry, transcranial Doppler measurement of cerebrovascular velocities, electroencephalography, and evoked potentials.

IV

Induction of Anesthesia

Intravenous induction of anesthesia via a large-bore cannula allows rapid loss of consciousness, reduces the risk of coughing, and permits the use of other drugs to ensure minimal change in transmural pressure (mean arterial pressure [MAP] – ICP). Aneurysmal rupture on induction is associated with high mortality, and acute aggressive reductions in ICP and hypertension are important risk factors. MAP should be maintained close to the patient's normal preoperative level. Stimulation with hypertension should be anticipated and prevented, especially from laryngoscopy, intubation, and the application of skull pins. Intravenous or topical lidocaine, β-blockers, short-acting opiates, or intravenous induction agents can be used. Poorer-grade patients with intracranial hypertension may benefit from mild hyperventilation.

Maintenance

Inhalational or total intravenous techniques are suitable for cerebral aneurysm surgery. Short-acting drugs such propofol, fentanyl, remifentanil, or sufentanil are commonly used in a total intravenous technique. Inhalational agents can be used in association with mild hypocapnia to avoid cerebral vasodilation. Colloid or glucose-free crystalloid solutions, or a mixture of both, should be administered to maintain normal to high intravascular volume.

There is substantial local variation in the specifics of intraoperative management, and such variations should be established by discussion with the surgical team. Methods to reduce the volume of intracranial contents, such as mannitol, moderate hyperventilation, and drainage of cerebrospinal fluid, may adversely alter transmural pressure and should therefore be delayed until the dura is open or be initiated slowly. Temporary proximal occlusion of the parent (feeding) vessel is often performed to facilitate dissection and clipping. The patient's blood pressure may be augmented to improve collateral circulation. Cooling the patient and administration of barbiturates, propofol, and extra doses of mannitol may extend the duration of occlusion, but human evidence is lacking. Controlled hypotension before application of the permanent clip is less favored now because of the risk for regional cerebral ischemia. Once the aneurysm has been clipped, normotension or mild hypertension is permitted to improve cerebral perfusion. However, in patients with significant myocardial dysfunction or other unruptured aneurysms, normotension is preferred.

Management of Intraoperative Aneurysm Rupture

Aneurysms that rupture before being secured surgically may be diagnosed by an abrupt onset of hypertension or bradycardia, sometimes associated with dilated pupils. Treatment is directed at maintaining CPP. Management requires active communication with the surgeon.

Survival depends on rapid control of the bleeding. Actions likely to help include

- Ventilation with 100% oxygen
- Transient induction of hypotension
- Restoration of intravascular volume
- Administration of thiopental or propofol to produce burst suppression, which reduces CBF and perhaps bleeding and may also produce "brain protection"
- Hyperosmolar therapy in the form of mannitol (0.5 to 1 g/kg) or hypertonic saline (2 mL/kg of 5% NaCl) to treat brain swelling
- Cooling to 33° C

17

Emergence

At the end of uneventful aneurysm surgery, patients should be extubated with a minimum of coughing or blood pressure fluctuation. Uncontrolled hypertension or hypotension requires treatment to prevent adverse cerebral or cardiac sequelae. Blood pressure control is important for patients with unruptured aneurysms.

Postoperative Anesthetic Care

Neurovascular patients should be managed in a neurosurgical high-dependency or intensive care unit to ensure continued hemodynamic monitoring, adequate oxygenation, optimum fluid and electrolyte management, and early detection of complications such as vasospasm. Analgesics, including small doses of opiates, may be used to treat postoperative pain. Failure to fully emerge from anesthesia after a suitable time has elapsed for drug metabolism should prompt a search for a neurologic cause.

ARTERIOVENOUS MALFORMATIONS

An AVM is an abnormal collection of dysplastic vessels. Seventy-five percent are supratentorial. The vascular mass normally has a center (nidus) surrounded by dilated draining veins. In the nidus, blood flows directly from dilated arteries to veins with no intervening capillary bed or neural parenchyma. AVMs are congenital lesions and are usually manifested before the age of 40 as cerebral hemorrhage (most common), seizures, symptoms of a mass effect, raised ICP, or neurologic signs secondary to cerebral ischemia (steal effect).

The use of cerebral angiography or magnetic resonance imaging (or both) is diagnostic. An associated aneurysm can be seen in up to 10% of patients. Treatment options for AVMs include

- Surgical excision
- Endovascular embolization
- Stereotactic radiosurgery

Surgical outcome is related to AVM grade, which takes into account size, eloquence of adjacent brain, and pattern of venous drainage (Table 17-4).

Anesthetic management of patients undergoing surgical resection of an AVM follows the same general principles as outlined for SAH. In the preoperative assessment, the presence of an associated aneurysm should be noted, as well as symptoms suggestive of cerebral ischemia or a mass effect. It is helpful to recognize that most AVMs are high-flow, low-resistance shunts whose mean transmural pressure is much less than MAP. Hence, rupture is not related to acute rises in MAP unless the AVM is small and there is higher pressure within the feeding artery. Moreover, large shunts can produce ischemia in non-autoregulating surrounding brain tissue. Therefore, during induction, blood pressure control is essential to avoid rupturing an associated aneurysm or inducing ischemic changes in hypoperfused areas.

During AVM surgery, severe intraoperative bleeding can occur and may be associated with malignant cerebral edema. Care should be taken to avoid any rise in venous pressure. The decision to use deliberate hypotension to decrease blood loss while possibly risking ischemia or predisposing to venous outflow thrombosis must be made after discussion with the surgical team.

Table 17-4   Spetzler-Martin Grading System for Arteriovenous Malformations

Graded Feature	Score
Size	
Small (<3 cm)	1
Medium (3-6 cm)	2
Large (>6 cm)	3
Eloquence of adjacent brain	
Noneloquent	0
Eloquent	1
Pattern of venous drainage	
Superficial only	0
Deep	1

From J Neurosurg 1986; 65:476-483.

Hyperemic complications that can lead to cerebral edema or hemorrhage are responsible for most of the postoperative mortality and morbidity. Hyperemia and its consequences can be caused by

- Normal perfusion pressure breakthrough—believed to be due to loss of autoregulation in previously hypoperfused brain tissue unable to deal with restored normal perfusion.
- "Occlusive hyperemia"—venous outflow obstruction produced by surgical ligation of veins in adjacent normal brain or in the AVM with incomplete occlusion of arterial feeders. Rebleeding may also occur from an inaccessible or unidentified residual AVM. In the postoperative period, hypertension should be avoided and treated with β-blockers or some other suitable agent. Because the risk of seizures after this surgery is 40% to 50%, patients may need prophylactic anticonvulsants.

KEY POINTS

- Nontraumatic SAH usually occurs after 40 years of age.
- The 30-day mortality is approximately 50%.
- In addition to central nervous system disturbances, SAH may cause significant cardiovascular and pulmonary complications, as well as fluid and electrolyte imbalances that need to be optimized before surgical or endovascular treatment.
- Perioperative control of blood pressure is crucial to prevent rebleeding or ischemia secondary to vasospasm.
- Inhalational or total intravenous techniques are suitable for anesthesia during cerebral aneurysm surgery.
- An AVM is an abnormal collection of dysplastic vessels. Up to 10% of patients have an associated aneurysm.
- During AVM surgery, uncontrollable venous hemorrhage is a significant risk.
- Hyperemic complications leading to cerebral edema or hemorrhage are responsible for most of the postoperative morbidity and mortality.

FURTHER READING

Brown RD Jr, Flemming KD, Meyer FB, et al: Natural history, evaluation, and management of intracranial vascular malformations. Mayo Clin Proc 2005; 80:269-281.

Drake CG: Report of world federation of neurological surgeons committee on a universal subarachnoid haemorrhage grading scale. Journal of Neurosurgery 1988; 68:985-986.

Feigin VL, Findlay M: Advances in subarachnoid haemorrhage. Stroke 2006; 37:305-308.

Fisher CM, Kistler JP, Davis JM: Relation of cerebral vasospasm to subarachnoid haemorrhage visualised by CT scanning. Neurosurgery 1980; 6:1-9.

Hunt WE, Hess RM: Surgical risk as related to time of intervention in the repair of intracranial aneurysms. Journal of Neurosurgery 1968; 28:14-20.

Manno EM: Subarachnoid haemorrhage. Neurol Clin 2004; 22:347-366.

Molyneux A, Kerr R, Yu L-M, et al: International subarachnoid aneurysm trial (ISAT) of neurosurgical clipping versus endovascular coiling in 2143 patients with ruptured intracranial aneurysms. Lancet 2005; 366:809-817.

Patel AB, Johnson DM: Endovascular treatment of neurovascular disorders. Mount Sinai J Med 2004; 71:29-41.

Spetzler RF, Martin NA: A proposed grading system for arteriovenous malformations. Journal of Neurosurgery 1986; 65:476-483.

Warner DS, Laskowitz DT: Changing outcome from aneurysmal subarachnoid haemorrhage. Anesthesiology 2006; 104:629-630.

Webb ST, Farling PA: Survey of arrangements for anaesthesia for interventional neuroradiology for aneurysmal subarachnoid haemorrhage. Anaesthesia 2005; 60:560-564.

Wijdicks EF, Kallmes DF, Manno EM, et al: Subarachnoid haemorrhage: Neurointensive care and aneurysm repair. Mayo Clin Proc 2005; 80:550-559.

IV

Chapter 18

Anesthesia for Posterior Fossa Lesions

Rosemary Ann Craen • Hélène Pellerin

The posterior fossa contains structures responsible for vital control of the respiratory and cardiovascular systems and therefore presents unique challenges to the anesthesiologist.

PATHOLOGY

Tumors are the most common posterior fossa lesions requiring surgical intervention. In children, posterior fossa tumors account for approximately 60% of all brain tumors. In the adult population, posterior fossa tumors are less frequent and include acoustic neuroma; metastases, mainly from the lung and breast; meningioma, and hemangioblastoma, which may be associated with polycythemia and occult pheochromocytoma.

Acoustic neuroma is a benign lesion arising from the vestibular portion of cranial nerve VIII in the cerebellopontine angle and can cause hearing loss, tinnitus, vertigo, and hemifacial spasm. Small acoustic neuromas can be removed via a retromastoid approach. Large ones involve a suboccipital approach, which can be a long procedure but is intended to preserve facial and cochlear nerve function.

Chiari malformations are divided into two types based on anatomic features. Chiari I is characterized by descent of the cerebellar tonsils into the cervical spinal canal and causes cough-induced headache, nuchal pain, and lower cranial nerve dysfunction in young adulthood. Chiari II malformation is a more complex abnormality in which the inferior vermis herniates through the foramen magnum, and it may be associated with spina bifida, hydrocephalus, and syringomyelia. Lower cranial nerve dysfunction can cause stridor, respiratory distress, dysphagia, and aspiration. Spasticity and quadriparesis are progressive if left untreated. Even with aggressive treatment,

18

119

Table 18-1	Characteristics to Look for during the Preoperative Evaluation
Signs of raised intracranial pressure	Altered state of consciousness
	Nausea and vomiting
	Papilloedema
Signs of brainstem dysfunction	Altered respiratory pattern
	Sleep apnea
Signs of cranial nerve dysfunction	Dysphagia
	Absent gag reflex
	Changes in phonation
Signs of cerebellar dysfunction	Ataxia
	Dysmetria

the condition is fatal in 30% of symptomatic infants. Both Chiari malformations are treated by suboccipital craniectomy and upper cervical laminectomy. Treatment of the associated hydrocephalus may require a shunt.

It is hypothesized that small vessels, most commonly arteries, compressing the roots of a cranial nerve may cause neuralgia. Trigeminal neuralgia, or tic douloureux, is the most common syndrome. Patients have paroxysmal episodes of excruciating and lancinating pain over the ipsilateral trigeminal distribution. Surgical decompression of the cranial nerves is performed with identification of an offending arterial vessel loop or, less frequently, a vein, tumor, or vascular malformation. Removing the offending lesion or placing a muscle pad or Teflon sponge between the artery and root entry zone often produces relief of pain. Patients with these conditions should have their chronic pain syndrome evaluated to guide pain management postoperatively.

PREOPERATIVE EVALUATION

In addition to the usual preoperative assessment, a detailed neurologic examination is crucial to guide perioperative management (Table 18-1).

Patients with posterior fossa lesions, especially in the presence of raised intracranial pressure (ICP), are more sensitive to sedatives and analgesics, and these agents should be used with caution if given preoperatively.

POSITIONING

Posterior fossa surgery can be performed in the prone, semiprone, or park bench position and, less commonly, in the sitting position. These positions and their perioperative implications are described in Chapter 15.

INTRAOPERATIVE MANAGEMENT

Monitoring

Routine monitors include electrocardiography, pulse oximetry, capnography, temperature, urinary catheter, and neuromuscular blockade. An intra-arterial catheter allows close monitoring of systemic blood pressure and cerebral perfusion pressure and assessment of Pa_{CO_2}. The decision to insert a central venous line should be dictated

Table 18-2	Treatment of Intracranial Hypertension

Head-up position
Free venous drainage
Hyperventilation
Reduce volatile anesthetic
Change to intravenous anesthetic
Give mannitol
Consider drainage of cerebrospinal fluid

by the patient's medical status, the size and the nature of the pathology, the expected degree of blood loss, and the risk for venous air embolism (VAE). Electrophysiologic monitoring should be tailored to the site of surgery and the location of the lesion.

Evidence suggests that changes in the respiratory pattern may be more sensitive to brainstem manipulation than changes in hemodynamics. Accordingly, the use of spontaneous ventilation may be appropriate in rare circumstances. However, a significant degree of hypercapnia may be needed for spontaneous ventilation to occur under general anesthesia, and the risk of VAE occurring is increased with spontaneous ventilation.

Induction and Maintenance

No specific anesthetic technique has been shown to be the most effective. Goals of anesthesia include maintenance of cerebral perfusion pressure and avoidance of coughing, straining, and hemodynamic instability. Techniques that decrease ICP and facilitate brain relaxation should be used to ensure the best surgical conditions (Table 18-2).

There is some question about whether mannitol is as effective in decreasing raised ICP in the infratentorial compartment as in the supratentorial compartment. However, it is still recommended that raised ICP be treated with posterior fossa lesions. Drainage of cerebrospinal fluid may be necessary and is possible through a burr hole often made before the skin incision.

If neurophysiologic monitoring is used, an appropriate anesthetic technique that provides the least interference should be applied. Electromyography of cranial nerve VII is often performed during cerebellopontine angle surgery and requires the avoidance of muscle relaxants.

18

Arrhythmias

Cardiac arrhythmias are common during manipulation of the brainstem. Bradycardia is the most frequent arrhythmia and usually subsides with cessation of the stimulus. Treatment with glycopyrrolate, atropine, or ephedrine may be indicated. Severe hypertension reflecting pain is often associated with manipulation of the cranial nerve entry zone during microvascular decompression.

Emergence

The aim of emergence should be early awakening to allow evaluation of neurologic function. Preoperative neurologic dysfunction, the nature and extent of the surgery, and the degree of airway and tongue edema should be considered before extubation (Table 18-3). A "leak test" around the endotracheal tube with the cuff deflated is used by some. Delaying extubation to allow the edema to resolve may be an option. Extubation with a tube exchanger in place is another option. Hypertension should

Table 18-3 Features to Look for during Evaluation before Extubation

Level of consciousness
Airway and gag reflex
Face and tongue edema
Airway edema
Regular respiratory pattern
Stable vital parameters

be avoided in the early postoperative phase because it contributes to postoperative brain edema and increases the risk for postoperative intracranial hemorrhage.

Scalp blocks or infiltration of the incision with local anesthetics at the end of surgery, or both, will reduce the need for postoperative opiates.

VENOUS AIR EMBOLISM

Factors that increase the risk for VAE include an operative site above the level of the heart and the presence of noncollapsible veins. Both are usually present during posterior fossa surgery, especially in the sitting position. The incidence of VAE in posterior fossa surgery has been reported to be 30% to 75% in the sitting position and 10% to 15% in the prone or park bench position. However, the incidence of hemodynamically significant VAE is only 8% to 15% and 3% to 5%, respectively. If air entrainment is stopped immediately after detection, the effects can be short-lived and insignificant with low morbidity.

The pathophysiology of VAE can be explained by an elevation in pulmonary vascular pressure leading to impaired gas exchange, hypoxemia, and CO_2 retention. Mechanical obstruction of pulmonary capillaries and increased intrapulmonary shunting result in a decrease in end-tidal CO_2 tension (P_{ETCO_2}). Bronchoconstriction may occur, and further air entrainment will lead to progressive decreases in cardiac output, hypotension, arrhythmias, and myocardial ischemia or failure. The sudden entry of a large bolus of air into the right heart can have a dramatic effect by causing an airlock that blocks the right ventricular outflow tract and leads to cardiac arrest or cardiovascular collapse.

The presence of a patent foramen ovale (PFO) increases the risk for paradoxical air embolism in which air travels to the systemic circulation through an intracardiac shunt and results in myocardial and cerebral ischemia. PFO has been found to be present in 25% of the adult population. It is recommended that any patient scheduled for surgery in the sitting position undergo echocardiography to rule out PFO. However, the sensitivity of echocardiography is low for the detection of PFO (<50%). Therefore, the risk for intraoperative paradoxical air embolism must always be considered, although the clinically observed incidence is low (<2%). A less invasive test to preoperatively detect PFO is the use of transcranial Doppler (TCD) ultrasound. However, the sensitivity and specificity of TCD in detecting PFO are comparable to that of echocardiography.

Monitoring

Precordial Doppler ultrasonography is the standard monitor, and the probe is placed along the right parasternal border at the fourth intercostal space. It can detect as little as 0.25 mL of air. Transesophageal echocardiography (TEE) is the most sensitive of all

Table 18-4 Prevention of Venous Air Embolism

Decrease the gradient between the heart and the site of surgery
Maintain normovolemia to hypervolemia
Apply bone wax during surgery
Avoid positive end-expiratory pressure

Table 18-5 Treatment of Venous Air Embolism

Notify the surgeon to flood the surgical site
Lower the operative site
Stop N_2O administration
Give 100% O_2
Perform aspiration through a central venous line
Consider compression of the jugular veins
Provide cardiopulmonary support (fluids, pressors, inotropes)

monitors and can detect paradoxical embolism. However, it is less readily available, is more invasive, and requires special expertise, and its safety with prolonged use in the presence of neck flexion is not well established. In addition, it is still uncertain whether the use of intraoperative TEE for detection of VAE decreases morbidity. Capnography will show an abrupt decrease in P_{ETCO_2}, whereas an increase in end-tidal nitrogen tension (P_{ETN_2}) is more specific for VAE but can be difficult to monitor. Pulmonary artery pressure monitoring is as sensitive as capnography. Monitors that measure the decrease in blood pressure and cardiac output are the least sensitive. In summary, precordial Doppler ultrasound and capnography (P_{ETCO_2}) remain the recommended monitors for VAE during posterior fossa surgery and should allow detection before significant clinical signs occur.

Preoperative Considerations

Table 18-4 outlines simple preventive steps to avoid VAE. To aspirate air, the right heart multiorifice central venous catheter should be positioned 2 cm below the junction of the superior vena cava and the atrium and the single-orifice catheter positioned 3 cm above this junction. Good placement can be confirmed by radiography, monitoring of intravascular pressure, portable ultrasound, or intravascular electrocardiography, in which the presence of a biphasic P wave will confirm midatrial placement of the tip of the catheter or the proximal orifice if a multiorifice catheter is used. The key, however, is to have a well-established plan for monitoring and treatment of VAE, as well as good communication between the surgeon and anesthesiologist.

Treatment

Notifying the surgeon to prevent further air entrainment is the first step in treatment (Table 18-5). The jugular veins can be compressed temporarily to increase venous blood pressure. The addition of positive end-expiratory pressure to the ventilator settings should be avoided because it can increase right atrial pressure and potentiate the risk for paradoxical embolism by reversing the gradient between the atria.

18

CONCLUSION

Anesthesia for posterior fossa surgery requires an understanding of the anatomy and pathophysiology involved. Perioperative management includes preoperative evaluation, especially of the brainstem and for the presence of cerebellar and cranial nerve dysfunction, meticulous attention to positioning of the patient, and adequate monitoring for the prevention of VAE. Careful assessment of the patient before extubation and good control of blood pressure are of paramount importance.

KEY POINTS

- Preoperative neurologic evaluation is crucial to guide perioperative management.
- Severe neck flexion and rotation should be avoided.
- The sitting position increases the risk for VAE.
- Prevention is the cornerstone in the management of VAE.
- Delayed extubation should be considered if brainstem/cranial nerve injuries are anticipated.
- Good blood pressure control in the postoperative period is important.

FURTHER READING

Engelhardt M, Folkers W, Brenke C, et al: Neurosurgical operations with the patient in sitting position: Analysis of risk factors using transcranial Doppler sonography. Br J Anaesth 2006; 96:467-472.

Manninen PH, Cuillerier DJ, Nantau WE, Gelb AW: Monitoring of brain stem function during vertebral basilar aneurysm surgery: The use of spontaneous ventilation. Anesthesiology 1992; 77:681-685.

Porter JM, Pidgeon C, Cunningham AJ: The sitting position in neurosurgery: A critical appraisal. Br J Anaesth 1999; 82:117-128.

Sloan TB: Monitoring the brain and spinal cord. Int Anesthesiol Clin 2004; 42(2):1-23.

IV

Chapter 19

Anesthesia for Epilepsy Surgery

Martin Smith

Pathophysiology	**Intraoperative Management**
Antiepileptic Therapy	Electrophysiologic Effects of Anesthetic Agents
Indications for Surgery	Anesthetic Technique
Preoperative Assessment	**Postoperative Care**

Epilepsy is a common disorder that occurs in 0.5% to 1.0% of the population, but a diagnosis of epilepsy will be made in around 3% of people at some time in their lives. Epilepsy is a chronic and disabling neurologic condition characterized by recurrent seizure activity. Despite considerable progress in the medical management of epilepsy and the development of new antiepileptic drugs, therapy remains problematic. Freedom from seizures cannot be achieved with medication (including multiple therapy) in about 30% of patients, and in others, seizure control is possible only at the expense of intolerable side effects. Surgery is an alternative and increasingly favorable option for this group of patients.

PATHOPHYSIOLOGY

Epilepsy is a symptom rather than a disease and may be long-standing or develop de novo secondary to another pathology (Table 19-1). Under normal circumstances electrical activity is well controlled within the brain, but in epileptic patients, regulatory functions are altered. A group of neurons develop the capacity to produce spontaneous burst discharges, which are recognized as interictal spikes on the electroencephalogram (EEG). Failure of normal inhibitory processes permits spread of these spike discharges to surrounding areas, and uncontrolled neuronal firing and electrophysiologic and clinical seizure activity result. Changes in membrane flux, impaired γ-aminobutyric acid (GABA)-mediated synaptic inhibition, and alterations in local neurotransmitter levels have been implicated in this complex process.

Epilepsy may be usefully classified into generalized and partial types (Table 19-2). Generalized seizures involve both hemispheres and are characterized by an initial loss of consciousness. Partial epilepsy occurs when the initial discharge is limited to one area of the brain. Simple partial seizures are caused by a localized discharge, and there is no impairment of consciousness. In complex partial seizures, the initial focal discharge spreads widely with secondary loss of consciousness. This is the most common seizure disorder and includes temporal lobe epilepsy (TLE).

Table 19-1 Causes and Risk Factors for Epilepsy

Birth/neonatal injuries
Genetic defects
Head injury
Tumors
Infection of brain/meninges
Metabolic disorders
Drug/alcohol abuse
Cerebrovascular disease
Degenerative disease of the brain
Demyelinating disease

Table 19-2 Classification of Epilepsy

Generalized Epilepsy
Generalized absence—petit mal
Generalized tonic-clonic—grand mal
Myoclonic
Tonic/atonic—drop attacks
Partial Epilepsy
Complex partial—temporal lobe epilepsy
Simple partial

ANTIEPILEPTIC THERAPY

The choice of antiepileptic medication is determined by the seizure type, seizure history, age of the patient, and side effects (Table 19-3). Monotherapy is sufficient to control seizures in many patients, but some require the addition of second- or third-line agents (see also Chapter 38).

INDICATIONS FOR SURGERY

Surgery is indicated for patients with a discrete epileptic focus whose seizures are drug resistant or who suffer severe medication-related side effects. TLE is particularly responsive to surgical intervention and extended temporal lobectomy, including amygdalohippocampectomy, is likely to offer significant benefit for such patients. Excision of discrete lesions (such as tumors or small vascular lesions) that are causing seizures is also a useful treatment option.

PREOPERATIVE ASSESSMENT

The pattern, type, and frequency of seizures should be noted. Coexisting medical problems are frequently encountered. Antiepileptic drug levels should be measured and attention given to the potential side effects of therapy (Table 19-3). Drugs are usually continued into the perioperative period, with doses adjusted to ensure adequate plasma levels. Premedication with a benzodiazepine is acceptable in most

Table 19-3   Antiepileptic Drugs: Indications and Side Effects

Drug	First-Line Indication	Side Effects
Carbamazepine	Complex partial, simple partial, generalized tonic-clonic	Rash, sedation, thrombocytopenia, leukopenia, cholestasis, hyponatremia
Ethosuximide	Petit mal	Rash, drowsiness, ataxia, irritability, nausea, abdominal discomfort, anorexia, diarrhea
Gabapentin	Simple partial, complex partial	Behavioral changes, weight gain
Lamotrigine	Second-line therapy	Insomnia, rash, Stevens-Johnson syndrome
Levetiracetam	Second-line therapy	Behavioral problems
Phenobarbital	Complex partial and second-line therapy	Rash, sedation, megaloblastic anemia, folate deficiency
Phenytoin	Grand mal, complex partial, generalized tonic-clonic	Rash, gingival hypertrophy, ataxia, megaloblastic anemia, Stevens-Johnson syndrome
Sodium valproate	Grand mal, generalized tonic-clonic	Tremor, weight gain, alopecia, thrombocytopenia, abnormal liver enzymes, hepatic
Topiramate	Second-line therapy	Behavioral effects, weight loss, kidney stones, rash, hypohidrosis
Vigabatrin	Second-line therapy	Sedation, irritability, psychosis, weight gain

patients but should be avoided if intraoperative recording of interictal spike activity is planned.

INTRAOPERATIVE MANAGEMENT

Special considerations during anesthesia for epilepsy surgery include the potential to record intraoperative cerebral electrical activity, activation of the epileptic focus, and facilitation of intraoperative cortical mapping.

In some patients it is necessary to monitor intraoperative spike activity via a small grid electrode placed over the cortex. Such monitoring is called electrocorticography (ECoG) and allows mapping of the epileptic focus and aids planning of resection margins. ECoG can be satisfactorily performed in most patients during general anesthesia by choosing techniques that have minimal effects on normal or epileptiform electrocerebral activity. In others, particularly those in whom resection margins might impinge on eloquent areas, ECoG is best combined with functional cortical mapping and the use of local anesthesia and sedation (see Chapter 20). However, the increasing sophistication of imaging allows accurate preoperative localization of areas of epileptogenesis and normal brain function, and in association with the tendency toward smaller focal resection and the questionable value of ECoG and cortical mapping in relation to seizure outcome, the indications for local anesthesia and sedation are changing. There has been a trend toward increased use of tailored general anesthesia with techniques, particularly in the United Kingdom, that have minimal effect on ECoG. Knowledge of the effects of anesthetic agents on the EEG allows rational selection of the anesthetic technique.

Electrophysiologic Effects of Anesthetic Agents

The action of anesthetic agents on the EEG is complex. Paradoxically, many agents that have been reported to cause clinical seizure activity also possess anticonvulsant action, and this effect is dose related. Low doses generally have proconvulsant action and higher doses have anticonvulsant activity. Thiopental is an anticonvulsant at clinical doses and is frequently used to control seizures. Methohexital and etomidate activate the EEG and should be avoided in epileptic patients. However, they are sometimes used intraoperatively in small doses to activate seizure foci. Propofol has been shown to activate the EEG in TLE and produce seizures and opisthotonos in nonepileptic patients. However, it is also used as an anticonvulsant and is widely used to treat status epilepticus resistant to other therapies. Propofol has a profound dose-dependent effect on the EEG and causes activation at small doses and burst suppression (anticonvulsant action) at higher (clinical) doses. Diazepam and other benzodiazepines have well-known anticonvulsant activity and are widely used in the treatment of seizures. The effects of inhalational agents on the EEG are also dose dependent. Epileptiform activity is suppressed by low-dose isoflurane, and an isoelectric EEG is produced at 2 minimum alveolar concentration (MAC). Sevoflurane and desflurane have isoflurane-like effects, but high-dose enflurane, in contrast, has convulsant activity that is exaggerated in the presence of elevated arterial carbon dioxide partial pressure ($Paco_2$). Dose-dependent changes on the EEG occur with the use of nitrous oxide, with anticonvulsant effects predominating at higher inspired concentrations.

Anesthetic Technique

The majority of epilepsy surgery can be performed safely under general anesthesia with continued ability to make excellent intraoperative electrophysiologic recordings. General anesthesia has many benefits, including provision of optimal operating conditions by the ability to control $Paco_2$ and blood pressure, assurance of immobility, and unawareness by the patient of the whole procedure. However, intraoperative cortical mapping with speech and language assessment is not possible.

Epilepsy surgical teams differ substantially in their comfort and familiarity with different anesthetic effects. Therefore, detailed discussion needs to occur in advance. The general anesthetic techniques used during epilepsy surgery are similar to those used for any intracranial procedure, with special attention paid to the choice of anesthetic agent if intraoperative ECoG is indicated. Careful titration of the end-tidal concentration of a volatile agent in combination with moderate doses of a short-acting opioid allows a depth of anesthesia to be maintained that does not interfere with ECoG while minimizing the risk of awareness. Alternatively, anesthesia may be maintained by propofol and remifentanil infusion, although the effect of this combination on ECoG has not yet been fully characterized. To avoid the potential confounding effects of hypnotics, some groups prefer an opioid–nitrous oxide anesthetic with regional block of the scalp, which may be supplemented with dexmedetomidine. Neuromuscular blockade should be maintained during the lighter stages of anesthesia necessary for ECoG, and monitoring of neuromuscular function is essential because of interactions between muscle relaxant and antiepileptic drugs. Blood pressure may be controlled by incremental opioid or β-adrenoceptor blockade, or both. In patients in whom intraoperative spike activity is not observed, it may be necessary for the anesthetist to administer proconvulsant anesthetic drugs. Small doses of methohexital, etomidate, thiopental, propofol, and alfentanil have all been successfully used for this purpose.

IV

Table 19-4	Risk Factors for Perioperative Seizures
Anesthetic Factors	
Proconvulsant anesthetic agents (e.g., methohexital, enflurane)	
Light anesthesia	
Hypocapnia/hypercapnia	
Hypoxemia	
Metabolic Factors	
Hypoglycemia	
Hyponatremia/hypernatremia	
Hypocalcemia	
Hypomagnesemia	
Uremia	
Neurosurgical Factors	
Postcraniotomy hematoma	
Previous poorly controlled epilepsy	

Intraoperative seizures during general anesthesia are rare but can occur for a variety of reasons (Table 19-4). They may be masked by neuromuscular blockade, but unexpected tachycardia, hypertension, or increases in end-tidal CO_2 are suspicious warning signs. The diagnosis can be confirmed by ECoG. An intravenous bolus of propofol or thiopental, followed by deepening of anesthesia, is usually sufficient to bring seizures under control.

POSTOPERATIVE CARE

After surgery, the patient should be managed in a neurosurgical intensive care or high-dependency unit and invasive monitoring continued into the postoperative period. The risk for seizures is increased in the immediate few hours after surgery, with the potential for progression to status epilepticus. Seizures may be precipitated by metabolic changes, hypercapnia, drugs, or the underlying epilepsy (Table 19-4). A surgical cause of recurrent postoperative seizures, such as a hematoma, should be excluded by computed tomography. Seizures should be treated aggressively to avoid cerebral damage and to prevent progression to status epilepticus (see Chapter 38). Because of a prolonged duration of action when given after other sedative/anesthetic drugs, benzodiazepine administration may limit the ability to carry out a postictal neurologic assessment. Propofol and thiopental are useful alternatives, and small doses rapidly and effectively terminate postoperative seizures and ensure swift recovery. Plasma levels of long-acting antiepileptic drugs should be checked and top-up doses administered as required. Recurrent seizures in the postoperative period may require the introduction of adjuvant therapy.

KEY POINTS

- The side effects and interactions of antiepileptic medications must be taken into account.
- Anesthetic agents should be chosen carefully to allow intraoperative recording of epileptiform activity.
- Surgical treatment is associated with a risk for intraoperative and postoperative seizures.

19

FURTHER READING

Chapman M, Smith M, Hirsch N: Status epilepticus. Anaesthesia 2001; 56:648-659.

Herrick IA, Gelb AW: Anesthesia for temporal lobe epilepsy surgery. Can J Neurol Sci 2000; 27:S64-S67.

Kofte W, Templehoff R, Dasheiff R: Anesthesia for epileptic patients and for epilepsy surgery. In Cottrell JE, Smith DS (eds): Anesthesia for Neurosurgery. St Louis, CV Mosby, 2001.

Marson A, Ramaratnam S: Epilepsy. Clin Evid 2005; 13:1588–1607.

Modica PA, Tempelhoff R, White PF: Pro- and anticonvulsant effects of anaesthetics (Part 1). Anesth Analg 1990; 70:303-315.

Modica PA, Tempelhoff R, White PF: Pro- and anticonvulsant effects of anaesthetics (Part 2). Anesth Analg 1990; 70:527-543.

Smith M. Anaesthesia for epilepsy surgery. In Shorvon S, Perucca E, Fish D, Dodson E (eds): The Treatment of Epilepsy. Oxford, Blackwell Science, 2004.

IV

Chapter 20

Perioperative Management of Awake Craniotomy

Martin Smith

Indications for Awake Craniotomy	**Intraoperative Anesthesia Management**
Background	Airway Control
Preoperative Assessment	Intraoperative Problems
Cortical Mapping	**Postoperative Care**

General anesthesia for craniotomy has many benefits for the neurosurgeon, including provision of optimal operating conditions by the ability to control the arterial partial pressure of carbon dioxide ($Paco_2$) and blood pressure, as well as assurance of immobility. The advantage for the patient is, of course, unawareness of the whole procedure. Although most craniotomies are performed under general anesthesia, resection of a mass or epileptogenic lesion close to vital areas of the brain, including those responsible for speech and motor activity, might, under certain circumstances, be more appropriately performed with an "awake" procedure. This permits intraoperative cortical mapping and assessment of memory and language.

Awake procedures are well established in the United States, the majority being performed under local anesthesia with sedation or with true asleep-awake-asleep techniques. In the United Kingdom there has historically been reluctance by both neurosurgeons and patients to participate in awake intracranial procedures, but this is changing as the potential benefits are being clarified and improved anesthetic techniques are being developed. Awake craniotomy is demanding for the neurosurgeon and neuroanesthetist and requires a high degree of motivation by the patient.

INDICATIONS FOR AWAKE CRANIOTOMY

Awake craniotomy for epilepsy surgery is well established, and awake surgery for tumor surgery, particularly for resection of mass lesions near eloquent areas of the brain, is gaining in popularity. Stereotactic and deep brain stimulator procedures (for Parkinson's disease or other movement disorders) can also be carried out in awake patients (Table 20-1).

BACKGROUND

The technique of awake craniotomy has developed over many years and includes local anesthesia alone or, more commonly, a combination of local anesthesia with sedation or general anesthesia and intraoperative wake-up. Although the advent of

Table 20-1   Indications for Awake Neurosurgery

Epilepsy surgery
Stereotactic surgery
Functional neurosurgery, e.g., deep brain stimulation for Parkinson's disease
    and other movement disorders
Resection of mass lesions in eloquent areas of the brain

neuroleptanesthesia offered some improvement in the technique in the early days, the introduction of short-acting agents, such as propofol and remifentanil, has given the neuroanesthetist the ability to titrate sedation and analgesia more reliably and thus deliver controllable sedation and achieve rapid wake-up.

PREOPERATIVE ASSESSMENT

Careful preoperative assessment and explanation are essential for success of this technique. It is crucial that the anesthetist develop a good rapport with the patient and give a detailed explanation of the procedure. In addition to routine preoperative considerations, the anesthetist must decide whether the patient is sufficiently cooperative to participate in the procedure and able to lie still and flat for the duration of the operation.

CORTICAL MAPPING

Electrical stimulation of the cortex allows recognition of motor, sensory, and speech areas and, when combined with neuropsychological assessment, determination of language areas. Cortical mapping assists the neurosurgeon in determining resection margins and is particularly important for dominant-hemisphere mass lesions where optimal tumor resection can be performed with minimal risk of postoperative neurologic deficits. Despite the use of cortical mapping, the majority of neurosurgeons prefer to complete the entire resection with the patient awake so that any infringement on eloquent areas can be recognized immediately.

During epilepsy surgery, intraoperative electrocorticography (ECoG) may be used to identify the extent of the epileptogenic focus and, when used in combination with sensorimotor mapping, allows safe resection of epileptic foci whose margins impinge on eloquent areas. Although awake techniques minimize the effects of anesthetic agents on ECoG, modern tailored general anesthetic techniques also permit adequate performance of ECoG (see Chapter 19).

INTRAOPERATIVE ANESTHESIA MANAGEMENT

All members of the team must be briefed in advance so that a calm atmosphere prevails in the operating room. Routine invasive cardiovascular monitoring is performed with local anesthesia and a urinary catheter inserted if the procedure will be prolonged. Because the procedure can last several hours, the patient should be positioned comfortably on a well-padded table before institution of sedation or anesthesia. The head is best supported with a three-pin fixator applied with local anesthesia to prevent head movement during surgery and maximize airway control

IV

during the sedation phase. Surgical drapes are positioned to allow continuous access by the anesthetist to the patient and airway while preserving a sterile field for the neurosurgeon.

Techniques available for awake craniotomy include local anesthesia alone, local anesthesia and sedation, or true asleep-awake-asleep techniques with the use of general anesthesia and intraoperative wake-up. Some procedures, such as stereotactic brain biopsy or insertion of deep brain stimulators, may be carried out entirely under local anesthesia with minimal sedation, but more complex procedures, particularly those requiring craniotomy, are better suited to a combined technique.

Whichever technique is chosen, provision of adequate local anesthesia using regional, field, and dural blocks is essential. Because the skin, scalp, pericranium, and periosteum of the outer table of the skull all have extensive sensory innervation, subcutaneous infiltration with local anesthetic in the manner of a field block or over specific sensory nerve branches effectively blocks afferent input from all layers of the scalp. The skull can be drilled and opened without discomfort to the patient because it has no sensation itself. However, the dura has extensive innervation and must be anesthetized by a local anesthetic nerve block around the nerve trunk running with the middle meningeal artery, as well as by a field block around the edges of the craniotomy. Relatively large doses of local anesthetic may be required, and therefore caution must be exercised to avoid toxicity.

When the patient is comfortable, intravenous sedation or general anesthesia is administered as appropriate. For sedation techniques, a small bolus of propofol followed by a titrated or target-controlled infusion works well. Patient-controlled sedation techniques with propofol have also been described. Incremental doses of a short-acting opioid (such as fentanyl) can be titrated against the respiratory rate, but vigilance is required to prevent respiratory depression or apnea. Remifentanil infusion is a safe and widely used alternative to fentanyl. Dexmedetomidine, a highly specific α_2-adrenoreceptor agonist, has been successfully used as an adjunct during awake craniotomy to provide sedation and analgesia sufficient to complete cortical mapping and tumor resection. An antiemetic agent should be administered to minimize nausea during awake craniotomy, particularly nausea caused by traction on the temporal lobe during epilepsy surgery. True asleep-awake-asleep techniques generally involve the use of total intravenous anesthesia, usually with propofol and remifentanil, and in many ways differ from sedation techniques only in the doses of drugs administered. A depth-of-anesthesia monitor may be used to guide the depth of sedation and anesthesia during the asleep phase.

20

Airway Control

Some asleep-awake-asleep techniques use conventional airway devices that are removed during the awake phase and reinserted after reinstitution of sedation/anesthesia. Techniques using endotracheal intubation and awakening without removal of the endotracheal tube (removing the ability to test speech), extubation, and reintubation with an endotracheal tube and methods using placement, removal, and replacement of a laryngeal mask airway (LMA) or cuffed oropharyngeal airway have been described. The use of an endotracheal tube or LMA allows assisted ventilation and control of $Paco_2$ during the asleep phase if required. However, in the context of awake craniotomy, airway instrumentation is not without problems. There is a risk of coughing during removal of the endotracheal tube or LMA, which is a significant problem when the dura is open. Furthermore, it can be difficult to reinsert the endotracheal tube or LMA after the reintroduction of anesthesia.

Table 20-2   Complications of Awake Craniotomy

Uncooperative patient
Cardiovascular (hypertension, hypotension, tachycardia)
Excessive sedation
Respiratory depression
Loss of control of the airway
Brain swelling
Seizures
Pain
Local anesthetic toxicity

Because of these potential risks, techniques that avoid airway instrumentation during the sedation/asleep phase have been developed. A soft nasopharyngeal airway, inserted through one nostril after preparation of the nasal mucosa with 25% cocaine paste, can remain safely in place throughout the procedure. It also has the advantage of allowing monitoring of end-tidal carbon dioxide by attachment of a sidestream carbon dioxide monitoring device into the end of the airway. Oxygen may be administered via the contralateral nostril. Emergency airway intervention is only rarely needed (<1%) with this technique, and this risk is reduced further if opioids are avoided during the sedation phase. However, patients with significant obesity are at greater risk, and formal airway control may be appropriate in this patient group.

Intraoperative Problems

Awake procedures have very low complication rates (Table 20-2) and are generally well tolerated by patients. However, because of the reluctance of some patients to undergo awake procedures, the depth of sedation required can be associated with an increased risk for complications. Oversedation results in a disinhibited uncooperative patient and may also lead to respiratory depression and associated brain swelling because of elevated levels of $Paco_2$. Although airway management is generally uneventful, the use of sedation inevitably runs the risk of airway obstruction and apnea, and facilities for emergency airway control should be available. The possibility of seizures also exists, particularly during electrical cortical stimulation. Seizures should be terminated rapidly, and application of a small bolus of propofol (20 to 40 mg) or iced saline spray to the cortex by the surgeon is usually adequate. Hypertension, hypotension, and tachycardia are more common during awake techniques than during general anesthesia. These hemodynamic changes can be appropriately treated when recognized early and rarely result in adverse outcomes. Arterial $Paco_2$ often rises during the sedation phase of awake procedures, but unless significant respiratory depression occurs, it is not associated with significant complications. Patients with lesions causing a substantial mass effect are most at risk for $Paco_2$-related brain swelling, whereas those undergoing epilepsy or functional surgery are rarely affected.

POSTOPERATIVE CARE

Care after surgery is determined by the neurosurgical procedure, and there are no special requirements from the anesthetic technique itself. After awake craniotomy, patients are fully alert and cooperative in the immediate postoperative period, and

IV

prolonged stay in a high-dependency area may not be necessary. Adequate analgesia should be provided before the effect of the local anesthetic wears off.

KEY POINTS

- Adequate operating conditions are essential.
- Airway control during the sedation phase is vital.
- Awake craniotomy is associated with a risk of seizures.
- Patient cooperation is important during awake craniotomy.

FURTHER READING

Berkenstadt H, Perel A, Hadani M, et al: Monitored anesthesia care using remifentanil and propofol for awake craniotomy. J Neurosurg Anesthesiol 2001; 13:246-249.
Hans P, Bonhomme V, Born J, et al: Target-controlled infusion of propofol and remifentanil combined with bispectral index monitoring for awake craniotomy. Anaesthesia 2000; 55:255-259.
Herrick I, Craen R, Gelb A, et al: Propofol sedation during awake craniotomy for seizures: Electrocorticographic and epileptogenic effects. Anesth Analg 1997; 84:1280-1284.
Manninen P, Balki M, Lukitto K, Bernstein M: Patient satisfaction with awake craniotomy for tumor surgery: A comparison of remifentanil and fentanyl in conjunction with propofol. Anesth Analg 2006; 102:237-242.
Sarang A, Dinsmore J: Anaesthesia for awake craniotomy—evolution of a technique that facilitates awake neurological testing. Br J Anaesth 2003; 90:161-165.
Skucas A, Artru A: Anesthetic complications of awake craniotomies for epilepsy surgery. Anesth Analg 2006; 102:882-887.
Smith M: Anaesthesia for epilepsy surgery. In Shorvon S, Perucca E, Fish D, Dodson E (eds): The Treatment of Epilepsy Oxford, Blackwell Science, 2004.

20

Chapter 21

Anesthesia for Stereotactic Surgery

Pekka O. Talke

Technical Aspects	Anesthetic Considerations
Fixed–Head Frame Stereotactic Neurosurgery	**Risks**
Frameless Stereotactic Neurosurgery	**New Directions**
Procedures Performed with Stereotactic Neurosurgery	

Stereotactic neurosurgery is used to treat and diagnose a wide variety of diseases of the nervous system. The word "stereotactic" is derived from the *stereos*, meaning three dimensional, and *tactus*, meaning to touch. Modern stereotactic neurosurgery is based on the use of three-dimensional localization of specific areas of the human nervous system acquired by neuroradiologic imaging techniques. Though initially developed almost a century ago, stereotactic neurosurgery became popular only in the 1970s with the development of better neuroimaging techniques. In the 1990s, further advances in imaging technology and electrophysiologic techniques dramatically increased the role of stereotactic neurosurgery in treating movement disorders.

TECHNICAL ASPECTS

Fixed–Head Frame Stereotactic Neurosurgery

Most commonly, stereotactic neurosurgery is performed with a stereotactic system that includes a head frame that is fixed to the patient's skull. In this technique, the first step is application of the head frame, which is typically performed by the neurosurgeon, who applies local anesthetic to four areas of the scalp of the sedated patient, whereupon the stereotactic head frame is secured to the patient's skull with four pins. The patient's head is then imaged in the computed tomography (CT) or magnetic resonance imaging (MRI) scanner. Based on these images, the neurosurgeons or neuroradiologists (or both) calculate the coordinates for the area of interest and plan the most appropriate location for the craniotomy (burr hole) trajectory through the brain.

In the operating room the stereotactic head frame is attached to the operating room table so that it remains in a fixed position. After infiltration of the skin of the craniotomy site with local anesthetic, a skin incision is made, followed by the burr hole. Once the dura is opened, the instruments (a biopsy needle, microrecording electrode, radiofrequency probe, etc.) can be advanced to the area of interest. After the procedure the scalp is closed with a few sutures and the stereotactic frame is removed from the patient's head.

Stereotactic radiosurgery is a means of delivering a single high dose of radiation in one session. Stereotactic radiosurgery also involves the application of a stereotactic head frame and neuroradiologic imaging. However, the procedure is not performed in the operating room and does not involve a skin incision. A stereotactic frame is required and imaging is used to plan a three-dimensional radiation target, most commonly a metastatic tumor or arteriovenous malformation (AVM). In the radiation suite the head frame is attached to the radiation device and radiation is delivered, after which the head frame is removed.

Frameless Stereotactic Neurosurgery

For these procedures no stereotactic head frame is used. The patient's head is first imaged in an MRI scanner with special markers (fiducials) pasted onto the scalp. In the operating room the patient's head is secured to the operating room table with three-point pin fixation that includes a neuronavigation reference attachment. Using a special pointer, the fiducials on the patient's head will be cross-referenced with the MR images, which will be used to direct the image-guided procedure.

PROCEDURES PERFORMED WITH STEREOTACTIC NEUROSURGERY

Stereotactic neurosurgery includes several very different surgical techniques to treat a wide variety of diseases of the nervous system. Some of the more commonly performed procedures include (1) deep brain stimulator (DBS) implants for movement disorders (Parkinson's disease [PD] and primary dystonia), (2) stereotactic radiosurgery, and (3) brain biopsy.

Parkinson's disease is a chronic, progressive neurologic disorder characterized by tremor, bradykinesia, postural instability, and rigidity. Currently, bilateral stimulation of the subthalamic nucleus with a DBS is one of the most effective treatments of advanced PD. One or two electrodes are implanted in the subthalamic nucleus to allow deep brain stimulation at high frequency, which suppresses the rigidity associated with PD. The stimulating electrodes may be placed under the guidance of intraoperative microelectrode recordings in a mildly sedated patient or by placing the electrodes during general anesthesia with only stereotactic techniques.

Patients first undergo head frame placement followed by MRI as described earlier. In the operating room the therapeutic target is located by stereotactic and neurophysiologic microelectrode recording techniques and intraoperative functional testing (usually movement of the limbs). Once the permanent lead is placed, the head frame is removed, general anesthesia is induced for the lead extension, and a pulse generator/battery is situated in the upper part of the chest. When bilateral electrodes are implanted, both can be controlled separately by a single pulse generator.

Dystonia consists of a group of movement disorders characterized by involuntary movement and sustained contraction of muscles leading to a distorted posture. Dystonia may affect only certain regions of the body or may be generalized. In addition to medication, primary dystonia in particular may be treated by selective destruction (pallidotomy) or high-frequency stimulation of nerve cells in the globus pallidus or subthalamic nucleus. Although the optimal therapeutic target to treat dystonia is not known, the globus pallidus, thalamus, and subthalamic nucleus have been targeted successfully. Because bilateral pallidotomy is associated with significant adverse effects, DBS implantation has been used more recently to treat dystonia. Deep brain stimulation has significant advantages over pallidotomy because it is reversible,

21

> **BOX 21-1** *Definitions*
>
> *Pallidotomy* is surgical destruction, most often by a heated probe, of a small number of brain cells within the globus pallidus internus, which helps control voluntary movements. Pallidotomy is most commonly performed to control involuntary movements or rigidity.
>
> *Thalamotomy* is surgical destruction of a small number of brain cells within the thalamus. The thalamus is part of the nerve pathways that control intentional movement. Thalamotomy is most commonly performed to control involuntary movements and tremor.

provides a safe bilateral approach, and affords continuous access to the therapeutic target. However, such stimulation in patients with dystonia is associated with lead failure and requires frequent battery changes.

Pallidotomy, thalamotomy, or DBS placement in the globus pallidus, thalamus, or subthalamic nucleus involves stereotactic surgery with a head frame (Box 21-1). The procedure, which follows steps similar to those for DBS insertion, is often performed in awake patients to allow assessment of neurologic responses to test stimulation. However, patients with severe dystonia may require general anesthesia.

Stereotactic *radiosurgery* was pioneered by Leksell in the 1950s. It combines neurosurgical stereotactic localization and immobilization techniques with radiation physics to distribute high levels of energy to an imaging-defined target while delivering as little radiation to surrounding brain as possible. The procedure can be performed on an outpatient basis and is associated with minimal morbidity and no mortality. Stereotactic radiosurgery is used to treat brain tumors (specifically metastases), AVMs, meningiomas, trigeminal neuralgia, and acoustic neuromas. Advances in neuroradiology imaging techniques and dose-planning software have improved patient outcomes with this technique. Stereotactic radiosurgery has been shown to improve survival, quality of life, and tumor control in patients with brain tumors.

Brain biopsy of difficult-to-access, deep lesions is often performed with stereotactic neurosurgical techniques. Biopsy is normally done in the operating room with a head frame or a frameless system. During the procedure a biopsy needle is inserted into the area of interest under stereotactic guidance as described previously. A biopsy sample is usually sent to pathology to verify that appropriate tissue has been obtained before removing the stereotactic frame. The procedure is minimally invasive and relatively brief and is performed under sedation or general anesthesia.

ANESTHETIC CONSIDERATIONS

Stereotactic neurosurgery is performed for many nervous system diseases and procedures, so anesthetic considerations are mainly related to the specific procedure, which may differ from center to center, and to the patient's frequent coexisting diseases. The literature is extremely limited on anesthetic considerations related to stereotactic neurosurgical procedures. Because many of the procedures require intraoperative neurophysiologic testing of an awake patient, the main goals of anesthesia are to alleviate anxiety and make the patient comfortable for procedures that are sometimes lengthy. Analgesia for the scalp is provided by local infiltration of anesthetic or nerve blocks, or both.

Mild sedation (midazolam) and local anesthesia may be used for head frame placement, with no additional sedation required for the imaging. In the operating room, sedation is provided with either propofol or dexmedetomidine infusion where available, which may be supplemented with lose doses of fentanyl or remifentanil. During lead placement and functional testing no anesthetics or sedatives are administered. Systolic blood pressure is maintained below 140 mm Hg with labetalol in an attempt to reduce the incidence of intracranial bleeding. General anesthesia through a laryngeal mask airway is used for lead extension and generator placement.

Poor access to the airway because of the head frame is one of the main considerations during deep brain stimulation, and a strategy for airway management should be in place before beginning the procedure. Sedation-induced airway compromise is to be avoided. Deep brain stimulation is usually done in a semisitting position, so intraoperative air embolism is a potential complication and should be detected rapidly and treated.

Although arterial carbon dioxide cannot be controlled during awake procedures, hypocapnia should be avoided during general anesthesia to prevent the brain (target) from shifting relative to the awake MR image.

Little has been published on the effect of general anesthesia on microelectrode recordings during deep brain stimulation. Empirically, propofol-based anesthesia or sedation and, in the United States, propofol- and dexmedetomidine-based sedation appear to allow adequate recording.

Some dystonic patients are not able to have adequate neuroradiologic imaging performed without deep sedation or general anesthesia. Because of the head frame application we prefer to use general anesthesia.

Intracranial bleeding is always a possibility during invasive stereotactic neurosurgery. The team should be able to recognize such an event and have a plan for treatment depending on the severity of the bleeding.

Most patients with movement disorders have their medications reduced and may be more symptomatic perioperatively. In patients with tremor severe enough to interfere with noninvasive blood pressure monitoring, intra-arterial blood pressure measurements should be considered.

RISKS

The risks of stereotactic neurosurgery vary depending on the procedure and experience of the team. Stereotactic radiosurgery has minimal morbidity and no mortality, whereas the more invasive techniques are associated with higher risk.

The most frequent risks associated with deep brain stimulation are hardware related (broken/misplaced lead), infections that require removal of the system, seizures, airway obstruction, perioperative intracranial hemorrhage (2% to 4%), and air embolism. Intracranial hemorrhage may be manifested as confusion, agitation, or coma. Air embolism in an awake patient may cause irregular breathing, gasping for air, coughing, and chest pain and may lead to pulmonary edema.

NEW DIRECTIONS

Stereotactic neurosurgery has expanded dramatically during the past 15 years. However, many questions are still unanswered, such as the best target for deep brain stimulation for different movement disorders and the ideal location and size of basal ganglia lesions to treat movement disorders. Meanwhile, new techniques are being used, such as stereotactic application of radiotherapeutics and biologicals (gene therapy) and real-time MRI-guided DBS placement. Computer-assisted surgery, robotics, and further improvements in imaging techniques will move this field of neurosurgery forward.

21

KEY POINTS

- Stereotactic neurosurgery is used to treat and diagnose a wide variety of diseases of the nervous system.
- Stereotactic neurosurgery is based on the use of three-dimensional localization of specific areas of the human nervous system acquired by neuroradiologic imaging techniques.
- Most commonly, stereotactic neurosurgery is performed with a stereotactic system that includes a head frame fixed to the patient's skull.
- Stereotactic radiosurgery is a means of delivering a single high dose of radiation in one session and is frequently used to treat metastatic brain tumors.
- Bilateral stimulation of the subthalamic nucleus with a deep brain stimulator is one of the most effective treatments of advanced Parkinson's disease.
- Pallidotomy or deep brain stimulation of the globus pallidus is a common treatment of dystonia.
- Many stereotactic neurosurgery procedures are performed under mild sedation, without general anesthesia.

FURTHER READING

Benabid AL, Chabardes S, Seigneuret E: Deep-brain stimulation in Parkinson's disease: Long-term efficacy and safety—what happened this year? Curr Opin Neurol 2005; 18:623-630.

Goetz CG, Poewe W, Rascol O, et al: Evidence-based medical review update: Pharmacological and surgical treatments of Parkinson's disease: 2001 to 2004. Mov Dis 2005; 20:523-539.

Okun MS, Vitek JL: Lesion therapy for Parkinson's disease and other movement disorders: Update and controversies. Mov Disord 2004; 19:375-389.

Suh JH, Vogelbaum MA, Barnett GH: Update of stereotactic radiosurgery for brain tumors. Curr Opin Neurol 2004; 17:681-686.

Tagliati M, Shils J, Sun C, et al: Deep brain stimulation for dystonia. Exp Rev Med Devices 2004; 1:33-41.

IV

Chapter 22

Anesthesia for Pituitary Surgery

Ram Adapa • Arun K. Gupta

ANATOMY

Location

The pituitary gland is located in the pituitary fossa, a bony depression in the base of the skull (sella turcica). Of importance, the lateral wall of the sella is related to the cavernous sinus, carotid artery, and third, fourth, and sixth cranial nerves.

Histologic Cell Types

The pituitary gland consists of two distinct lobes with differing embryologic origins. The anterior lobe, which develops from the ventral edges of the neural tube, has at least five different types of cells that secrete different hormones. There are also nonfunctional "null" cells that can give rise to nonfunctioning pituitary tumors. The posterior lobe, which develops as a downgrowth from the floor of the third ventricle, is made up of nonhormonal cell types that store and release hormones (vasopressin and oxytocin) secreted from the hypothalamus.

PHYSIOLOGY

The hormones secreted by the different cell types of the anterior pituitary and their effects on target tissues and other endocrine glands are summarized in Tables 22-1 and 22-2.

22

Table 22-1 Hormones Secreted by Different Cell Types of the Anterior Pituitary

Cell Type	Population with Tumor in the Anterior Pituitary (%)	Hormone Secreted	Hypothalamic Feedback	Clinical Disease
Somatotrophs	50	Growth hormone (GH)	GH-releasing hormone (GHRH) Somatostatin (inhibitory)	Acromegaly
Lactotrophs	10-25	Prolactin	Prolactin-releasing hormone (PRH) Prolactin-inhibiting hormone (dopamine)	Prolactinoma
Corticotrophs	15	Adrenocorticotropic hormone (ACTH)	Corticotropin-releasing hormone (CRH)	Cushing's disease
Thyrotrophs	5-10	Thyroid-stimulating hormone (TSH)	Thyrotropin-releasing hormone (TRH)	Hyperthyroidism
Gonadotrophs	10	Follicle-stimulating hormone (FSH), luteinizing hormone (LH)	LH-releasing hormone (LHRH)	

Table 22-2 Effects of Hormones on Target Tissues and Other Endocrine Glands

Hormone	Target Tissue	Clinical Effect
Growth hormone	Various tissues	Stimulation of bone and cartilage growth Increase protein synthesis and lipolysis, decrease insulin sensitivity (through insulin-like growth factor I [IGF-I])
Prolactin	Breast tissue	Milk secretion
Adrenocorticotropic hormone (ACTH)	Adrenal gland	Increased secretion of cortisol
Thyroid-stimulating hormone (TSH)	Thyroid	Increased blood flow to the thyroid Stimulates iodine binding to the thyroid Increased synthesis and release of triiodothyronine (T_3), thyroxin (T_4)
Follicle-stimulating hormone (FSH), luteinizing hormone (LH)	Gonadal tissues	Ovarian follicle maturation Ovulation and spermatogenesis Secretion of testosterone

Feedback Mechanisms

Secretion of hormones by the anterior pituitary is under control of the hypothalamus. The hypophyseal portal system carries arterial blood containing hypothalamic hormones to the anterior pituitary. These hormones either inhibit or stimulate release of hormones from the anterior pituitary (see Table 22-1).

Increased levels of insulin-like growth factor I (IGF-I) cause somatostatin to be secreted from the hypothalamus and also decrease the secretion of growth hormone (GH) from the anterior pituitary. Similarly, thyroid hormones decrease secretion of thyrotropin-releasing hormone (TRH) and thyroid-stimulating hormone (TSH) in a feedback loop, and cortisol decreases secretion of corticotropin-releasing hormone (CRH) and adrenocorticotropic hormone (ACTH).

PITUITARY PATHOLOGY

Pituitary tumors account for 10% to 15% of all intracranial neoplasms, tend to be benign, and are occasionally found as incidental postmortem findings (10% to 25% of autopsies) or unrelated to the condition being investigated (incidentalomas). These adenomas have a peak incidence in middle age and can be microadenomas or macroadenomas (tumors ≤1 cm in size).

CLINICAL FEATURES

Tumors of the anterior pituitary can be "functioning" or "nonfunctioning"; functioning tumors are often initially manifested by symptoms of hormonal excess. Prolactin-secreting tumors are the most common type of functioning pituitary adenomas; however, their mass effect is probably more significant. Prolactin secretion can also be increased with nonfunctioning tumors, which can compress the pituitary stalk and reduce the transfer of dopamine to the anterior pituitary, thereby decreasing the inhibitory influence of the hypothalamus.

Other common manifestations include the following:

Mass effect, more common with macroadenomas, which tend to occur later. The effect can be localized, with optic chiasmal or oculomotor nerve lesions. Larger tumors can also obstruct the outflow pathway of cerebrospinal fluid (CSF) and result in a generalized mass effect and symptoms of raised intracranial pressure (ICP).

Pituitary hypofunction. Intrasellar growth of a tumor can result in compression of adjacent normal pituitary tissue, which can cause pituitary hypofunction. Other causes include previous radiotherapy or surgery in the area or hemorrhage into the pituitary gland.

Nonspecific symptoms, including infertility and epilepsy. These symptoms can occasionally be the initial features of macroadenomas.

PREOPERATIVE DIAGNOSIS AND MANAGEMENT

Diagnosis of pituitary disorders is often delayed by lack of awareness and the subtle onset of symptoms and signs, and it hence relies on a combination of clinical suspicion, elevated hormone levels, and imaging techniques. Magnetic resonance imaging (MRI) is technically superior in the identification of microadenomas, whereas computed tomography (CT) is better at detection of bony invasion.

Management of Specific Tumors

Prolactinomas

Elevated plasma prolactin levels in the absence of dopamine antagonist intake should raise suspicion of a prolactin-secreting tumor. Medical therapy in the form of dopaminergic agonists such as bromocriptine and cabergoline constitutes the first line of management. Surgery is reserved for the few who cannot tolerate the drug effects or for those with progression of visual symptoms despite medical therapy.

Growth Hormone–Secreting Tumors

An elevated IGF-I level in combination with an elevated random GH level and failure of suppression of GH secretion after an oral glucose load is diagnostic of acromegaly. GH-secreting tumors tend to be resistant to medical therapy, and surgery with radiotherapy is the usual line of management.

Adrenocorticotropic Hormone–Secreting Tumors

Diagnosis of these tumors is complex, and identification of the source of hormonal excess typically follows a pathway similar to the one described in Figure 22-1. Management of these patients is usually surgical, with or without associated radiotherapy (especially in children). Bilateral adrenalectomy with subsequent hormonal replacement can result in Nelson's syndrome (browning of the skin because of excess ACTH production) with a risk of compression of structures surrounding the enlarging pituitary gland.

Thyroid-Stimulating Hormone– or Follicle-Stimulating/Luteinizing Hormone–Secreting Microadenomas

These tumors are diagnosed on the basis of elevated hormone levels, and the primary treatment is surgical, as is the case with nonfunctional macroadenomas.

Preoperative Assessment

Preoperative assessment of patients scheduled for pituitary surgery should focus on the identification and management of (1) raised ICP and (2) the effects of hormonal hypersecretion.

Mass Effect

Symptoms such as headache, nausea, and vomiting in the presence of papilledema should raise suspicion of raised ICP, and anesthetic management should be appropriately altered to avoid any maneuver that raises ICP. It should be noted that focal deficits such as bitemporal hemianopia and quadrant defects might occur in the absence of raised ICP.

Syndromes of Hormonal Hypersecretion

ACROMEGALY

The clinical manifestations of excess GH secretion that are of particular concern to anesthesiologists are upper airway, cardiac, and respiratory involvement. Upper airway changes include macroglossia, prognathism with malocclusion, and hypertrophy of the laryngeal soft tissue, epiglottis, and aryepiglottic folds leading to a reduction in size of the glottic opening. Hoarseness should prompt investigation for laryngeal involvement or recurrent laryngeal nerve injury. Indirect laryngoscopy and imaging techniques have been recommended to identify potentially difficult airways. A history suggestive of obstructive sleep apnea (OSA) should also be sought inasmuch as nearly 70% of acromegalic individuals have either a peripheral or, more uncommonly, a central form of

OSA. This is also manifested in lung function tests, where flow-volume loops suggestive of extrathoracic obstruction are more common than impaired gas exchange.

Cardiac disease is the most common cause of death in patients with untreated acromegaly. Cardiac effects include left ventricular hypertrophy with or without hypertension, interstitial myocardial fibrosis and resultant cardiomyopathy, small-vessel coronary artery disease, supraventricular tachyarrhythmias, and disorders of conduction. Electrocardiographic changes consisting of ST depression and T-wave abnormalities are common.

Impaired glucose tolerance and diabetes mellitus occur in up to 25% of patients with acromegaly.

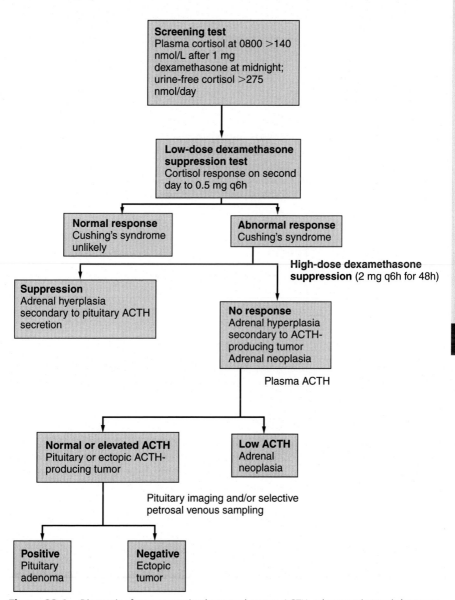

Figure 22-1 Diagnosis of tumors causing hormonal excess. ACTH, adrenocorticotropic hormone.

Table 22-3 Multisystem Manifestations of Cushing's Syndrome	
Organ Systems Affected	**Clinical Features**
Cardiorespiratory	Hypertension
	Increased sensitivity to endogenous and exogenous vasopressors
	Left ventricular hypertrophy and strain
	Congestive cardiac failure
	Obstructive sleep apnea
Electrolyte imbalance	Hypokalemia, hypernatremia
Endocrine	Diabetes mellitus
Musculoskeletal	Osteoporosis, aseptic necrosis of the hip, vertebral crush fractures, proximal myopathy, capillary fragility
Miscellaneous	Obesity, polycythemia, decreased wound healing, thin skin, gastroesophageal reflux

CUSHING'S SYNDROME

Many of the multisystem manifestations of Cushing's syndrome are important to anesthesiologists (Table 22-3). Coexisting hypertension is common and usually multifactorial: increased cardiac output, increased activation of the renin-angiotensin system through enhanced hepatic production of angiotensinogen, and reduced synthesis of vasodilatory prostaglandins. The increased sensitivity to exogenous and endogenous vasoconstrictors is due to increased expression of type I angiotensinogen II receptors and enhanced inositol triphosphate production in vascular smooth muscle.

Preoperative Optimization of Hormonal Function

Perioperative Steroid Supplementation

Historically, all patients undergoing elective pituitary surgery received hydrocortisone at anesthetic induction and two additional divided doses postoperatively for 24 hours, followed by a tapering dose thereafter. Dose regimens vary depending on the specialist center. Patients with Cushing's syndrome may receive either dexamethasone (which causes minimal interference with serum cortisol levels) or no additional perioperative steroids, along with regular repeated assays of serum cortisol and steroid replacement only if indicated by a low serum cortisol level.

Preoperative Control of Thyroid Function

Though rare, thyrotropic pituitary adenomas are often more locally invasive, carry the potential for blood loss, and may be susceptible to medical therapy (antithyroid medication, somatostatin analogues). For these reasons, hyperthyroidism is aggressively treated in these patients before elective pituitary surgery.

INTRAOPERATIVE CONSIDERATIONS

Surgical Approach

The traditional surgical approach to pituitary tumors has relied on transnasal or transseptal transsphenoidal access to the sella. Optimal removal of larger tumors and decompression may require a craniotomy. Newer techniques such as the endoscopic endonasal approach have allowed superior visualization of both the sellar and suprasellar components of these tumors. Opening of the diaphragma sellae is also possible and allows decompression of the optic apparatus under direct visualization. This approach has the added benefit of minimizing patient discomfort, decreasing the incidence of diabetes insipidus (DI), and allowing early patient discharge.

A lumbar intrathecal catheter is occasionally inserted to aid visualization of the adenoma by manipulation of CSF pressure. Increasing CSF pressure pushes the tumor down toward the surgeon. Air is also occasionally injected via the catheter to delineate the mass fluoroscopically, thus contraindicating the use of nitrous oxide intraoperatively. A drain can also be used postoperatively if the dura has been breached during surgery.

Anesthetic Management

Topical preparation of the nasal mucosa is usually performed by the surgeon before the start of surgery. The choice of drug varies, but xylometazoline is frequently used because of its safety profile, longer duration of action, and efficacy.

Airway Management

Preoperative airway assessment and Mallampati grading of the airway have been shown to be relatively poor indicators of a difficult airway in acromegalic patients. The soft tissue enlargement and overgrowth of the upper airway can make airway management difficult. This situation may require the use of airway adjuncts and alternative techniques to secure the airway. Direct laryngoscopy may require the use of a long blade. In the event of an anticipated difficult intubation, awake fiberoptic intubation may be a prudent option. Insertion of an laryngeal mask airway (LMA) may likewise prove to be difficult because of the enlarged tongue, as may the use of fiberoptic laryngoscopy.

Cushing's syndrome is also associated with phenotypic features related to the difficult airway, such as obesity. Hence, caution should be exercised during induction of anesthesia in such patients. A throat pack is normally inserted after endotracheal intubation to minimize aspiration of blood during a transsphenoidal approach and must be removed before extubation.

22

Choice of Drugs

Intravenous and inhalational techniques have both been used successfully for transsphenoidal surgery. Adherence to the general principles of neurosurgical anesthesia is more crucial to a successful outcome than the choice of drugs. However, the use of short-acting drugs allows rapid awakening at the end of surgery. Remifentanil is particularly useful during the periods of intense stimulation that occurs during transsphenoidal surgery.

Positioning of the Patient

Patients are usually positioned supine with the head up for either transsphenoidal surgery or subfrontal craniotomy.

Monitoring

In addition to basic standard monitoring, invasive arterial pressure monitoring should be considered in patients with coexisting cardiac disease or Cushing's syndrome. The choice of artery for cannulation should be dictated by the presence or absence of carpal tunnel syndrome (more common in acromegaly) and the Allen test. Central venous pressure monitoring is indicated only in patients with severe cardiorespiratory comorbidity.

Visual evoked potentials (VEPs) are used in some centers; however, the sensitivity of VEPs to anesthetic agents, the high incidence of false-positive and false-negative results, and the relative lack of evidence of postoperative improvement in visual acuity have all prevented more widespread use of VEPs in pituitary surgery.

POSTOPERATIVE CARE

Emergence from anesthesia should ideally be smooth and rapid to prevent dislodgement of nasal packs or stents and also to allow early neurologic assessment. Airway obstruction is not uncommon in the early postoperative period and is usually due to blood in the nasopharynx or airway morphology in acromegaly. Meticulous attention should be maintained in this period to ensure airway patency. Patients with OSA can benefit from a period of stay in a high-dependency area. Transsphenoidal surgery is associated with moderate postoperative pain, which is usually controlled with a mild opiate. Craniotomy can be associated with more severe pain, and delivery of morphine by patient-controlled analgesia (PCA) is often very helpful. Postoperative nausea and vomiting are common after pituitary surgery, and routine prophylactic antiemetics can reduce the undesirable effects of vomiting in this patient population.

COMPLICATIONS

Transsphenoidal surgery is usually associated with minimal blood loss. However, the proximity of the cavernous sinus and the internal carotid artery means that there is significant potential for massive and potentially fatal blood loss. Cavernous sinus injury is more common and can result in prolonged venous oozing. Though rare, injury to the carotid artery can be fatal, and deliberate hypotension can be used to improve visualization and surgical access. Persistent leakage of CSF from the operative site is also a potential complication, and a Valsalva maneuver may be used toward the end of surgery to help identify such leakage. A patch of muscle taken from the thigh and inserted into the pituitary fossa is sometimes used to minimize the risk of leakage.

Subfrontal pituitary surgery carries all the risks that are associated with craniotomy. In particular, the incidence of trauma to surrounding structures, frontal lobe ischemia, postoperative anosmia, and seizures is greater with the open approach.

Hormonal Complications

Hypernatremia or hyponatremia may occur postoperatively, the diagnosis and treatment of which are described in Chapter 37.

Transient DI causing hypernatremia is common after transsphenoidal surgery and generally occurs in the first 24 to 48 hours. Hyponatremia can be caused by either the syndrome of inappropriate antidiuretic hormone (SIADH) secretion or rarely by the cerebral salt wasting syndrome (CSWS). Most often, however, it is caused by fluid overload or excessive secretion of antidiuretic hormone.

IV

KEY POINTS

- Patients who are to undergo pituitary surgery commonly have signs and symptoms of hormonal hypersecretion. These syndromes have significant anesthetic implications and require careful preoperative evaluation and perioperative management.
- Preoperative assessment of these patients should include examination to identify a potentially difficult airway. Intubation may be difficult, and fiberoptic laryngoscopy and other adjuncts could be required.
- Perioperative steroid supplementation is routinely administered because most patients have maximal baseline steroid secretion and do not cope well with stressful states.
- Transsphenoidal or endonasal approaches to pituitary tumors have largely superseded intracranial procedures because they are safer and require a shorter hospital stay; however, they can be associated with significant complications of their own.
- Postoperative disorders of salt and water balance (SIADH, DI, CSWS) can occur frequently; careful management of fluid balance and repeated laboratory measurements should be adequate for most patients.

FURTHER READING

Anaesthetic complications of acromegaly. Br J Anaesth 2000; 84:179-182.

In Diseases of the adrenal cortex. (eds) Harrison's Principles of Internal Medicine, 14th ed. New York, McGraw-Hill, 1998.

Nemergut EC, Dumont AS, Barry UT, Laws ER. Perioperative management of patients undergoing transsphenoidal pituitary surgery. Anesth Analg 2005; 101:1170-81.

Pituitary disease and anaesthesia. Br J Anaesth 2000; 85:3-14.

Seidman PA, Kofke WA, Policare R, Young M. Anaesthetic complications of acromegaly. Br J Anaesth 2000; 84:179-82.

Smith M, Hirsch NP. Pituitary disease and anaesthesia. Br J Anaesth 2000; 85:3-14.

Williams GH, Dluhy RG. Diseases of the adrenal cortex. In: Harrison's Principles of Internal Medicine-14th edition. Ed: Fauci A, Braunwald E, Isselbacher K, et al. McGraw Hill, 1998:Chapter 332.

22

Chapter 23

Anesthesia for Patients with Head Injury

Sarah Yarham • Anthony Absalom

Classification	**Intraoperative Management**
Pathophysiology	**Complications**
Morphology of Injury	**Postoperative Management**
Indications for Surgical Management	
Preoperative Management	
History	
Physical Examination	
Investigations	

Head injury has a dramatic impact on the health of the nation: it accounts for 15% to 20% of deaths in people aged 5 to 35 years and is responsible for 1% of all adult deaths.

CLASSIFICATION

The Glasgow Coma Scale (GCS) is used as a guide to the severity of head injury. In the following classification the GCS score refers to the score observed after hypovolemia, hypoxia, and drug and alcohol effects have been corrected:

- Mild head injury (GCS score of 13 to 15)
- Moderate head injury (GCS score of 9 to 12)
- Severe head injury (GCS score less than 9)

Severe head injury accounts for 5% of the total number of patients with head injury who arrive at the hospital. It has an associated mortality of nearly 25%—most deaths occur in young people in whom associated life-threatening injuries contribute to the adverse outcome.

PATHOPHYSIOLOGY

Primary brain injury is irreversible. It occurs at the moment of impact and involves immediate neuronal damage from axonal shearing. After the initial injury, secondary injury may result from hypoxia, hypotension, and intracranial hypertension, all of

Table 23-1   Systemic and Intracranial Causes of Secondary Brain Injury

Systemic Causes	Intracranial Causes
Hypotension	Intracranial hypertension
Hypoxia	Edema
Hypoglycemia/hyperglycemia	Vasospasm
Acidosis	Seizures
Sepsis	Infection
Hyperthermia	
Coagulopathy	
Anemia	

which cause cerebral ischemia (Table 23-1). Secondary injury can thus be attenuated or prevented by appropriate medical intervention. Systemic and central nervous system monitoring must be used to allow early detection and prompt treatment of factors that may cause or exacerbate secondary injury. This is a principle that should follow the patient from the prehospital setting, during transfer, in the operating room, and in the intensive care unit.

MORPHOLOGY OF INJURY

Hemorrhagic contusions are superficial, multiple bilateral areas of hemorrhage that usually affect the gray matter of the temporal and frontal lobes. The computed tomography (CT) image is characterized by a "salt and pepper" appearance because of interspersed hemorrhage and edema. The contusions are better delineated by magnetic resonance imaging.

Intracerebral hematomas, in contrast to contusions, usually affect the white matter or basal ganglia and are differentiated from contusion by demarcation between normal and injured brain. They can be a cause of delayed neurologic deterioration but usually have a good prognosis unless a marked mass effect is present. An intracerebral hematoma should be suspected in all patients with a skull fracture (25% risk for an intracerebral hematoma).

Subdural hematomas (SDHs) are caused by tearing of cortical bridging veins between the dura and pia mater. They appear crescent shaped on CT and occur most commonly in the inferior frontal and anterior temporal lobes. SDH is classified as acute (<3 to 4 days old, hyperdense appearance on CT), subacute (4 to 20 days old, isodense), and chronic (>20 days old, hypodense). A poor outcome is more likely if the SDH is bilateral or accumulates rapidly or if there is a delay of more than 4 hours in surgical management (acute SDH).

Extradural hematomas are caused by injury to the middle meningeal artery (secondary to skull fracture) in 90% of cases. The remaining 10% are caused by venous sinus laceration. The parietal and parietotemporal areas are affected, and the CT appearance consists of biconvex lenticular lesions between the skull and dura. The bleeding is arterial, so the onset of coma may be rapid, and it is therefore important to minimize the interval between injury and surgery. Because the underlying brain may not be significantly injured, there may be a lucid period before the onset of neurologic symptoms. Outcomes are generally worse with poorer levels of consciousness at the time of surgery.

23

Diffuse injuries represent a continuum of brain damage produced by increasing levels of acceleration-deceleration injury. Concussion represents the least severe end of the spectrum. Diffuse axonal injury generally has a poor outcome and is characterized by small bilateral nonhemorrhagic lesions affecting the lobar white matter, corpus callosum, and upper brainstem; it is classified as mild (coma for 6 to 24 hours), moderate (coma for >24 hours without decerebrate posturing), or severe (coma for >24 hours with decerebrate posturing).

Traumatic arterial and venous injuries (such as dissection, fistula formation, and pseudoaneurysm) are diagnosed by means of angiography. These injuries may be associated with subarachnoid hemorrhage and secondary vasospasm.

INDICATIONS FOR SURGICAL MANAGEMENT

The following neurologic injuries or sequelae require urgent neurosurgical intervention:

- *Skull fractures.* If the fracture is depressed to a greater depth than the skull thickness or the fracture is compound and the dura torn, surgical reduction is required.
- *Intracranial mass lesions.* Greater than a 5-mm midline shift or basal cistern compression on CT is a sign of imminent transtentorial herniation.
- *Acute subdural and extradural hematomas.* Such hematomas should be evacuated within 2 to 4 hours of injury to maximize prospects for recovery.
- *Intracerebral hematoma.* The decision to operate is guided by the patient's clinical condition and intracranial pressure (ICP). Urgent surgical management may be required for large temporal lobe lesions (risk of transtentorial herniation) and posterior fossa collections (risk of brainstem compression).
- *Refractory intracranial hypertension.* Decompressive craniectomy may be required. There is no consensus for this indication for surgery, but an ongoing multicenter randomized controlled trial is currently in progress.

PREOPERATIVE MANAGEMENT

IV

The initial resuscitation and transfer of patients are dealt with in detail in Chapter 33. It is important to remember that a successful surgical outcome is dependent on prevention of secondary insult from the time of injury. In addition, 40% of patients with a severe head injury will have another life-threatening injury, and hypotension is rarely due to the head injury at an early stage. Polytrauma victims with a head injury often require anesthesia for urgent treatment of other life-threatening (but non-neurologic) injuries, which should be managed in priority order.

History

An account of the acute injury and the GCS score at the scene and subsequently are essential information for assessment of the patient. It is important to note any associated injuries and whether there have been any problems with cardiorespiratory instability. All fluid and drug therapy should be recorded. The AMPLE mnemonic can assist by eliciting key facts during anesthetic assessment (A = allergies, M = medications currently used, P = past medical history, L = last meal, E = events/environment related to the injury). The past medical history is particularly relevant in patients with SDH because significant comorbidity is often present.

Physical Examination

The primary survey (airway, breathing, circulation) should be repeated along with reassessment of neurologic function in terms of GCS score and pupil size and reactivity. Any further resuscitation should be carried out while preparing the patient for the operating theater.

The cervical spine must be cared for appropriately when moving patients. Spinal injury is found in 2% to 5% of patients with severe head injuries and should be assumed to be present until the spine has been cleared in accordance with local practice guidelines.

Investigations

As for any neurosurgical patient, it is important to pay particular attention to tests of clotting function and ensure that cross-matched blood is available. Additional investigations relevant to trauma patients (such as a chest radiograph, electrocardiogram, complete blood count, and urea and electrolyte studies) should have been carried out according to advanced trauma life support protocols and the results noted.

INTRAOPERATIVE MANAGEMENT

Baseline monitoring should include electrocardiography, pulse oximetry, and capnography. Invasive hemodynamic monitoring is essential—invasive arterial pressure monitoring allows assessment of beat-to-beat variation in blood pressure and enables blood sampling, and central venous pressure monitoring helps optimize intravascular volume and fluid balance. Arterial blood gases, blood glucose, electrolytes, hematocrit, and coagulation should be monitored throughout the anesthesia.

The aims of intraoperative management are similar to those for elective craniotomy, with some notable additions:

- Because cerebral edema is likely, a target cerebral perfusion pressure (CPP) greater than 60 mm Hg should be maintained.
- Commencement of vasopressors or inotropes may be required.
- Excessive hyperventilation should be avoided and $Paco_2$ maintained at 4.0 to 4.5 kPa (30 to 35 mm Hg).

23

Total intravenous anesthesia with a combination of propofol and remifentanil is widely used. The beneficial effects of propofol on oxygen metabolism, ICP, and flow-metabolism coupling are discussed in Chapter 8. Sevoflurane (in concentrations <1 minimum alveolar concentration) is considered to be the volatile agent of choice. Nitrous oxide should be avoided. Patients should be paralyzed with neuromuscular blocking agents and be provided adequate analgesia, particularly if other painful injuries are present.

As for all neurosurgical patients, normovolemia, a hematocrit appropriate for the patient's age and underlying medical condition, and a normal blood glucose level should be maintained. In trauma patients, hypovolemia is likely to be due to blood loss from associated injuries. Current evidence suggests that hypertonic saline (5%) solutions may be most beneficial to restore intravascular volume in head-injured patients because CPP is maintained with a reduction in cerebral edema. This may have particular relevance to pediatric practice. Hypotonic and glucose-containing solutions should be avoided. Although moderate hypothermia to 33° C has not been shown to improve outcome, it is important to maintain core body temperature below 37° C and avoid hyperthermia.

COMPLICATIONS

- Sudden and massive local brain swelling develops in up to 20% of patients with acute SDH at the time of clot removal. This swelling should be treated by increased ventilation (to ensure an $Sjvo_2$ of >50%), diuretics (mannitol or 5% saline, or both), and removal of cerebrospinal fluid. Administration of thiopental or propofol to achieve EEG burst suppression should be considered. Swollen brain tissue may need to be retracted (leading to further brain injury) or resected.
- Surgical decompression of markedly elevated ICP may be associated with sudden profound hypotension requiring very aggressive management.
- Penetrating brain injuries may be associated with profuse bleeding, usually from venous sinuses.
- Post-traumatic seizures occur in 15% of patients with severe head injuries. They may initially be manifested perioperatively and are treated with phenytoin for at least 1 week after injury.

POSTOPERATIVE MANAGEMENT

Postoperative management is dependent on the preoperative GCS score and the presence of other injuries. Patients with ongoing impaired levels of consciousness may require continued sedation and ventilation with monitoring and management of ICP. When multiple injuries requiring further surgery are present, it may be prudent to elect to maintain sedation until definitive surgery has been performed. It is, however, difficult to monitor neurologic status in these patients.

After tracheal extubation, patients should be monitored closely in a high-dependency setting for neurologic deterioration. It is possible to have postoperative increases in ICP because of local swelling or development of a new lesion. This occurs most commonly after evacuation of an intracerebral hematoma.

KEY POINTS

- Secondary injury must be avoided. The anesthetic technique must allow early detection and prompt treatment of factors that may exacerbate such injury.
- CPP must be maintained at greater than 60 mm Hg.
- The principles of anesthesia for patients with head injury apply from the time of the injury, including transfer from the scene to a neurosurgical center and the perioperative period.
- Associated injuries in polytrauma patients can cause significant physiologic derangements. In particular, chest injuries may cause hypoxia, as well as hypotension (secondary to blood loss, myocardial contusion, or acute valvular lesions).
- Postoperative high-dependency or intensive care with ICP monitoring and assessment of neurologic status is essential.

FURTHER READING

Jackson R, Butler J: Hypertonic saline. Best evidence topic report. Emerg Med J 2004; 21:80-81.
The Royal College of Surgeons of England Trauma Committee: A position paper on the acute management of patients with head injury. Ann R Coll Surg Engl 2005; 87:323-325.

Chapter 24

Anesthesia for Spinal Surgery

Mary C. Newton

Preoperative Assessment	**Positioning**
Induction and Maintenance of Anesthesia	**Spinal Cord Monitoring**
Spinal Cord Perfusion	**Postoperative Management**
Airway	Treatment of Postoperative Pain
Maintenance of Anesthesia	

Most spinal surgery is performed to relieve compression of the spinal cord or a nerve root, to remove tumor, or to provide vertebral stabilization and prevent secondary neurologic damage. A reduction in the bore of the vertebral spinal or root canals (spinal stenosis) can occur in many conditions, and some patients have congenitally narrow canals. Osteophytic projections at the intervertebral joints (cervical spondylosis) are the most common problem. Tumor, infection, trauma, disc protrusion, and rheumatoid arthritis are less common causes of canal stenosis. In some of these conditions (notably trauma, infection, tumor, and rheumatoid arthritis), the cord may also be at risk, with vertebral instability causing or threatening a reduction in volume of the spinal or root canals. Many patients have significant comorbidity.

PREOPERATIVE ASSESSMENT

Although a general systematic history and physical examination are required, specific information relevant to the surgical procedure and associated pathology is also necessary.

Respiratory reserve must be carefully assessed, especially in patients with significant scoliosis, spinal cord injury, and rheumatoid arthritis. Patients who have significant respiratory compromise (<15 mL/kg vital capacity) may require respiratory support postoperatively. Baseline pulmonary function tests and arterial blood gas analysis may be required.

Cardiovascular instability may be present as a result of autonomic hyperreflexia in patients with spinal cord injury. If present, triggering stimuli should be avoided (see Chapter 32). Cardiovascular compromise may occur in patients with muscular dystrophy and severe scoliosis. Hypertensive patients should have their blood pressure well controlled to ensure optimal spinal cord perfusion intraoperatively. Consideration should be given to omitting angiotensin-converting enzyme and angiotensin II inhibitors to minimize the risk for severe hypotension perioperatively.

Neurologic deficits need to be documented preoperatively. Cervical spine trauma (especially trauma high in location) is associated with an appreciable incidence of traumatic brain injury. If posterior spinal surgery is planned after a significant recent brain injury, it may be prudent to monitor intracranial pressure perioperatively.

Hematologic evaluation is important. Many patients will be taking antiplatelet agents such as nonsteroidal anti-inflammatory drugs (NSAIDs). Medications affecting the clotting process should be stopped preoperatively to allow clotting to return to normal. This is particularly important with anterior cervical spinal surgery, where hematoma formation may compromise the airway postoperatively or a small amount of bleeding may result in spinal cord compression. Adequate blood must be available at all times for transfusion.

Regarding *other systems*, patients with cervical pathology may have long-standing problems with swallowing postoperatively and will benefit from the preoperative creation of a percutaneous gastrostomy. Patients with rheumatoid arthritis may be taking immunosuppressant drugs that may cause renal or hepatic impairment.

Physical examination must include careful assessment of the airway. Many patients have a predictably difficult airway, and cervical spine rigidity or deformity may make face mask ventilation and laryngoscopy difficult. Cervical spine trauma is associated with a significant incidence of maxillofacial injury (see Chapter 25).

All *imaging* must be reviewed to quantify the degree of any cord compression. Imaging in trauma cases should exclude injury to major vessels.

INDUCTION AND MAINTENANCE OF ANESTHESIA

Spinal Cord Perfusion

The anesthetic technique must ensure adequate spinal cord perfusion at all times, although there is little evidence to suggest an optimal perfusion pressure. However, maintenance of normotension may require pressor agents, and hypotension should be corrected quickly.

Several large-bore venous cannulas are essential if there is the potential for heavy blood loss. Invasive blood pressure monitoring is important when spinal cord compression is significant or maintenance of adequate spinal cord perfusion is of particular concern. Central venous pressure should be monitored when significant blood loss is anticipated.

The use of a cell saver device should be considered if massive blood loss is a possibility. Perioperative hemodilution or the use of aprotinin (or both) may also reduce transfusion requirements. Some vascular tumors are amenable to preoperative embolization. Abnormal clotting needs to be corrected promptly.

Airway

In patients with a difficult airway, secondary neurologic damage must be avoided during intubation (see Chapter 25).

Preservation of normothermia with warming devices is important because hypothermia is common when large areas of the patient are exposed intraoperatively. Temperatures lower than 36° C increase the risk for postoperative infection.

Maintenance of Anesthesia

The choice of agents for maintenance of anesthesia may be limited by the intraoperative monitoring of somatosensory evoked potentials (SSEPs) or motor evoked potentials (MEPs) (see Chapter 44). Propofol and opioid infusion allows spinal cord monitoring by both motor and sensory evoked potentials. Sensory evoked potential monitoring can be performed with low-dose volatile agents.

IV

POSITIONING

Careful positioning of the neck is important during every stage of anesthesia, especially in patients with cord compression at the cervical level. In general, neck flexion is more detrimental than extension. The Trendelenburg position should be avoided because spinal cord perfusion may be further compromised by high venous pressure.

Sufficient personnel (five for an unstable spine) are required to move the patient in a controlled manner to maintain correct alignment of the vertebral column and keep intravenous lines and so forth in place.

If the risk of damage to the cervical spinal cord is considered to be high during positioning, some may chose to perform an awake fiberoptic intubation and position the patient awake in the prone position. If no new neurologic symptoms occur, the position is maintained and anesthesia is induced. Most centers favor positioning the patient under general anesthesia with immediate radiologic screening to confirm correct spinal column alignment or prepositioning and postpositioning SSEPs or MEPs, or both.

Surgery involving the posterior spinal column and spinal cord is performed with patients in the prone position. They should be positioned on a special mattress or support that allows free movement of the abdomen with ventilation. In practice, there is invariably some restriction that becomes more significant in the obese. An increase in intra-abdominal pressure results in inferior vena cava compression and contributes to reduced cardiac output. Preloading with crystalloid/colloid at induction reduces the impact of this complication. It is important to measure blood pressure as soon as possible after "proning" so that hypotension may be treated promptly.

The patient's neck must be positioned well clear of the mattress in the prone position. Impedance of venous and lymphatic drainage of the face and neck may result in swelling sufficient to cause airway obstruction. If significant facial/neck swelling is noted postoperatively, extubation should be delayed until it resolves. Independent of the site of surgery, the final position of the neck should be as neutral as possible and excessive rotation avoided.

Visual field defects are a rare but serious complication after surgery in the prone position. The most common cause is ischemic optic neuropathy, in which arterial hypotension or increased intraocular pressure (or both) result in inadequate blood flow to the optic nerve. Visual field defects also result from central retinal artery occlusion caused by direct pressure on the globe from a misplaced head ring and other items. Intraoperative use of the Mayfield head clamp has reduced the incidence of these problems. Corneal damage can be avoided by placing a waterproof covering over the eyes.

Care must be taken to avoid stretching of the brachial plexus if a patient's arms need to be positioned beside the head to facilitate imaging during prone thoracic/lumbar surgery.

The anterior thoracic spine is accessed via a thoracotomy and one-lung anesthesia is required. The brachial plexus and common peroneal and ulnar nerves of the dependent limbs are most vulnerable to damage and must be free of compression to prevent any injury. Judicious fluid replacement will minimize the risk for re-expansion pulmonary edema.

SPINAL CORD MONITORING

SSEPs have been widely used to monitor spinal cord function intraoperatively in the past 10 years. More recently, experience has been gained with monitoring MEPs for spinal cord surgery (see Chapter 44).

24

Table 24-1 Maneuvers to Consider If Cord Injury Is Suggested by Intraoperative Spinal Cord Monitoring

Inform the surgeon immediately (who may alter traction/instrumentation, etc.)
Correct hypoxia
Consider increasing blood pressure to normal or supranormal levels
Correct hypovolemia
Correct anemia (hemoglobin >8 g/dL)
Consider methylprednisolone (NASCIS III regimen)
Consider anesthetic effect, especially if using high concentration of volatile/total intravenous anesthetic agent
Check the patient's position (e.g., has neck flexion increased?)
Consider technical problems with recording

NASCIS, National Acute Spinal Cord Injury Study.

Although the sensory tracts being monitored with SSEPs are close to the motor tracts, their blood supply is different, and it is therefore possible for a patient to have a motor deficit postoperatively despite "normal" SSEP recordings intraoperatively (anterior spinal artery syndrome). Whenever possible, MEPs should be monitored, especially with spinal cord tumors and where there is a high risk of motor impairment.

The depth of anesthesia should be as stable as possible to enable reliable interpretation of changes in the amplitude and latency of signals. Anesthetic agents, particularly volatile agents, can have a significant effect on both types of evoked potentials, but potentials are usually unaffected by "standard" doses of opioids and propofol. The "wake-up" test is rarely used because it has been superseded by SSEPs and MEPs. It can still be useful in difficult cases, however.

Signal changes suggestive of cord injury should "trigger" immediate corrective measures (Table 24-1). Consideration should be given to commencing high-dose methylprednisolone in line with the National Acute Spinal Cord Injury Study III recommendations if the signals do not return to baseline with the aforementioned maneuvers.

IV POSTOPERATIVE MANAGEMENT

Postoperative complications should be anticipated. With careful planning and preventive measures, most should be avoidable.

After cervical spine fusion a previously "easy" airway may subsequently be difficult. This problem should be considered when planning tracheal extubation. If the operative approach has combined surgery on the anterior and posterior cervical spine in one procedure, the patient should remain intubated overnight to allow any airway edema (which may be concealed) time to resolve. In general, extubation should be considered only when there is an audible low-pressure leak (<20 cm H_2O) around the deflated cuff of the tracheal tube.

Cervical collars should be avoided in the immediate postoperative period because they may conceal the development of anterior cervical hematoma and potential airway obstruction. Any suspicion of airway obstruction must be treated as a matter of urgency.

Some patients will require stay in an intensive care unit for respiratory or hemodynamic management, or both. Wherever possible, intubated patients should be lightly sedated to assist in toleration of the tracheal tube while enabling cooperation with accurate neurologic assessment. Any "new" postoperative motor deficit warrants consideration of immediate return to the operating room, without delaying for a magnetic resonance imaging study, to exclude cord compression secondary to a hematoma. This should be done in conjunction with prompt resuscitation of the cord (see earlier) and commencement of high-dose methylprednisolone.

Treatment of Postoperative Pain

Spinal surgery, especially posterior operations, accounts for some of the most painful neurosurgical procedures. Pain relief should be adequate to allow early mobilization and expectoration.

Balanced analgesia with the *regular* administration of paracetamol (acetaminophen), an NSAID, and an opioid (either intravenously or orally) is often required together with the ability to receive additional opioid as required. Many surgeons do not allow NSAIDs to be prescribed because of concern that they impair bone fusion. There is no level 1 evidence in humans to support this contention, however.

Epidural analgesia is not without risk in patients after spinal surgery. A "new" neurologic deficit must never be attributed to the effect of the epidural until a pathologic cause has been excluded. This will necessitate stopping the local anesthetic infusion to facilitate prompt surgical assessment.

Acute neuropathic pain may respond well to a short course of dexamethasone. If likely to persist for some time, specific neuropathic analgesic agents such as amitriptyline and gabapentin should be started. The preemptive use of gabapentin, dexmedetomidine, or ketamine has also been reported to reduce pain significantly.

KEY POINTS

- Many patients with disease of the cervical spine have difficult airways.
- Maintenance of spinal cord perfusion pressure must be ensured at all stages of anesthesia.
- Careful positioning is essential to optimize operating conditions and prevent injury (especially to the eyes).
- Many procedures have the potential for massive blood loss.
- Postoperative pain may be severe and must be well managed to facilitate early mobilization.

24

FURTHER READING

Bandolier Extra: NSAIDs, coxibs, smoking and bone. March 2004.
Pandey CK, Navkar DV, Giri PJ, et al: Evaluation of the optimal preemptive dose of gabapentin for postoperative pain relief after lumbar diskectomy: A randomized, double-blind, placebo-controlled study. J Neurosurg Anesthesiol 2005; 17:65-68.
Raw DA, Beattie JK, Hunter JM: Anaesthesia for spinal surgery in adults. Br J Anaesth 2003; 91:886-904.

Chapter 25

Airway Management and Cervical Spine Disease

Ian Calder

Cervical disease may make all airway techniques, from face mask to tracheostomy, difficult to perform, but it is probably true to say that more anxiety is generated over the *possibility* of damage to the spinal cord than the *probability* of difficult airway management.

The consequences of cervical disease for airway management are not evenly distributed throughout its length. Disease of the *occipito-atlanto-axial (OAA) complex* has greater effect than does disease at lower levels.

THE OCCIPITO-ATLANTO-AXIAL COMPLEX AND AIRWAY MANAGEMENT

The range of movement available at the OAA complex is of particular interest to anesthetists because of the following:

1. *"Head tilt" is required for basic airway management.* Interestingly, cervical spine disease has not emerged as a risk factor in investigations of difficult face mask ventilation. It is probable that patients who might have been a problem were excluded by being selected for awake intubation. Severe flexion deformity will render face mask application impossible. However, when a face mask can be applied, ventilation may be difficult but rarely impossible.
2. *Extension at the OAA complex is useful for direct laryngoscopy.* During direct laryngoscopy, angulation is most marked at the OAA complex and there is little movement at levels below C2 (Figs. 25-1 and 25-2). Difficult laryngoscopic rates of 40% and 7% were observed in a study of patients with cervical spine disease when disease affected the OAA complex and below C3, respectively.
3. *Mouth opening is related to OAA extension.* Ninety-five percent of subjects whose heads are fixed in a neutral position have an interincisor distance of less than 37 mm (95% confidence limit, 29 to 37 mm). An observation of reduced interincisor distance or a Mallampati III grade should raise suspicion of poor OAA movement.

IV

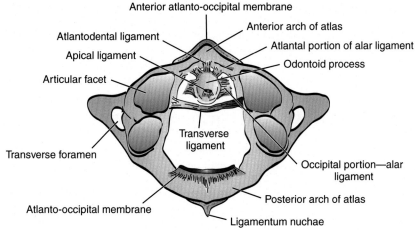

Figure 25-1 Axial section of the atlas vertebra. (Reproduced from Crosby ET: Airway management in adults after cervical trauma. Anesthesiology 2006; 104:1293-1318 by kind permission of the author and Lippincott Williams & Wilkins, Inc.)

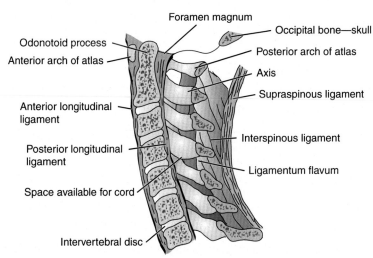

Figure 25-2 Sagittal section of the cervical spine. (Reproduced from Crosby ET: Airway management in adults after cervical trauma. Anesthesiology 2006; 104:1293-1318 by kind permission of the author and Lippincott Williams & Wilkins, Inc.)

4. *The atlantoaxial articulation is unstable.* In this well-known complication of several diseases, the direction of subluxation is most commonly anterior. Rotational dislocation occurs mainly in children in association with upper respiratory tract infections and results in a "wry neck" deformity (Grisel's disease). Diseases associated with atlantoaxial instability include rheumatoid arthritis, Down's syndrome, mucopolysaccharidoses, infections (notably tuberculosis), and Klippel-Feil deformity.

5. *Unfortunately, a reliable noninvasive clinical method of detecting significantly reduced OAA mobility remains elusive.* It appears that compensation at subaxial cervical segments can obscure poor OAA movement, so measurements of craniocervical movement are unreliable. Poor separation of the posterior elements of the OAA complex on lateral radiographs in the neutral or flexed position is a good predictor of difficult laryngoscopy.

CERVICAL STENOSIS AND CERVICAL INSTABILITY

Reduction of the space available for the spinal cord or nerve roots is commonly the cause of neurologic disease. Encroachment on the vertebral canal by arthritic osteophytes or pannus, disc protrusion, or thickening of the ligaments may result in canal "stenosis." Abnormal movement of the vertebrae as a result of instability may also reduce the space available for the cord. Spinal disease may have implications for spinal cord blood supply because the vertebral artery runs through the bones of the cervical spine.

Definition of an "Unstable" Cervical Spine

An all-embracing definition of instability has to include situations in which the spine may not show obvious abnormality for months or years but will eventually become seriously deformed. The condition of a spine described as unstable may vary from complete disruption to an abnormality that has little immediate significance (Table 25-1).

The "Unstable" Spine and Airway Management

This issue remains contentious. There is no good evidence that points to any particular method of airway management as being the most or least favorable in terms of neurologic outcome. Resolution of this issue is unlikely because of the multifactorial nature of neurologic deterioration in cervical spinal disease and the unfeasibly large numbers of patients who would have to be entered into a trial. It needs to be emphasized that many case reports of suspected spinal cord injury after airway management have involved patients with *stable* spines. Several points can be made:

1. There are ethical difficulties in comparative investigations of cervical movement and angulation in at-risk patients. Unstable cadaver preparations or simulated cervical rigidity studies are all that we have available, which obviously precludes investigation of "awake" procedures.
2. Studies of unstable cadaver spine models have suggested that basic airway management techniques, such as "jaw thrust," can cause as much or more displacement or angulation as any of the other airway maneuvers. It can be argued that if this is so, discussion of which laryngoscopic or intubation technique causes the least movement under general anesthesia is somewhat academic.
3. Studies in patients with real or simulated cervical spine disease have found that devices such as the Bullard, GlideScope, or Airtraq laryngoscopes, lightwands, or Bonfils endoscope offer better visualization of the glottis with less cervical movement but generally take longer to achieve intubation than direct (Macintosh) laryngoscopy does.

IV

Table 25-1   Definitions of Instability

General

"Loss of the ability under normal physiologic loads to maintain relationships between vertebrae in such a way that there is neither initial nor subsequent damage to the spinal cord or nerve roots and there is neither development of incapacitating deformity or severe pain"—White and Panjabi, 1990

Radiologic Measurements

Translation
   C1-C2: Anterior atlantodental interval (ADI) >5 mm, posterior ADI <13 mm
   C2-T1: >3.5 mm between points on adjacent vertebrae
Angulation
   >11 degrees between vertebrae
These values have been widely used, but there is poor correlation between radiographic abnormality and neurologic symptoms and signs

Integrity of the Anterior and Posterior Spinal Columns

The spine can be thought of as two columns (anterior and posterior); anterior column disruption tends to make the spine unstable in extension, and posterior column damage favors instability in flexion

4. Studies in cadavers have suggested that the least movement and angulation occur when a flexible fiberoptic technique is used, but absolute differences in terms of millimeters or degrees are small and the clinical significance is unknown.
5. Surveys of opinion among anesthesiologists in the United States have found that a majority would choose a flexible fiberoptic technique in patients at risk for spinal cord injury. However, some of the practitioners espousing this view admit that they doubt their competence with a flexible endoscope. Serious complications have followed attempted flexible endoscopic intubation, and it is debatable whether a patient's interests are best served when an inexperienced endoscopist adopts an unfamiliar technique.
6. There is uncertainty about the cause of reported cases of neurologic deterioration after anesthesia. It has been suggested that airway management is a relatively unlikely culprit because it causes a relatively minor amount of cervical movement, tends to raise blood pressure (direct laryngoscopy), which should improve perfusion, and most importantly, is of short duration.
7. Spinal cord injury can follow cervical deformation in individuals with normal spines, and tolerance of malpositioning is reduced in abnormal spines. This suggests that an awake positioning technique is the most logical choice because the patient should be the best judge of a favorable position. However, surgical requirements may preclude the preferred position and awake techniques can lead to false-positive neurologic deterioration and false-negative results (the patient sustains an injury despite awake positioning). Many and probably the majority of experienced centers do not routinely position the patient while awake.

"Clearing" the Cervical Spine in Suspected Injury

Twenty-five percent to 50% of patients with a traumatic cervical spine injury have an associated head injury, so a common dilemma is the need to confirm or exclude a cervical injury in an unconscious patient. Although local practice varies, Table 25-2 summarizes the current position in the United Kingdom.

Table 25-2 Criteria for Stability after Cervical Trauma

Conscious Patient	Unconscious Patient
Alert, no distracting injuries No midline pain Normal movement No neurologic abnormalities	Plain radiographs are inadequate The combination of plain films and computed tomography is adequate to diagnose bony *and* ligamentous instability Magnetic resonance imaging is not required for the exclusion of instability

Neurologic deterioration after a traumatic cervical spine injury is a worrying and ill-understood phenomenon. Approximately 5% of patients admitted with traumatic cervical injury will deteriorate neurologically. Most deteriorate early (24 hours), some are delayed (1 to 7 days), and occasional patients undergo late deterioration (weeks—subacute post-traumatic ascending myelopathy).

What Is Good Airway Management Practice in Cervical Spine Disease?

The current position is that there is no clear evidence that airway management has any significant influence on neurologic outcome, but adequately powered trials have not been and are unlikely to be conducted. Again, several points can be made:

1. It is likely that secondary injury attributable to hypoxia and hypotension influence spinal cord outcome in the same way as in cerebral injury. In emergencies this consideration militates for rapid intubation, which in most practitioners' hands means direct laryngoscopy.
2. When airway management is performed in suspected unstable patients, the practice of manual in-line stabilization (MILS) is currently a standard of care. However, because establishment of an airway is of paramount importance to the patient, MILS must be relaxed if necessary.
3. If direct laryngoscopy is undertaken in a patient with potential or actual instability, it is a useful practice to combine it with the use of a gum-elastic bougie so that only the least amount of glottic exposure consistent with insertion of the bougie need be obtained. There can be no place for persisting with attempts at intubation if direct laryngoscopy is difficult. This means that practitioners undertaking airway management should be competent in techniques other than direct laryngoscopy.

Flexible Fiberoptic Intubation— Current Technique

Flexible fiberoptic endoscopy is well tolerated by conscious patients, so this technique remains the "gold standard" when the chance of difficult direct laryngoscopy or face mask ventilation is obviously high. However, endoscopy is not risk free and is not suitable for all patients.

IV

Practical Points

1. In the author's view, practitioners should accustom themselves to endoscopy while standing at the side of the patient. This position (with the patient in a semi-sitting pose) is the most appropriate when the patient is awake, and practitioners should accustom themselves to the endoscopic appearances by also using this position in anesthetized patients.
2. It has been suggested that endoscopy is in some way enhanced by keeping the portion of the endoscope exterior to the patient straight. In the author's experience, this is unnecessary, leads to operator fatigue, and is an illogical requirement when using a flexible instrument.
3. Under general anesthesia, the oral route is usually appropriate. An intubation airway such as the Berman or Ovassapian can be helpful. After failed direct laryngoscopy or in other situations in which blood or secretions are interfering with vision, endoscopy through a laryngeal mask airway (LMA) is an excellent rescue technique. The "classic" LMA is the easiest to use for this purpose. One should use either an Aintree catheter technique, a 6.0-mm Flexilum (size 3 or 4 LMA), or a 6.5-mm Flexilum with a size 5 LMA after cutting 5 cm from the shaft of the LMA.
4. In an awake patient the nasal route is usually easiest because gagging and biting are avoided.
5. Glottic closure reflexes must be adequately obtunded. Complete airway obstruction and glottic damage have followed attempted awake fiberoptic intubation. Lidocaine can be used liberally (up to 9 mg/kg) in a "spray as you go" technique. Threading an epidural catheter (with the end cut off above the multiorifice section) partway down the suction channel of the endoscope allows easy injection of the lidocaine. A drying agent such as glycopyrrolate, 0.2 mg, makes topicalization more effective.
6. An infusion of remifentanil is very useful during awake endoscopy and intubation. A dilute solution (10 to 20 μg/mL) should be used so that infusion rates can be changed quickly. Infusion rates between 0.05 and 0.15 μg/kg/min are effective. A small dose of midazolam (1 mg) can be administered if amnesia is required.
7. A target-controlled infusion (1 to 2 μg/kg/min) of propofol is also a successful technique of sedation, with low-dose ketamine (0.25 mg/kg) used for analgesia. Dexmedetomidine with or without low-dose ketamine is also used.
8. Small-diameter, flexible tubes are easiest to pass, and multiple rotations to "spiral the tube in" are often helpful.

KEY POINTS

- Disease of the OAA complex makes difficult laryngoscopy likely, but detection of immobility of the OAA complex by clinical examination is unreliable.
- Instability of the cervical spine is hard to define and of varying clinical importance.
- There is a risk of spinal cord injury during anesthesia, and it is not confined to the cervical region. The cause is uncertain. Injury has been reported in both stable and unstable spines.
- Flexible fiberoptic intubation remains the most useful alternative to direct laryngoscopy in cervical spine disease, but it has not been proved to be safer in terms of neurologic outcome.

FURTHER READING

Calder I, Picard J, Chapman M, et al: Mouth opening—a new angle. Anesthesiology 2003; 99:799-801.

Crosby ET: Airway management in adults after cervical spine trauma. Anesthesiology 2006; 104:1293-1318.

Machata AM, Gonano C, Holzer A, et al: Awake nasotracheal fiberoptic intubation: Patient comfort, intubating conditions, and hemodynamic stability during conscious sedation with remifentanil. Anesth Analg 2003; 97:904-908.

McCleod ADM, Calder I: Spinal cord injury and direct laryngoscopy—the legend lives on. Br J Anaesth 2000; 84:705-709.

Morris CG, McCoy W, Lavery GG: Spinal immobilization for unconscious patients with multiple injuries. BMJ 2004; 329:495-499.

Nolan JP, Wilson ME: Orotracheal intubation in patients with potential cervical spine injuries. An indication for the gum elastic bougie. Anaesthesia 1993; 48:630-633.

Sawin PD, Todd MM, Traynelis VC, et al: Cervical spine motion with direct laryngoscopy and orotracheal intubation. An in vivo cinefluoroscopic study of subjects without cervical abnormality. Anesthesiology 1996; 85:26-36.

Turkstra TP, Craen RA, Pelz DM, Gelb AW: Cervical spine motion: A fluoroscopic comparison during intubation with lighted stylet, GlideScope, and Macintosh laryngoscope. Anesth Analg 2005; 101:910-915.

Urakami Y, Takennaka I, Nakamura M, et al: The reliability of the Bellhouse test for evaluating extension capacity of the occipitoatlantoaxial complex. Anesth Analg 2002; 95:1437-1444.

IV

Chapter 26

Carotid Endarterectomy

Amit Prakash • Derek T. Duane

Surgical Technique, Cross-Clamping, and Monitoring of Cerebral Perfusion	**Anesthetic Technique** General Anesthesia Regional Anesthesia
Preoperative Management	**Postoperative Considerations**

Significant narrowing of the internal carotid artery (ICA) causes up to 20% of all strokes. Of the patients who suffer this condition, approximately a third die, a third recover, and a third experience residual neurologic impairment. Carotid endarterectomy (CEA) is a validated surgical procedure that can reduce the risk for stroke in patients recently symptomatic with transient ischemic attacks or nondisabling stroke because of severe (70% to 99%) ICA stenosis. The benefit of CEA over medical treatment is uncertain when the stenosis is either 50% to 69% and symptomatic or 60% to 99% and asymptomatic. Although CEA can be beneficial, the risk of stroke or death within 30 days of the operation can be as high as 8%, with cardiovascular complications accounting for almost 50% of the mortality. Recently, there has been great interest in carotid angioplasty and stenting for carotid stenosis, and evidence suggests that it can be as safe and effective as CEA in selected patients.

SURGICAL TECHNIQUE, CROSS-CLAMPING, AND MONITORING OF CEREBRAL PERFUSION

During surgery for CEA, the carotid artery is clamped above and below the diseased area. The atheromatous plaque is meticulously removed, followed by closure. Cross-clamping risks hypoperfusion and ischemic damage to the ipsilateral cerebral hemisphere, especially if cross-flow through the circle of Willis is insufficient. Therefore, monitoring the adequacy of cerebral blood flow is common, although the benefit has not been validated in prospective randomized trials. The following modalities are frequently used:

- Clinical assessment
- Stump pressure
- Electroencephalography
- Somatosensory evoked potentials
- Transcranial Doppler ultrasonography
- Near-infrared cerebral oximetry

PREOPERATIVE MANAGEMENT

Most patients who undergo CEA suffer primarily from cardiovascular and cerebrovascular disease, although some will also have chronic obstructive pulmonary disease or diabetes. They are usually hypertensive, have some degree of ischemic heart disease, and are frequently receiving medical treatment for these conditions. A detailed history plus examination of the cardiac, respiratory, and neurologic systems is performed to assess the degree of impairment of organ function and facilitate the optimization of medical therapy for all coexisting conditions. Baseline investigations should include a complete blood count, electrolyte studies, coagulation profile, 12-lead electrocardiograph, and a chest radiograph. Echocardiography may be valuable in patients with severe ischemic heart disease, poor exercise tolerance, or valvular heart disease. Patients who are breathless while lying flat or suffer frequent episodes of angina are unsuitable candidates for a regional anesthetic technique. All patients should be given a comprehensive explanation of the anesthetic and analgesic plan, including the risks and complications of any local anesthetic procedure. Aspirin is administered preoperatively to reduce the risk for postoperative stroke, and premedication with a short-acting benzodiazepine is usually sufficient to achieve anxiolysis in the majority of patients.

ANESTHETIC TECHNIQUE

General Anesthesia

General anesthesia has the advantages of ensuring a motionless patient, creating optimal surgical conditions, and allowing greater control over cerebral perfusion by manipulating arterial carbon dioxide and cerebral metabolism. Before induction, monitoring should include electrocardiography with ST-segment analysis, pulse oximetry, and blood pressure measurement. Noninvasive, rapidly cycling blood pressure measurements may suffice during induction in patients with minimal cardiovascular disease, but invasive monitoring should be used intraoperatively in all. A smooth intravenous induction with minimal hemodynamic fluctuations (<20% of preoperative values) is desirable. Maintenance of anesthesia is achieved by inhalational agents and short-acting opioids given as a bolus or a total intravenous anesthetic technique with propofol and remifentanil. Shorter-acting nondepolarizing muscle relaxants (rocuronium, atracurium, vecuronium) are appropriate.

Ventilation to normocapnia is recommended to avoid cerebral vasoconstriction with hypocapnia and generation of a "steal" phenomenon with hypercapnia. Bleeding is rarely a problem in these cases because exposure of the major vessels allows surgical control. Therefore, modest amounts of intraoperative fluids in the form of glucose-free crystalloid solutions are commonly used. Before carotid cross-clamping, systemic heparinization with up to 5000 IU is achieved. Once the arteries are clamped, mean arterial blood pressure (MAP) may increase without intervention. However, it should be manipulated with the use of vasoactive agents to ensure adequate blood flow through the circle of Willis. The minimum MAP target should equate with the patient's treated preoperative value, whereas the maximum MAP should generally not exceed 20% of this value. Ensuring cerebral perfusion is imperative, but care must be taken to not induce myocardial ischemia with excessive increases in afterload. Bradycardia and hypotension may occur because of surgical interference with the carotid sinus; however, infiltration of local anesthetic around this area commonly resolves this problem.

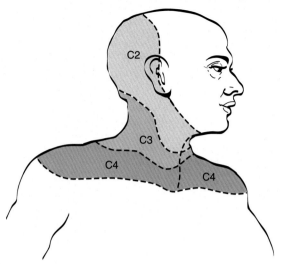

Figure 26-1   Anatomy of the cervical dermatomes. (From Stoneham MD, Knighton JD: Regional anesthesia for carotid endarterectomy. Br J Anaesth 1999; 82:910-919.)

Once surgery is complete, emergence and extubation should be managed actively. The aim is to wake the patient rapidly yet smoothly and maintain hemodynamic stability. Hypertension, tachycardia, and excessive coughing may induce myocardial ischemia or disrupt tissue and vessel anastomoses and thereby promote bleeding into the wound. Lidocaine, β-blockers, vasodilators, and opioids may be used to blunt these responses, together with judicious timing of extubation.

Regional Anesthesia

Advantages of a local anesthetic technique include simple and direct evaluation of the patient's neurologic status, better perioperative hemodynamic stability, reduced requirements for intraoperative shunts, shorter hospital stay, and an overall decrease in complications. Whether a general or local anesthetic technique has any effect on morbidity and mortality is still unsettled. A prospective trial comparing general anesthesia with local anesthesia (the GALA trial) is presently in progress to answer this question.

Surgery for CEA is best performed under a combination of a deep and superficial cervical plexus block (CPB) to produce anesthesia of the C2 to C4 dermatomes (Fig. 26-1). Local infiltration, especially of the carotid sheath, may also be necessary during the procedure. The deep cervical plexus is blocked first because these nerves lie on the transverse processes of the cervical vertebrae approximately 1.5 to 3 cm from the skin. A single injection at C3 or C4 or a three-injection technique (C2 to C4) can be performed. Location of the landmarks is crucial. Three points at intervals of approximately 1.5 cm are marked on a line drawn from the mastoid process (C1) to the level of the cricoid cartilage (C6), 1 cm posterior to the posterior border of the sternocleidomastoid (SCM) muscle (Fig. 26-2). A 22-gauge short-beveled needle is then inserted at each level and aimed slightly posteriorly and caudad until the transverse process is encountered or paresthesia is elicited. Using an immobile needle technique, 3 to 5 mL of local anesthetic is injected after careful aspiration.

In conjunction with the deep block, a superficial CPB is commonly performed. From the midpoint of the posterior border of the SCM muscle, up to 20 mL of local

26

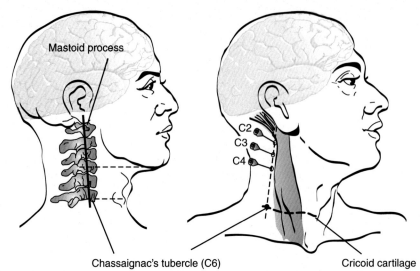

Figure 26-2 Landmarks for deep cervical plexus blockade. (From Cousins MJ, Bridenbaugh PO [eds]: Neural Blockade in Clinical Anesthesia and Management of Pain, 3rd ed. Philadelphia, Lippincott Williams & Wilkins, 1996.)

anesthetic is injected in a subcutaneous plane in a cranial and caudad direction (Fig. 26-3). To block the afferent branches of the facial nerve, the inferior border of the mandible can be infiltrated to reduce pain secondary to surgical retraction.

Patients undergoing CPB require the same level of monitoring as for general anesthesia, and light sedation up to the point of cross-clamping can be obtained with the infusion of remifentanil or propofol. Neurologic deficits and increasing confusion occurring anytime after cross-clamping can be treated by increasing MAP and administering high oxygen concentrations.

The success of local anesthesia for CEA is very much dependent on a patient's ability to lie flat, keep still, and cooperate during surgery. This is better ensured by careful selection, adequate information, minimal surgical draping, short duration of surgery, and constant presence of the anesthetist for reassurance. Complications can arise when performing CPB and include intravascular or subarachnoid local anesthetic injection leading to seizures, loss of consciousness, and cardiovascular collapse and blockade of the phrenic nerve, sympathetic chain (Horner's syndrome, nasal congestion), recurrent laryngeal nerve (hoarseness), and glossopharyngeal nerve (dysphagia).

POSTOPERATIVE CONSIDERATIONS

Patients should be transferred to the postanesthetic care unit in the head-up position, where all monitoring, including transcranial Doppler ultrasonography, should be re-established. Hypertension should be treated quickly with commonly used agents (β-blockers, vasodilators) because it may lead to wound hematoma and airway compromise and possibly worsen a hyperperfusion syndrome. Hypotension should also be prevented if neurologic deficits are apparent, but consideration must be given to the possibility that the cause may be cardiac in origin. Any deterioration in the patient's level of consciousness, signs of limb weakness, or speech difficulty may herald the occurrence of emboli, ICA thrombosis, or rarely, cerebral hemorrhage.

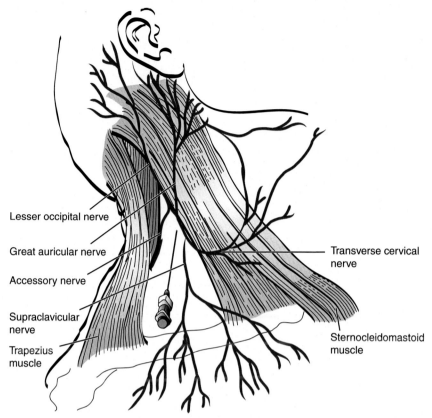

Figure 26-3   Landmarks for superficial cervical plexus blockade. (From Cousins MJ, Bridenbaugh PO [eds]: Neural Blockade in Clinical Anesthesia and Management of Pain, 3rd ed. Philadelphia, Lippincott Williams & Wilkins, 1996.)

Urgent cerebral angiography or surgical re-exploration (or both) are needed to treat carotid occlusion or significant residual stenosis, whereas the use of dextran solutions may reduce embolic phenomena. Other surgical complications that may occur include dysfunction of cranial nerves VII, IX, X, and XII.

KEY POINTS

- Patients undergoing CEA have an approximately 5% risk of stroke or death.
- Cardiovascular complications are the major cause of mortality.
- CEA can be performed under regional or general anesthesia.
- Maintenance of hemodynamic stability should be a prime concern.
- Appropriate monitoring may be used for assessing the adequacy of cerebral perfusion.
- Tight blood pressure control is important during the recovery period.

26

FURTHER READING

Abir F, Barkhordarian S, Sumpio BE: Efficacy of dextran solutions in vascular surgery. Vasc Endovasc Surg 2004; 38:483-491.

Findlay JM, Marchak BE, Pelz DM, et al: Carotid endarterectomy: A review. Can J Neurol Sci 2004; 31:22-36.

GALA trial (General Anaesthesia vs. Local Anaesthesia for Carotid Endarterectomy). Available at http://www.dcn.ed.ac.uk/gala/main_frame.htm.

Krenn H, Deusch E, Jellinek H, et al: Remifentanil or propofol for sedation during carotid endarterectomy under cervical plexus block. Br J Anaesth 2001; 87:637-640.

Rerkasem K, Bond R, Rothwell PM: Local versus general anaesthesia for carotid endarterectomy. Cochrane Database Syst Rev 2004; 2. CD000126.

Rothwell PM, Eliasziw M, Gutnikov SA, et al: Analysis of pooled data from the randomised controlled trials of endarterectomy for symptomatic carotid stenosis. Lancet 2003; 361:107-116.

Rowed DW, Houlden DA, Burkholder LM, Taylor AB: Comparison of monitoring techniques for intraoperative cerebral ischaemia. Can J Neurol Sci 2004; 31:347-356.

Santamaria G, Britti RD, Tescione A, et al: Comparison between local and general anaesthesia for carotid endarterectomy: A retrospective analysis. Minerva Anesthesiol 2004; 70:771-778.

Stoneham MD, Knighton JD: Regional anaesthesia for carotid endarterectomy. Br J Anaesth 1999; 82:910-919.

IV

Chapter 27

Anesthesia for Interventional Neuroradiology

Chanhung Z. Lee • William L. Young

In this chapter we primarily discuss anesthetic management for major interventional neuroradiology (INR) procedures, including treatment of cerebral aneurysm, carotid stenosis, ischemic stroke, and brain arteriovenous malformations. INR may be broadly defined as treatment of central nervous system (CNS) disease via endovascular access for the purpose of delivering therapeutic agents, including both drugs and devices. Because of rapid advancement in INR, anesthesiologists are increasingly being involved in this arena.

PREANESTHETIC CONSIDERATIONS

Baseline blood pressure and cardiovascular reserve should be assessed carefully, especially when blood pressure manipulation and perturbations are anticipated. Preoperative calcium channel blockers for prophylaxis against cerebral ischemia may make patients prone to hypotension. These agents or transdermal nitroglycerin are sometimes used to lessen the incidence of catheter-induced vasospasm.

For procedures managed with an unsecured airway, routine evaluation of the potential ease of laryngoscopy in an emergency situation should take into account the fact that direct access to the airway may be limited by table or room logistics. The possibility of pregnancy in female patients and a history of adverse reactions to radiographic contrast agents should be explored.

MONITORING AND VASCULAR ACCESS

Secure intravenous access should be available with adequate extension tubing to allow drug and fluid administration at a maximal distance from the image intensifier during fluoroscopy. Access to an intravenous or arterial catheter can be difficult when the patient is draped and the arms are restrained at the sides; connections should be secure. Infusion of anticoagulant, primary anesthetics, or vasoactive agents should be through proximal ports with minimal dead space.

For intracranial procedures and postoperative care, beat-to-beat arterial pressure monitoring and blood sampling can be facilitated with an arterial line. A side port of the femoral artery introducer sheath can be used, but the sheath may be removed immediately after the procedure. For patients who require continuous blood pressure monitoring postoperatively, it is convenient to have a separate radial arterial blood pressure catheter.

In addition to standard monitors, a pulse oximetry probe can be placed on the great toe on the leg that will receive the femoral introducer sheath to provide an early warning of femoral artery obstruction or distal thromboembolism. Because a significant volume of heparinized flush solution and radiographic contrast material is often used, bladder catheters assist in fluid management, as well as patient comfort.

ANESTHETIC TECHNIQUE

The choice of anesthetic technique varies among centers, with no clear superior method identified. Rapid recovery from anesthesia is often required for neurologic testing.

Intravenous Sedation

Many neuroangiographic procedures, though not painful per se, can be psychologically stressful. Careful padding of pressure points and working with the patient to obtain final comfortable positioning may assist in the patient's ability to tolerate a long period of lying supine and motionless and thus decrease the requirement for medication.

A variety of sedation regimens is available, and specific choices are based on the experience of the practitioner and the goals of anesthetic management. Frequently used agents include intermittent midazolam and fentanyl, low-dose propofol (25 to 75 μg/kg/min), remifentanil (0.03 to 0.1 μg/kg/min), or dexmedetomidine (0.3 to 0.7 μg/kg/hr). Common to all intravenous sedation techniques is the potential for upper airway obstruction. Placement of nasopharyngeal airways may cause troublesome bleeding in patients receiving anticoagulants and is generally avoided.

General Anesthesia

There is an increasing trend toward the use of general endotracheal anesthesia, which is particularly attractive for control of motion during imaging, including temporary periods of apnea, especially in small children and uncooperative adults. The specific choice of anesthetic is guided primarily by other cardiovascular and cerebrovascular considerations. Total intravenous anesthetic techniques or combinations of inhalational and intravenous methods may optimize rapid emergence. A theoretical argument could be made for eschewing the use of N_2O because of the possibility of introducing air emboli into the cerebral circulation, but there are no data to support this.

ANTICOAGULATION

Careful management of coagulation is required to prevent thromboembolic complications during and after the procedures. Generally, after a baseline activated clotting time (ACT) is obtained, intravenous heparin (70 U/kg) is given to a target prolongation of two to three times baseline. Heparin can then be administered continuously or as an intermittent bolus with hourly monitoring of the ACT. Occasionally, a patient may be refractory to attempts to achieve adequate anticoagulation. Switching from bovine to porcine heparin or vice versa should be considered. If antithrombin III deficiency is suspected, administration of fresh frozen plasma may be necessary. At the end of the procedure, heparin may need to be reversed with protamine.

Antiplatelet agents (aspirin, ticlopidine, and the glycoprotein IIb/IIIa receptor antagonists) are increasingly being used for management of cerebrovascular disease, as well as for rescue from thromboembolic complications. It is difficult to monitor the effect of these drugs because there is no accurate bedside test of platelet aggregation. Because of the long effective duration of action, rapid reversal of antiplatelet activity can be achieved only by platelet transfusion. Concomitant heparin use may synergistically predispose to hemorrhage.

DELIBERATE HYPOTENSION

The two primary indications for induced hypotension are to test cerebrovascular reserve in patients undergoing proximal vessel occlusion, and to slow flow in an artery feeding a brain arteriovenous malformation before injection of glue. The most important factor in choosing a hypotensive agent is the ability to safely and expeditiously achieve the desired reduction in blood pressure while maintaining the patient physiologically stable. The choice of agent should be determined by the experience of the practitioner, the patient's medical condition, and the goals of the blood pressure reduction in a particular clinical setting. Agents and maneuvers that have been used include increasing depth of anesthesia, sodium nitroprusside, nitroglycerin, labetalol, and esmolol. Intravenous adenosine has been used to induce transient cardiac pause and may be a viable method of partial flow arrest.

DELIBERATE HYPERTENSION

During acute arterial occlusion or vasospasm, the only practical way to increase collateral blood flow may be augmentation of collateral perfusion pressure by raising systemic blood pressure. The circle of Willis is a primary collateral pathway in the cerebral circulation. However, in as many as 21% of otherwise normal subjects, the circle may not be complete.

The extent to which blood pressure has to be raised depends on the condition of the patient and the nature of the disease. Typically, systemic blood pressure is raised by 30% to 40% above baseline or until ischemic symptoms resolve. Phenylephrine is commonly the first-line agent and is titrated to achieve the desired level of blood pressure. The risk of causing hemorrhage into the ischemic area must be weighed against the benefits of improving perfusion, but augmentation of blood pressure in the face of acute cerebral ischemia is probably protective in most settings.

MANAGEMENT OF NEUROLOGIC AND PROCEDURAL CRISES

A well–thought-out plan, coupled with rapid and effective communication between the anesthesia and radiology teams, is critical for good outcomes.

The primary responsibility of the anesthesia team is to preserve gas exchange and, if indicated, secure the airway. Simultaneous with airway management, the first branch in the decision-making algorithm is for the anesthesiologist to communicate with the INR team and determine whether the problem is hemorrhagic or occlusive. In the setting of vascular occlusion, the goal is to increase distal perfusion by blood pressure augmentation with or without direct thrombolysis. If the problem is hemorrhagic, immediate cessation of heparin plus reversal with protamine is indicated. As an emergency reversal dose, 1 mg of protamine can be given for each 100 units of initial heparin dosage that resulted in therapeutic anticoagulation. The ACT can then be used to fine-tune the final protamine dose. Complications of protamine administration include hypotension, anaphylaxis, and pulmonary hypertension. With the advent of new long-acting direct thrombin inhibitors such as bivalirudin, new strategies for emergency reversal of anticoagulation will need to be developed.

Bleeding catastrophes are usually heralded by headache, nausea, vomiting, and vascular pain related to the area of perforation. Sudden loss of consciousness is not always due to intracranial hemorrhage. Seizures as a result of reactions to contrast material or transient ischemia and the ensuing postictal state can also result in an obtunded patient. In an anesthetized patient, the sudden onset of bradycardia or the endovascular therapist's diagnosis of extravasation of contrast material may be the only clues to a developing hemorrhage.

POSTOPERATIVE MANAGEMENT

Endovascular surgery patients should pass the immediate postoperative period in a monitored setting to watch for signs of hemodynamic instability or neurologic deterioration. Blood pressure control, either induced hypotension or induced hypertension, may be continued during the postoperative period. Complicated cases may first undergo computed tomography or some other type of tomographic imaging; critical care management may need to be extended during transport and imaging.

PROCEDURES FOR SPECIFIC CEREBROVASCULAR DISEASES

Intracranial Aneurysm

The two basic approaches to INR treatment of cerebral aneurysms are occlusion of the proximal parent arteries and obliteration of the aneurysmal sac. With publication of the International Subarachnoid Aneurysm Trial, coil embolization of intracranial aneurysms has become a routine first-choice therapy for many lesions in many centers. The aneurysmal sac may be obliterated with the use of coils and balloons. The anesthesiologist should be prepared for aneurysmal rupture and acute subarachnoid hemorrhage (SAH) at all times, either from spontaneous rupture of a leaky sac or from direct injury of the aneurysm wall by vascular manipulation.

Angioplasty may be used to treat symptomatic vasospasm secondary to aneurysmal SAH with correlating angiographic stenosis refractory to maximal medical therapy. It is also possible to perform a "pharmacologic" angioplasty by direct intra-arterial infusion of a vasodilator drug such as papaverine, but this has potential CNS toxic effects; other agents such as calcium channel blockers (nicardipine and verapamil) are also being used. Transient hypotension may occur as a result of these agents and will need to be treated.

Carotid Stenosis

Angioplasty plus stenting for the treatment of atherosclerotic disease involving the cervical and intracranial arteries is an area of intense activity and growing interest. The risk for distal thromboembolism is the major issue to be resolved in this procedure. Multiple ongoing trials are being conducted to compare the utility of stenting with various devices and carotid endarterectomy. It is likely that the use of stenting will continue to increase as favorable data supporting its safety and efficacy emerge.

Intravenous atropine or glycopyrrolate may be used in an attempt to mitigate against bradycardia, which frequently occurs with inflation of the balloon. Preparation for anesthetic management may include placement of transcutaneous pacing leads in patients with severe bradycardia or asystole from carotid sinus stimulation. Adverse effects of increasing myocardial oxygen demand need to be considered in antibradycardia interventions.

Potential complications include vessel occlusion, perforation, dissection, spasm, thromboembolism, occlusion of adjacent vessels, transient ischemic episodes, and stroke. Similar to carotid endarterectomy, there is about a 5% risk of symptomatic cerebral hemorrhage or brain swelling after carotid angioplasty. Although the cause of this syndrome is unknown, it has been associated with cerebral hyperperfusion, and it may be related to poor postoperative blood pressure control or severe stenosis.

Ischemic Stroke

In acute occlusive stroke, it is possible to recanalize the occluded vessel by superselective intra-arterial thrombolytic therapy. Thrombolytic agents can be delivered in high concentration via a microcatheter navigated close to the clot or combined with mechanical measures to disrupt the clot. Neurologic deficits may be reversed without any additional risk of secondary hemorrhage if treatment is completed within 4 to 6 hours after the onset of carotid territory ischemia and 24 hours in the vertebrobasilar territory. Although complications are rare, migration of the thrombus or emboli, injury to intracerebral vessels, and spontaneous hemorrhagic transformation are always possible. It could take place rapidly and be life threatening. Adequate preparation to handle any intracranial catastrophe may make a difference between an uneventful outcome and death.

Brain Arteriovenous Malformations

Arteriovenous malformations in the brain are typically complex lesions made up of a tangle of abnormal vessels (called the nidus), and they frequently contain several discrete fistulas served by multiple feeding arteries and draining veins. The goal of therapeutic embolization is to obliterate as many of the fistulas and their respective feeding arteries as possible. Embolization of brain arteriovenous malformations is usually an adjunct to surgery or radiotherapy, although in rare cases treatment results in total obliteration.

The cyanoacrylate glues offer relatively "permanent" closure of abnormal vessels. Passage of glue into a draining vein can result in acute hemorrhage; in smaller

27

patients, pulmonary embolism of glue may also occur. For these reasons, deliberate hypotension may increase the safety of glue delivery.

SUMMARY

Anesthesia management can help facilitate imaging and procedures in INR. Appropriate hemodynamic control is crucial for the success of many procedures and good patient outcome. Prompt communication with neuroradiologists is essential in managing catastrophic crises.

KEY POINTS

- Baseline blood pressure and cardiovascular reserve should be assessed carefully, especially when blood pressure manipulation and perturbations are anticipated.
- Maintaining patient immobility during the procedure will facilitate imaging.
- Careful management of coagulation is required to prevent thromboembolic and manage hemorrhagic complications during and after the procedure.
- Complications during endovascular instrumentation of the cerebral vasculature can be rapid and life threatening and require multidisciplinary collaboration.
- Signs of hemodynamic instability or neurologic deterioration need to be monitored in the postoperative period.

FURTHER READING

Fiorella D, Albuquerque FC, Han P, et al: Strategies for the management of intraprocedural thromboembolic complications with abciximab (ReoPro). Neurosurgery 2004; 54:1089-1098.

Harrigan MR, Levy EI, Bendok BR, et al: Bivalirudin for endovascular intervention in acute ischemic stroke: Case report. Neurosurgery 2004; 54:218-222. discussion 222-213.

Hashimoto T, Young WL, Aagaard BD, et al: Adenosine-induced ventricular asystole to induce transient profound systemic hypotension in patients undergoing endovascular therapy. Dose-response characteristics. Anesthesiology 2000; 93:998-1001.

Higashida RT, Meyers PM, Connors JJ 3rd, et al: Intracranial angioplasty & stenting for cerebral atherosclerosis: A position statement of the American Society of Interventional and Therapeutic Neuroradiology, Society of Interventional Radiology, and the American Society of Neuroradiology. AJNR Am J Neuroradiol 2005; 26:2323-2327.

Lee CZ, Litt L, Hashimoto T, et al: Physiological monitoring and anesthesia considerations of the acute ischemic stroke patient. J Vasc Interv Radiol 2004; 15(Suppl):S13-S19.

Molyneux A, Kerr R, Stratton I, et al: International Subarachnoid Aneurysm Trial (ISAT) of neurosurgical clipping versus endovascular coiling in 2143 patients with ruptured intracranial aneurysms: A randomised trial. Lancet 2002; 360:1267-1274.

Pelz D, Andersson T, Soderman M, et al: Advances in interventional neuroradiology 2005. Stroke 2006; 37:309-311.

Phatouros CC, Higashida RT, Malek AM, et al: Carotid artery stent placement for atherosclerotic disease: Rationale, technique, and current status. Radiology 2000; 217:26-41.

See JJ, Manninen PH: Anesthesia for neuroradiology. Curr Opin Anaesthesiol 2005; 18:437-441.

IV

Chapter 28

Anesthesia and Sedation for Neuroimaging Outside the Operating Room

Jonathan P. Coles

Imaging Techniques	Safety Concerns within the Imaging Environment
Computed Tomography	
Gamma Camera Imaging, Single-Photon Emission Computed Tomography, and Positron Emission Tomography	Anesthesia and Sedation
	Magnetic Resonance Imaging and Spectroscopy
Interventional Neuroradiology	
Magnetic Resonance Imaging and Spectroscopy	

Neuroradiology is an expanding field that has seen the development of several diagnostic and interventional procedures for patients with a variety of neurologic disorders. These procedures are likely to involve increasing input from the neuroanesthetist and neurocritical care physician, with many patients requiring careful management during procedures carried out in sites remote from the normal operating theater or neurocritical care facility.

IMAGING TECHNIQUES

Computed Tomography

Computed tomography (CT) provides wide access to tomographic structural imaging. In addition, rapid sequential imaging after the administration of intravenous contrast material (CT perfusion) allows computation of cerebral blood flow (CBF) and cerebral blood volume (CBV) (Fig. 28-1), whereas imaging after the inhalation of 28% xenon (xenon CT) can be used to measure CBF. Image-guided stereotactic surgery uses imaging data to improve surgical planning and excision of intracranial lesions. A mechanical frame is attached to the patient's head, a CT scan is performed, and a computer calculates three-dimensional coordinates within the brain. In frameless stereotaxy the initial CT or magnetic resonance (MR) image is stored on computer and fixed points on the skull are mapped onto the image with a sensor wand.

Gamma Camera Imaging, Single-Photon Emission Computed Tomography, and Positron Emission Tomography

Single-photon emission CT uses conventional γ-emitting nuclear medicine isotopes with multiple detectors to generate tomographic images of CBF that are nonquantitative. Positron emission tomography is a research technique in which isotopes such as ^{15}O and ^{18}F

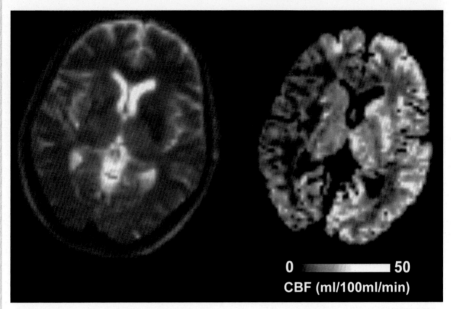

0 ▬▬▬▬▬▬ 50
CBF (ml/100ml/min)

Figure 28-1 Computed tomographic perfusion. T2-weighted magnetic resonance and cerebral blood flow images were obtained from a patient with an evolving right middle cerebral artery stroke. (Courtesy of Dr. Joe Guadagno, Addenbrooke's Hospital, Cambridge, UK.)

emit positrons. Annihilation of these positrons can be localized in space by pairs of gamma detectors and provides whole-brain quantitative imaging of many aspects of cerebral physiology, including CBF, CBV, and oxidative and glucose metabolism.

Interventional Neuroradiology

Flow-directed microcatheters are introduced into blood vessels via the femoral artery under local or general anesthesia and manipulated through the carotid or vertebral vessels. Digital technology results in images that are optimized by subtraction of bone and other nonvascular structures. After injection of a contrast agent, the resulting image of vascular anatomy can be saved as a "road map" image. The current image can be superimposed over this road map and used to aid manipulation and advancement of the microcatheter within the relevant cerebral vessel. This technique obviously requires the patient to remain immobile, although repeated injections can be used to update the road map image. A variety of devices and drugs, including microcoils, stents, balloons, glue, thrombolytics, and sclerosing and chemotherapeutic agents, can be introduced for diagnostic angiography, coiling or ablation of cerebral aneurysms and arteriovenous malformations, percutaneous transluminal angioplasty, or intravascular thrombolysis. Patients must remain immobile to ensure success and prevent complications such as rupture or intimal tearing of small vessels.

Interventional neuroradiology is described in more detail in Chapter 27.

Magnetic Resonance Imaging and Spectroscopy

Images are produced by using powerful static magnetic fields and intermittently oscillating radiofrequency electromagnetic fields that elicit signals from the nuclei of certain atoms. Magnetic field strengths are measured in units termed tesla (T). One

IV

tesla equals 10,000 gauss (G). The magnetic field strength at the surface of the earth is 0.5 to 1.5 G. Field strengths used in clinical magnetic resonance imaging (MRI) range from 0.05 to 3.0 T and tend to be based on cryogenic superconducting magnets, which are maintained at −273° C by immersion in liquid helium.

MRI combines high-resolution structural imaging with a variety of functional imaging tools. After the administration of an MRI contrast agent, images of vascular patency can be obtained (MR angiography), and rapid imaging can be used to generate images of cerebral perfusion. Evidence of cerebral ischemia and impending tissue necrosis can be determined with information obtained from both perfusion and diffusion-weighted imaging. MR spectroscopy provides in vivo biochemical analysis of a variety of important markers of cellular function, including lactate, N-methyl-d-aspartate, and glutamate.

Recent interest has focused on interventional MRI, which involves imaging of the patient in the course of surgical procedures on the brain. It allows surgeons to avoid critical structures and ensure that surgical resection of tumors is complete. In practice, surgery may continue during imaging and all surgical equipment has to be MRI compatible (*interventional* MRI), or surgery is periodically halted to allow imaging with a movable magnet after all MRI-incompatible surgical equipment has been removed (*intraventional* MRI). This distinction is of no consequence for anesthesia because anesthetic drug delivery and patient monitoring need to continue uninterrupted with both approaches.

SAFETY CONCERNS WITHIN THE IMAGING ENVIRONMENT

All the aforementioned techniques, excluding MRI, involve exposure to ionizing radiation. To limit exposure to staff members, the maximum distance possible should be maintained from the x-ray source. Lead glass shields, lead aprons, and thyroid shields should be used (together with radiation exposure badges in selected settings) to assess the cumulative radiation burden.

Although exposure to magnetic fields is generally thought to be safe, unnecessary exposure to high field strengths should be minimized. Exposure can be reduced by the use of custom-designed MRI monitoring equipment with slave patient monitor screens positioned outside the MR scanning room so that patient studies can be supervised from outside the 5-G line and away from the most intense noise produced by gradient fields.

Adverse incidents involving patients, equipment, and personnel continue to occur within MRI scanners, thus underlining the importance of users understanding the MRI environment and ensuring that safe practice is observed. The magnetic field within the scanning environment is based on a cryogenic superconducting magnet that is maintained at −273° C by emersion in liquid helium. The helium can boil off ("*quench*") rapidly if the temperature is allowed to rise. This has the potential to dilute room oxygen, and the cold vapor can cause frostbite and burns. Any loose ferromagnetic object can become a dangerous projectile and should not be taken into the MRI suite unless known to be safe. Even implanted ferromagnetic devices may move, and depending on their size and location, this may prove disastrous (e.g., intraocular foreign bodies and cerebral aneurysm clips). Patients with an intracranial aneurysm clip should not undergo MRI unless the clip has been documented to be nonferromagnetic or the patient has already been imaged at the same field strength with no problems. Even nonferromagnetic implants can result in significant image distortion or cause local burns as their temperature is increased in the presence of radiofrequency currents. Fatalities have been reported in patients

28

with cardiac pacemakers. The magnetic field causes the reed switch on pacemakers to stick and revert to a fixed-rate mode in which delivery of a pacing spike on the upstroke of a T wave can result in an R on T phenomenon and trigger ventricular fibrillation. Therefore, MRI is contraindicated in the presence of pacemakers and other implanted electronic devices unless it is known with absolute certainty that it will function safely. In the event of doubt, implants should be tested with a powerful hand-held magnet and checked against manufacturer's specifications. MRI units generally have a comprehensive checklist for patients and staff to complete to exclude the presence of implants. Monitoring devices are also potential hazards and should be thoroughly checked before moving into the magnetic field. Leads from such devices present a particular risk because induced currents may result in burns. Devices are described as *MRI safe* when they do not represent a risk to the patient and *MRI compatible* when they also continue to function in the MRI environment without degrading image quality.

Finally, the use of iodinated contrast agents in CT and angiographic procedures and MRI contrast agents such as gadopentetate dimeglumine (Gd-DTPA, Magnevist) is not without risk. In general, the incidence of serious side effects is low, but both agents may result in renal impairment or other adverse reactions.

Anesthesia and Sedation

Most diagnostic neuroradiologic procedures can be performed with sedation and local anesthesia as required. General anesthesia is sometimes required for children, extreme cases of anxiety and claustrophobia, failed sedation, patients with reduced consciousness, and those with movement disorders or learning difficulties. The choice of sedation or anesthesia for patients undergoing imaging depends on the stability of the patient concerned and the requirements of the neuroradiologist. High-dose sedation may be inappropriate in patients with concurrent medical disease and evidence of raised intracranial pressure. General anesthesia and airway protection are needed for prolonged and uncomfortable procedures and for critically ill patients requiring intermittent positive pressure ventilation. The anesthetic technique should aim to maintain stable cerebral physiology by optimizing cerebral perfusion and controlling intracranial pressure. Both volatile and intravenous anesthesia can be used, and the specific choice depends on the clinical circumstances.

IV

Patients should be carefully positioned on the narrow scanning table and thought given to the risk of equipment disconnection during table movement within the scanner. Patients must be adequately monitored during transport to the imaging facility and during the investigation or procedure. Despite the isolated and unfamiliar environment, minimal monitoring standards should apply:

- Circulatory function, including electrocardiogram, blood pressure, and auscultation of heart sounds or pulse oximetry
- Oxygenation, including an oxygen analyzer and pulse oximetry
- Ventilation if general anesthesia is induced, ideally by capnography
- Monitoring of patient temperature in the air-conditioned environment of the scanner room, where heat loss is rapid, even with short procedures

Magnetic Resonance Imaging and Spectroscopy

Although there are difficulties in the use of monitoring and other anesthetic equipment within the MRI suite, integrated monitoring and anesthetic systems based on technology developed for the MRI environment are widely available and represent

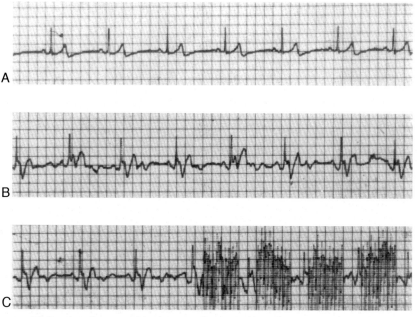

Figure 28-2 Interference with electrocardiographic (ECG) tracing during magnetic resonance imaging (MRI). The radiofrequency and gradient fields used in MRI induce currents within ECG leads. **A,** ECG tracing with the subject outside the magnet bore. **B,** ECG tracing with the subject in the magnet (note the ST-T changes). **C,** ECG tracing during operation of the imaging sequence. (Reproduced with permission from Coles JP, Menon DK: Anesthesia for neuroimaging and neurointerventional radiology. Anaesth Intensive Care Med 2004: 5:340-342.)

the standard of care. Nonetheless, even MRI-compatible devices should be given special attention to ensure their safe application. Intracranial pressure can be measured accurately via a ventriculostomy. Although several intraparenchymal sensors are MRI safe, they are not MRI compatible and result in image artifacts. Another difficulty concerns the distortion of electrocardiographic monitoring within the MRI environment. Changes occur in early T waves and late ST segments and mimic hyperkalemia or pericarditis, and radiofrequency currents produce electrocardiographic artifacts (Fig. 28-2).

28

KEY POINTS

- Neuroradiology is an expanding field that is likely to require increasing input from neuroanesthetists and critical care physicians.
- By using a variety of imaging techniques, both structural and functional data can be obtained and interventional procedures performed.
- All individuals involved in the management of patients undergoing neuroimaging and neurointerventional radiology must understand the principles of the techniques involved.
- Anesthesia and patient monitoring within the MRI environment are possible with dedicated MRI-compatible equipment in accordance with local guidelines.

FURTHER READING

Burnstein RM, Menon DK: Anaesthesia for Magnetic Resonance Imaging. In Matta BF, Menon DK, Turner JT (eds): Textbook of Neuroanaesthesia and Critical Care. London, Greenwich Medical Media, 2000, pp 411-425.

Coles JP: Imaging of cerebral blood flow and metabolism. Curr Opin Anaesthesiol 2006; 19:473-480.

Coles JP, Menon DK: Anaesthesia for neuroimaging and neurointerventional radiology. Anaesth Intensive Care Med 2004; 5:340-342.

Kanal E, Borgstede JP, Barkovich AJ, et al: American College of Radiology White Paper on MR Safety. AJR Am J Roentgenol 2002; 178:1335-1347.

Kanal E, Borgstede JP, Barkovich AJ, et al: American College of Radiology White Paper on MR Safety: 2004 update and revisions. AJR Am J Roentgenol 2004; 182:1111-1114.

Peden CJ, Menon DK, Hall AS, et al: Magnetic resonance for the anaesthetist. Part 2: Anaesthesia and monitoring in MR units. Anaesthesia 1992; 47:508-517.

The Association of Anaesthetists of Great Britain and Ireland. Provision of anaesthetic services in magnetic resonance units. Available at http://www.aagbi.org/pdf/mri.pdf.

Turner JM: Anaesthesia for neuroradiology. In Matta BF, Menon DK, Turner JT (eds): Textbook of Neuroanaesthesia and Critical Care. London, Greenwich Medical Media, 2000, pp 399-409.

IV

Chapter 29

Anesthesia for Neurosurgery in Infants and Children

Claire Brett

Preoperative Evaluation	Specific Procedures
Neurologic Assessment	Neurosurgical Procedures in the Newborn:
Associated Anomalies/Physiologic Status	Meningomyelocele Repair and
General Concepts	Ventriculoperitoneal Shunt Placement
Monitoring/Intravenous Access	Neurosurgical Procedures in Older Infants:
	Craniofacial Reconstruction
Intravenous Fluids	

Safe and effective neuroanesthesia for infants and children requires meticulous dissection of physiologic and clinical factors from two separate but interrelated viewpoints. First, the impact of age-related factors must be incorporated into the operative scheme, and second, neurosurgical procedures often have their own specific requirements (e.g., positioning, evoked potentials).

PREOPERATIVE EVALUATION

Neurologic Assessment

Symptoms and physical signs of increased intracranial pressure (ICP) should be evaluated in relation to the imaging studies. The risk for pulmonary aspiration secondary to vomiting is difficult to estimate, but the possibility should be borne in mind. Most patients treated with corticosteroids also receive an H_2 blocker. Electrolyte abnormalities may result from central nervous system dysfunction (e.g., diabetes insipidus or the syndrome of inappropriate antidiuretic hormone secretion) or from various therapies (e.g., diuretics, mannitol, corticosteroids), and management depends on rate of development, as well as the degree of the abnormality.

An embolic event is a particular risk during craniofacial procedures and craniotomies. In all newborns and patients with congenital heart disease, air (or other foreign material) may enter the systemic circulation from the right atrium or ventricle. In the newborn, the foramen ovale must be considered to be patent and is therefore a portal of entry of an embolus into the arterial circulation, even with an otherwise anatomically normal heart. More commonly, an embolus from a peripheral vein enters the right ventricle or the pulmonary circulation (or both), and major hemodynamic instability results from right-sided outflow obstruction.

Associated Anomalies/Physiologic Status

Immaturity of the cardiorespiratory, renal, and hepatic systems may significantly affect the response to and dose requirement for a variety of anesthetic agents, antibiotics, and antiseizure medications, as well as intravenous fluid delivery. The "normal for age" physiology and many laboratory values (hematocrit, clotting studies, electrolytes, creatinine clearance) vary significantly as a function of age, and trends should be reviewed in the patient's "flow sheets" before surgery to help define "normal" for a specific patient. Coexisting anomalies, current medications, and poor nutritional status exaggerate the complexity of normal immaturity.

General Concepts

The prolonged nature of many neurosurgical procedures may dramatically affect body temperature, increase risks for injury secondary to pressure/positioning, and usually requires an appropriate system to provide mechanical ventilatory support. These risks/requirements may be exaggerated in newborns and young infants. Meticulously securing the endotracheal tube is particularly critical, especially in the prone position, where secretions are most likely to disrupt the adhesive property of tape. Ensuring ideal positioning (i.e., midtrachea) is essential because repositioning of the endotracheal tube during surgery is challenging and risky. Appropriate sizes are indicated on Table 29.1 Inspiratory gases should be heated and humidified. Intravenous fluids and packed red blood cells (RBCs) should be warmed, heating blankets should be available for the bed, and the environmental temperature should be adjusted to minimize any decrease in body temperature.

MONITORING/INTRAVENOUS ACCESS

Noncomplex neurosurgery requires only routine monitoring, but typically during craniotomies and complex craniofacial reconstructions, blood pressure is monitored with an arterial catheter, which allows easy sampling of blood if necessary. A Foley catheter to monitor urine output helps guide intravenous fluid administration. Adequate intravenous access is imperative. However, the risks of inserting and maintaining a central line often outweigh any potential clinical value.

Intravenous Fluids

Adequate hydration/intravascular volume is essential, but conservative fluid delivery may minimize exacerbation of preexisting cerebral edema. Low creatinine clearance/tubular insufficiency combined with unique cardiorespiratory physiology in this age group further contributes to the complexity. In hemodynamically stable patients, the maintenance rate of crystalloid plus replacement of ongoing losses (blood, urine) with blood products introduced after about 10% of blood volume has been lost should avoid the administration of large volumes of crystalloid. Delivery of glucose is calculated separately from that of crystalloid to avoid both hypoglycemia and hyperglycemia. Beyond the neonatal period and in the absence of any metabolic requirements (e.g., diabetes, inherited metabolic disorders), glucose is avoided during neurosurgical procedures to prevent possible exacerbation of ischemic damage (Table 29-2).

Table 29-1 Intubation: Laryngoscopes/Endotracheal Tubes

Age	Endotracheal Tube (mm, Uncuffed/Cuffed)	Laryngoscope
Preterm	2.5	Miller 0
Newborn-1 month	2.5-3.0	Miller 1
1-6 months	3.0-3.5	Miller 1
6-12 months	3.5-4.0	Miller 1
1-3 years	4.0-4.5	Miller 1-2
3-5 years	4.5-5.0	Miller 2
	4.0-4.5	Macintosh 2
5-8 years	5.0-5.5	Miller 2
	4.5-5.0	Macintosh 2
8-10 years	5.5-6.0	Miller 2
	4.0-5.5	Macintosh 3
10-14 years	Variable	Variable

Summary

3.0 ETT for a newborn, 4.0 for a 1-year-old, 5.0 for a 5-year-old
Miller 1 for infants up to 1 year; Miller 2 for infants >1 to 2 years
Cuffed ETTs—decrease size by 0.5 mm

Table 29-2 Fluid Therapy

Calculating Intravenous Crystalloid: Four Components

Rehydration (based on history, physical examination, laboratory tests)
Maintenance
  A. 1-10 kg: 4 mL/kg/hr
  B. 10-20 kg: A (40 mL/hr) + 2 mL/kg/hr
  C. >20 kg: A + B (60 mL/hr) + 1 mL/kg/hr
Ongoing losses
"Special" (unusual requirements for glucose, K^+, Ca^{2+}, Na^+, colloid, blood products)

Calculating "Maintenance" Glucose: Newborn/Young Infant

5% dextrose at rates greater than maintenance may lead to hyperglycemia
  in a normal infant
  4 mg/kg/m: 240 mg/kg/hr
  5% dextrose: 50 mg/mL
Maintenance rate: 4 mL/kg/hr × 50 mg/mL = 200 mg/kg/hr

Calculating Allowable Blood Loss Preoperatively

$ABL = EBV \times [H_o - H_L]/[H_a]$

ABL, allowable blood loss; EBV, estimated blood volume (preterm, 90 mL/kg; term, 80 ml/kg); H_o, hemoglobin, observed; H_L, hemoglobin, lowest; H_a, hemoglobin, average.

SPECIFIC PROCEDURES

Two neurosurgical procedures provide the framework to apply these general principles to the operating room:

- Repair of a neural tube defect in a newborn
- Craniofacial reconstruction

Neurosurgical Procedures in the Newborn: Meningomyelocele Repair and Ventriculoperitoneal Shunt Placement

A defect in closure of the neural tube resulting in meningomyelocele/myelocele requires prompt surgical treatment in the first days after birth. The major risks associated with anesthetic care are those related to neonatal physiology. Electrolyte/acid-base balance, glucose, calcium, and hydration must be evaluated and, if necessary, monitored during surgery. Cardiorespiratory function may be "in transition" for several days after birth, so oxygenation and ventilation must be adapted to what is needed in the operating room.

The surgical procedure is related to the size of the lesion and its required treatment. A simple closure is often completed in less than 1 to 1.5 hours, but larger defects that require complex procedures (e.g., a flap) take longer. Preoperatively, the patient is usually maintained in a prone or lateral position to avoid pressure on the lesion. For positioning in the supine position during induction of anesthesia, a "donut"-shaped pillow can be used to avoid pressure on the fragile open neural tube. Similarly, intraoperative and postoperative management must allow safe prone/lateral positioning.

Most patients with a meningomyelocele (>70%) will require placement of a ventriculoperitoneal shunt, often in the first week of life. Because of nonfused sutures, increased ICP is rare in young infants who have hydrocephalus. Instead, the sutures are separated, the fontanelles may bulge, and macrocephaly eventually develops. Cardiovascular and respiratory status guides the need for a second anesthetic. No invasive monitoring is required during placement of a ventriculoperitoneal shunt unless associated medical/neurologic problems exist. Blood loss should be minimal; postoperative ventilatory support reflects preoperative status and unexpected intraoperative events.

Neurosurgical Procedures in Older Infants: Craniofacial Reconstruction

Craniosynostosis prevents growth of the skull perpendicular to the affected suture and results in compensatory growth in other areas. For example, premature closure of the sagittal suture arrests growth in the lateral direction, growth anteroposteriorly is accelerated, and scaphocephaly ("boat skull") develops. Craniosynostosis can be an isolated lesion (e.g., sagittal, coronal, metopic, or multiple craniosynostosis) or part of a malformation syndrome (chromosomal deletion or duplications, monogenic syndromes [e.g., Apert's, Crouzon's, or Pfeiffer's], or drug-associated syndromes [e.g., phenytoin, retinoic acid]). Syndromic craniosynostosis implies the possibility of multiple anomalies of major significance for both the surgeon and anesthesiologist.

Intracranial hypertension (raised ICP) is uncommon (less than 10%) in isolated craniosynostosis (higher with coronal than sagittal) but increases over time. In complex cranial deformities (e.g., Apert's, Crouzon's syndrome), as many as 50% of patients have elevated ICP, but these patients are not symptomatic.

Anesthesia for Single-Suture Synostosis

A strip craniectomy is the procedure most commonly performed to treat single fused sutures (e.g., sagittal, coronal). The procedures are performed during the first year of life, usually before 6 months of age. The following is a general scheme of an anesthetic plan for a 3- to 6-month-old infant for this procedure.

PREOPERATIVE EVALUATION

1. Clarify the surgical plan, including positioning (e.g., supine or prone).
2. Address anxieties of the family. Discuss anesthetic risk/plans and postoperative supportive care (pediatric intensive care unit [PICU], ventilatory support). Reassure the family that staff will provide updates during surgery. Discuss blood transfusion.
3. Premedication is unnecessary; parental presence for induction provides no advantage to the patient at this age (<6 months).

INTRAOPERATIVE COURSE

1. Noninvasive monitoring is sufficient in most cases.
2. Specific anesthetic agents/techniques are required rarely and can include inhaled agents, narcotics, propofol, and in some cases, muscle relaxants. Because ICP may be elevated, mild hyperventilation ($P_{CO_2} \cong 30$ mm Hg) should be initiated during induction and maintained throughout the procedure. Additional agents (mannitol, diuretics, barbiturates) may be introduced if further lowering of ICP is required. Some anesthesiologists choose to emphasize an inhaled agent (<0.75 minimum alveolar concentration [MAC]) and minimize the narcotic; others will choose a narcotic-based technique and add low doses of inhaled agent (<0.5 MAC).
3. Blood loss commonly ranges between 10% and 20% of blood volume. Dissection of the scalp/bone is the primary source of blood loss, aside from accidental trauma to the sagittal sinus or other large blood vessels. Transfusion depends on the baseline hematocrit, ongoing rate of blood loss, and cardiovascular status. The youngest infants do not tolerate blood loss, and most anesthesiologists follow a "mL of colloid for mL of blood loss" scheme. Infants older than 6 to 8 months may tolerate approximately a 10% blood loss before colloid is indicated.
4. The rate of crystalloid delivery depends on the volume of RBCs and other colloid delivered, cardiovascular status, and anticipated events.
   - Evaporative or "third-spacing" loss from the exposed surgical field or secondary to tissue trauma is minimal.
   - Maintenance crystalloid infusion rate is continued.
   - Blood loss not replaced with colloid is replenished with crystalloid at a volume two to three times the volume of blood loss.
   - The risks associated with blood transfusion must be weighed against the risks related to large volumes of intravenous fluid.
5. After a simple strip craniectomy, patients are usually monitored in the PICU postoperatively but generally do not require mechanical ventilatory support.

Anesthesia for Complex Synostosis

The two significant differences between simple and complex synostosis are

- Coexistent anomalies
- The complexity of the lesion and its surgical treatment

Surgery for syndromic craniosynostosis usually occurs into two phases:

- Frontocranial remodeling, performed at 3 to 4 months of age to avoid impairment of the rapid brain growth in the first year of life
- Advancing the midface, which is a separate procedure delayed until 3 to 4 years of age

The general technique for frontocranial remodeling involves a bicoronal incision and then reflection of the scalp forward off the skull onto the face. The affected bony areas are mobilized, removed and often split into several components, augmented, and remodeled. The remodeled bone is repositioned and fixed in place. Approaches are individualized.

The surgical approach to advancement of the midface involves various combinations of osteotomies:

- Le Fort I (maxillary underdevelopment)
- Le Fort II (lower maxilla and nose moved forward)
- Le Fort III (complete midface advancement—nose, maxilla, orbits)

Blood loss, injury to the endotracheal tube, and venous air embolism are well-described complications.

PREOPERATIVE EVALUATION

The profound alteration in body image associated with the surgery, the intense postoperative recovery, and the significant morbidity (and even mortality) should be discussed in the preoperative clinic. Preoperative assessment should evaluate the patient's cardiorespiratory, renal, hepatic, and neurologic status with particular emphasis on the following:

- Evidence of upper airway obstruction (e.g., snoring) and its complications (pulmonary hypertension).
- Past difficulty with airway management (poor neck mobility, previous experience with mask ventilation and intubation).
- Heart disease (surgical and medical treatment, complications), neurologic status (developmental delay, unexpected reaction to sedatives, seizure disorders, and treatment).
- Hematologic status (hematocrit, bleeding abnormalities, transfusion reactions, donor-designated blood).
- The possibility of tracheostomy, postoperative ventilation, extensive dressing, and fixation of the jaw should be discussed.
- The challenge of upper airway management may override the advantages of premedication or parental presence during induction. The risks associated with hypercapnia in patients with increased ICP must be considered.
- Laboratory orders are based on coexistent medical problems and the surgical plan. At a minimum, a complete blood count, platelet count, coagulation panel, and samples for the blood bank must be considered. Baseline arterial blood gas analysis may be required.

INTRAOPERATIVE COURSE

1. In addition to the routine noninvasive monitors and urinary catheter, monitoring/access should include
   - Intra-arterial blood pressure
   - Approximately two to three intravenous catheters
   - Possibly a central venous catheter
2. Aggressive administration of colloid/crystalloid fluid is required because the surgical dissection is extensive and can cause facial, neck, and scalp edema, which may require 12 to 48 hours of postoperative mechanical ventilation. Intermaxillary fixation adds to the indications for postoperative intubation. Instruments to release the fixation must be available at the patient's bedside

IV

before the patient leaves the operating room. Selection of anesthetic agents should take into consideration hemodynamic stability and the planned post-operative ventilation.

3. Blood loss can be enormous (two or more blood volumes), but with highly experienced surgeons, it usually ranges between 40% and 60% of blood volume. Some surgeons and anesthesiologists recommend "controlled hypotension" to decrease blood loss, but this technique is controversial, especially in young infants, in whom the range of cerebral autoregulation is less well defined than in adults. As the blood loss approaches the patient's blood volume, acid-base status, electrolytes, calcium, hemoglobin, and coagulation function must be monitored to respond appropriately to bleeding or hemodynamic instability.

4. The anesthetic regimen should incorporate strategies (i.e., hyperventilation, <1.0 MAC inhaled agent, mannitol, steroids) to minimize exacerbating increased ICP/decreased intracranial compliance.

5. Meticulous attention to maintaining body temperature is essential.

6. Parents should be available for intraoperative updates and consultation.

KEY POINTS

- Age-related factors, including blood pressure, heart rate, hematocrit, and fluid requirements, must be incorporated into the preoperative evaluation, intraoperative management, and postoperative care of infants and children.
- Newborns present specific challenges for anesthetic care because of their unique physiology associated with cardiorespiratory, renal, and hepatic immaturity.
- The psychological impact of surgery and anesthesia at various ages and the role of parental presence and premedication must be assessed.
- The effects of neurologic injury/abnormalities, including vomiting, electrolyte derangements, increased ICP, and side effects of therapeutic agents (e.g., mannitol, diuretics, corticosteroids), must be meticulously evaluated in the perioperative setting.
- Craniofacial procedures may demand extensive monitoring and supportive care as a result of significant blood loss, edema from surgical manipulation and intravenous fluids, and coexisting congenital anomalies. Postoperative intensive care should be considered.
- Heat loss may be significant during lengthy procedures in infants. Systems to prevent significant hypothermia must be incorporated into the intraoperative plan.

29

FURTHER READING

Bissonnett B, Sadeghi P: Anesthesia for neurosurgical procedures. In Gregory G (ed): Pediatric Anesthesia. Philadelphia, Churchill Livingstone, 2002, pp 381-422.

Krane EJ, Philip BM, Yeh KK, Domino KB: Anesthesia for pediatric neurosurgery. In Motoyama ED, Davis PJ (eds): Smith's Anesthesia for Infants and Children. Philadelphia, Mosby Elsevier, 2006, pp 651-684.

Volpe J: Brain tumors and vein of Galen malformations. In Neurology of the Newborn. Philadelphia, WB Saunders, 2001, pp 841-856.

Chapter 30

Anesthetic Considerations for Pediatric Neurotrauma

Monica S. Vavilala • Randall Chesnut

Epidemiology	Airway Management
	Anesthetic Technique
Patterns of Injury	Intravenous Access
Physiology and Pathophysiology	Intravenous Fluids
	Monitoring
Cerebral Metabolic Rate, Cerebral Blood	
Flow, and Cerebral Autoregulation	**Indications for Surgery**
Intracranial Pressure	
Inflicted Traumatic Brain Injury	**Summary**
Cervical Spine and Spinal Cord Injury	
Clinical Management	
Initial Assessment	
Cervical Spine Immobilization	

Pediatric neurotrauma (traumatic brain injury [TBI] and spinal cord injury [SCI]) is the leading cause of death in children older than 1 year. Significant disability is frequent after pediatric neurotrauma and often has a profound impact on functional long-term outcome.

EPIDEMIOLOGY

TBI should be considered in all children after trauma, particularly those with a suspicious mechanism of injury, loss of consciousness, multiple episodes of emesis, tracheal intubation, and extracranial injuries. Most children with multiple trauma have TBI, and most trauma deaths are associated with TBI. Motor vehicle–related crash (blunt trauma) is the most common mechanism of TBI, but in children younger than 4 years, 30% to 50% of TBI is caused either by falls or by inflicted TBI (iTBI). Ten percent to 15% of TBI is severe with an associated mortality rate of 50%. After TBI, mortality is lower in children than in adults (10.4% versus 2.5%), but certain factors predict worse outcomes (Table 30-1).

PATTERNS OF INJURY

Children are more susceptible to TBI because they have a larger head-to-body size ratio; thinner cranial bones that provide less protection to the intracranial contents; less myelinated neural tissue, which makes them more vulnerable to damage;

IV

Table 30-1	**Predictors of Poor Outcome after Pediatric Traumatic Brain Injury**

Age <4 years
Cardiopulmonary resuscitation
Multiple trauma
Hypoxia (Pao_2 <60 mm Hg)
Hyperventilation ($Paco_2$ <35 mm Hg)
Hyperglycemia (glucose >250 mg/dL)
Hyperthermia (temperature >38° C)
Hypotension (systolic blood pressure <5th percentile for age)
Intracranial hypertension (intracranial pressure >20 mm Hg)
Poor rehabilitation

and a greater incidence of diffuse injury and cerebral edema than occurs in adults. Children have a higher incidence of increased intracranial pressure (ICP) after TBI than adults do (80% versus 50%). Diffuse TBI is the most common type of injury and results in a range of injury severity from concussion to diffuse axonal injury and permanent disability. Diagnosis of TBI is primarily made by computed tomography (CT) of the brain and is associated with increased ICP. Patients with diffuse axonal injury may initially have a normal CT scan despite significant neurologic findings and increased ICP; repeat CT often shows secondary injury caused by cerebral edema. Similar to adults, acute treatment of pediatric TBI is directed at preventing secondary injury from systemic hypotension, hypoxia, hypocapnia, and hyperglycemia.

PHYSIOLOGY AND PATHOPHYSIOLOGY

Cerebral Metabolic Rate, Cerebral Blood Flow, and Cerebral Autoregulation

The global cerebral metabolic rate (CMR) for oxygen and glucose is higher in children than in adults (oxygen, 5.8 versus 3.5 mL/100 g brain tissue/min; glucose, 6.8 versus 5.5 mL/100 g brain tissue/min, respectively). Unlike adults, cerebral blood flow (CBF) changes with age and may be higher in girls than in boys. After TBI, CBF and $CMRO_2$ may not be matched, thereby resulting in either cerebral ischemia or hyperemia, but recent work has demonstrated that the incidence of cerebral hyperemia is only 6% to 10% and that $CMRO_2$ may be normal, low, or high after TBI.

Data suggest that healthy infants may autoregulate CBF as well as older children do during low-dose sevoflurane anesthesia. However, the long-held assumption that the lower limit of autoregulation (LLA) is lower in young than in older children may not be valid (same LLA range for younger and older children: 46 to 76 mm Hg). Because blood pressure increases with age, young children may be at increased risk for cerebral ischemia because of lower blood pressure reserve (mean arterial pressure − LLA). Similar to adults, the incidence of impaired cerebral autoregulation is higher after severe than after mild TBI (42% versus 17%), and children with impaired cerebral autoregulation early after TBI may have poor long-term outcomes. One potential explanation for this association may be hypotension, which is common after pediatric TBI and may lead to cerebral ischemia.

30

Intracranial Pressure

In adults, normal ICP is between 5 and 15 mm Hg as opposed to 2 to 4 mm Hg in young children. Unlike adults with relatively poor cranial compliance, infants with open fontanelles may be able to accommodate slow and small increases in intracranial volume by expansion of the skull. However, rapid expansion of intracranial volume, small as it may be, can explain the not uncommonly encountered rapid deterioration in infants after TBI. Management of increased ICP in children is similar to that in adults (Fig. 30-1). The indications for ICP monitoring and the treatment threshold for increased ICP are presented in Table 30-2.

Inflicted Traumatic Brain Injury

Most deaths after inflicted injury involve TBI. Children with iTBI commonly exhibit altered consciousness, coma, seizures, vomiting, or irritability. Histories are often lacking, and injuries out of proportion to the history or developmental milestone should alert clinicians to consider this diagnosis. Types of injuries include subdural hematoma, subarachnoid hemorrhage, skull fractures, and diffuse axonal injury with or without cerebral edema. Outcome is poor after iTBI.

Cervical Spine and Spinal Cord Injury

Children with an unknown mechanism of injury, multisystem trauma, TBI, or injury above the clavicle should be suspected of having cervical spine injury. The incidence of SCI is low (1%) because of greater flexibility of tissues than in adults. A motor vehicle crash is the most common cause, although sports injuries are a second common mechanism in adolescents. Half of all children with SCI die at the scene of the injury. Approximately half of children with cervical spine injury have concomitant TBI, and the presence of TBI increases the risk for spine injury. The role of high-dose steroids in pediatric SCI is unclear, but their use is not a standard of practice.

Sixty percent to 70% of cervical spine injuries occur in children older than 12 years. Young patients have injuries to the upper cervical spine, and this is related to the fulcrum of cervical motion (C1 to C3). In children older than 12 years, the fulcrum moves down to C5-C6. Complete plain radiographic assessment of the cervical spine includes an anteroposterior image, lateral views of the cervicothoracic junction, and odontoid views. Because of the increased proportion of upper cervical injuries in young children, adding cuts through C3 to the initial head CT scan should be considered. The spine cannot be "cleared" by radiographic examination alone. A child with normal cervical spine radiographs should be maintained in cervical spine immobilization until a thorough examination is performed.

In children, cervical spine fractures can occur without a neurologic deficit, and neurologic deficits can occur without a fracture. Neurologic deficit without fracture has been termed SCIWORA (spinal cord injury without radiologic abnormalities). SCIWORA was a diagnosis made in the pre–magnetic resonance imaging (MRI) era, and nowadays most children undergo MRI. SCIWORA can occur in the cervical or thoracic spine, and the onset of neurologic deficit is delayed in about a quarter of children with SCIWORA. Symptoms include brief sensory or motor deficits initially, with later onset of more severe signs. The majority of SCIWORA injuries appear to be due to flexion or hyperextension and are caused by stretching or disruption of ligaments without bony injury. Children with these injuries need to be treated with spine immobilization because recurrent injury can occur.

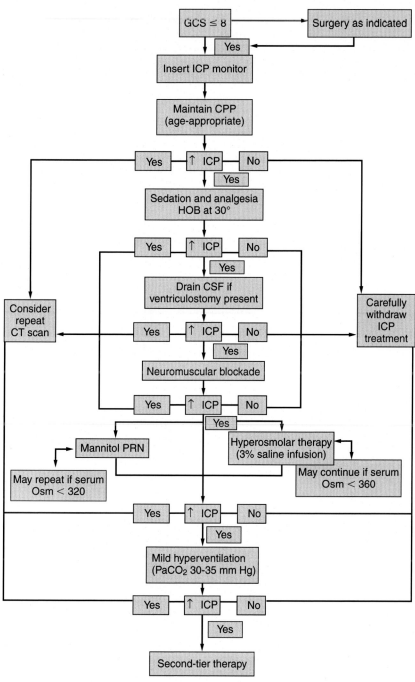

Figure 30-1 Intracranial pressure management algorithm. CPP, cerebral perfusion pressure; CSF, cerebrospinal fluid; CT, computed tomography; GCS, Glasgow Coma Scale score; HOB, head of bed; ICP, intracranial pressure; PRN, as needed. (Adapted from Guidelines for the acute medical management of severe traumatic brain injury in infants, children, and adolescents. Critical pathway for the treatment of established intracranial hypertension in pediatric traumatic brain injury. Pediatr Crit Care Med 2003; 4[3 Suppl]:S65-S67.)

30

Table 30-2 Select 2003 Brain Trauma Foundation Guidelines for the Management of Severe Brain Injury

Physiologic Parameter	Recommendations
Blood glucose	Avoid dextrose-containing solutions
	Keep blood glucose <200-250 mg/dL
Temperature	Avoid hyperthermia; cool patients to 36-37° C
	Hypothermia (32-34° C) may be considered for refractory ICP
CBF and $Paco_2$	Avoid mild/prophylactic hyperventilation ($Paco_2$ <35 mm Hg)
	Mild hyperventilation if acute brainstem herniation present
	Mild hyperventilation may be considered for refractory ICP
SBP	Hypovolemia should be corrected ASAP
	SBP should be maintained at least >5th percentile for age
	May be beneficial to maintain SBP in the normal range (>50th percentile)
CPP	Keep CPP >40 mm Hg
	CPP of 40-65 mm Hg may represent an age-related continuum for best treatment
ICP	Monitor if Glasgow Coma Scale score <9
	Treat ICP >20 mm Hg
	Ventriculostomy or intraparenchymal catheter
Hypertonic solutions	3% Saline, 0.1-1.0 mL/kg/hr
	Mannitol, 0.25-1.0 g/kg

CBF, cerebral blood flow; CPP, cerebral perfusion pressure; ICP, intracranial pressure; SBP, systolic blood pressure.

Adapted from Adelson PD, Bratton SL, Carney NA, et al. Guidelines for the acute medical management of severe traumatic brain injury in infants, children and adolescents. Pediatr Crit Care Med 2003; 4(3):Suppl.

CLINICAL MANAGEMENT

Initial Assessment

The initial approach to a traumatized child involves the primary and secondary surveys. Definitive care of all injuries is undertaken, and the principles outlined in the 2003 Brain Trauma Foundation guidelines for managing children with severe TBI (Table 30-2) are followed during general anesthesia. The Glasgow Coma Scale (GCS) score (modified for children) is the most commonly used neurologic assessment (Table 30-3). Discussed in the following sections are relevant issues specific to the different components of anesthetic management not described in Table 30-2.

Cervical Spine Immobilization

In infants younger than 6 months, the head and cervical spine should be immediately immobilized by using a spine board with tape across the forehead and blankets or towels around the neck. In infants 6 months or older, the head should be immobilized either in the manner just described or by using a small rigid cervical collar. Children older than 8 years require a medium-sized cervical collar. The use of rigid cervical collars is essential inasmuch as they prevent cervical distraction during laryngoscopy. Because children younger than 7 years have a prominent occiput, a pad placed under

Table 30-3	Glasgow Coma Scale and Modification for Young Children		
Glasgow Coma Scale	**Pediatric Coma Scale**	**Infant Coma Scale**	**Score**
Eyes			
Open spontaneously	Open spontaneously	Open spontaneously	4
Verbal command	React to speech	React to speech	3
Pain	React to pain	React to pain	2
No response	No response	No response	1
Best Verbal Response			
Oriented and converses	Smiles, oriented, interacts	Coos, babbles, interacts	5
Disoriented and converses	Interacts inappropriately	Irritable	4
Inappropriate words	Moaning	Cries to pain	3
Incomprehensible sounds	Irritable, inconsolable	Moans to pain	2
No response	No response	No response	1
Best Motor Response			
Obeys verbal command	Spontaneous or obeys verbal command	Normal spontaneous movements	6
Localizes pain	Localizes pain	Withdraws to touch	5
Withdraws to pain	Withdraws to pain	Withdraws to pain	4
Abnormal flexion	Abnormal flexion	Abnormal flexion	3
Extension posturing	Extension posturing	Extension posturing	2
No response	No response	No response	1

the thoracic spine provides neutral alignment of the spine and avoids the excessive flexion that may occur in the supine position. These two maneuvers are paramount in avoiding iatrogenic cervical spine injury.

Airway Management

The most important element during the primary survey phase is to establish an adequate airway. A lucid and hemodynamically stable child can be managed conservatively, but if the child has altered mental status, attempts should be made to establish the airway by suctioning the pharynx, performing chin-lift and jaw-thrust maneuvers, or inserting an oral airway. Children with a GCS score lower than 9 require tracheal intubation for airway protection and management of increased ICP. However, recent studies have not demonstrated any survival or functional advantage of prehospital tracheal intubation over prehospital bag-valve-mask ventilation in pediatric TBI. The most common approach to tracheal intubation remains direct laryngoscopy and oral intubation with cricoid pressure after induction of anesthesia, ventilation with 100% oxygen, and manual in-line stabilization without traction. Nasotracheal intubation is contraindicated in patients with basilar skull fractures. Fiberoptic bronchoscopy may not be available and often has poor resolution and suctioning capability. Moreover, it cannot be used in an agitated child.

Anesthetic Technique

Most recommendations regarding the choice of anesthetic technique and monitoring are extrapolated from data in adults, so anesthesiologists should be aware of the hemodynamic and physiologic recommendations given in Table 30-1.

30

Intravenous Agents

All intravenous sedative-hypnotic induction agents, including barbiturates, etomidate, and propofol, that are used to facilitate tracheal intubation are potent cerebral vasoconstrictors, cause coupled reductions in CBF and $CMRO_2$, and can decrease ICP. Opioids and benzodiazepines can be safely used to facilitate tracheal intubation but should be given in small doses. Ketamine should probably be used with caution in patients with TBI. Lidocaine is commonly administered as an anesthetic adjunct to prevent increases in ICP induced by laryngoscopy and tracheal intubation in patients whose hemodynamic instability precludes the use of large doses of sedative-hypnotic agents.

Volatile Agents

All inhalational agents are cerebral vasodilators, but less than 1 minimal alveolar concentration (MAC) of sevoflurane does not increase middle CBF velocity when compared with other agents. Consequently, sevoflurane may be the preferred volatile agent over isoflurane, desflurane, or halothane in pediatric TBI. Nitrous oxide can increase ICP.

Muscle Relaxants

Muscle relaxants have little effect on the cerebral circulation. Succinylcholine can be safely administered without causing an increase in ICP with or without a defasciculating dose of nondepolarizing muscle relaxant. Succinylcholine is a better choice than rocuronium if a difficult airway is a concern.

Intravenous Access

Obtaining vascular access in a traumatized child can be very challenging. A well-functioning 20-gauge or larger peripheral intravenous catheter will suffice for induction of anesthesia. The saphenous veins are commonly used. A second intravenous line should be started after induction. In emergency cases, if peripheral access is unsuccessful after two attempts, an interosseous line should be placed. Central venous catheters should be inserted by experienced personnel.

Intravenous Fluids

Unlike adults, children can become hypovolemic from scalp injuries and isolated TBI. Isotonic crystalloid solutions are commonly used during anesthesia and for cerebral resuscitation. Hypotonic crystalloids should be avoided, and the role of colloids is controversial. The use of hydroxyethyl starch is discouraged because of its role in exacerbating coagulopathy. Hypertonic saline, 0.1 to 1.0 mL/kg, may be used to lower ICP and improve cerebral perfusion pressure (CPP).

Glucose

Retrospective studies suggest that hyperglycemia (glucose, 200 to 250 mg/100 mL) is associated with a poor outcome.

Monitoring

Standard American Society of Anesthesiologists (ASA) monitors and invasive arterial blood pressure monitoring are recommended. Central venous pressure monitoring can be useful. An internal jugular line may be placed safely and used without increasing ICP. Retrograde jugular venous saturation monitoring can be useful to guide the degree of hyperventilation in patients with TBI but is not standard of care. ICP monitoring is useful during surgery involving extracranial injuries because CPP can be calculated, but any preexisting coagulopathy must be treated before monitor placement. Urine output must be monitored. It is unclear at this time whether hypothermia affords any benefit in children with TBI, but a multicenter randomized controlled trial in children is currently under way. Hourly arterial blood gas and coagulation test results need to be examined. ICP monitoring should be used to guide blood pressure management in children with TBI who are undergoing nonneurosurgical procedures.

Cerebral Hemodynamics (Intracranial Pressure and Blood Pressure)

The presence of the Cushing reflex and autonomic dysfunction might be the only indication of increased ICP. Although systolic blood pressure lower than the 5th percentile defines hypotension, in the absence of ICP monitoring and suspected increased ICP, supranormal systolic blood pressure may be needed to maintain CPP. At a minimum, mean arterial pressure should not be allowed to decrease below values normal for age by using vasopressors. At our institution, intravenous phenylephrine infusion is commonly used to treat hypotension and maintain CPP above 50 mm Hg.

INDICATIONS FOR SURGERY

Evidence-based practice guidelines have recently been published for the surgical management of TBI in general and for the surgical management of increased ICP in pediatric TBI in particular. Nevertheless, the indications remain controversial for many procedures. The major goal of surgery for TBI is to optimize the recovery of viable brain. Most operations involve the removal of mass lesions for the purpose of preventing herniation, intracranial hypertension, or alterations in CBF. In general, unless small and deemed to be probably venous, epidural hematomas should be evacuated in comatose patients. Subdural hematomas that are associated with herniation, are thicker than 10 mm, or produce a midline shift of greater than 5 mm should be removed. Indications for surgical treatment of intraparenchymal mass lesions include progressive neurologic deterioration referable to the lesion, signs of a mass effect on CT, or refractory intracranial hypertension. Penetrating injury may often be managed by local débridement and watertight closure if not extensive and there is minimal intracranial mass effect (as defined earlier). Patients with severe brain swelling as manifested by cisternal compression or a midline shift on CT or intracranial hypertension by monitor are potential candidates for decompressive craniectomy. The relatively increased incidence of diffuse swelling in the pediatric population makes children more frequent candidates for such treatment. Generous decompressive craniectomy with duraplasty should be considered when intracranial hypertension reaches or approaches medical refractoriness in salvageable patients in whom the elevation in ICP and its effects are thought to be the major threat to recovery. Unilateral craniectomy is appropriate for lateralized swelling; bifrontal decompression is selected for diffuse disease.

In general, surgical removal of mass lesions in comatose patients should be performed as early as safely feasible. Because this often involves incompletely resuscitated patients, close collaboration between surgery and anesthesia is critical. Bidirectional communication should be maintained regarding issues such as the stage of the procedure, anticipated and ongoing blood loss, systemic stability, and unanticipated events so that the procedure can be altered or even terminated if necessary.

SUMMARY

Pediatric TBI results in large societal costs. Therefore, efforts to improve outcome are extremely important. Although many general principles of managing pediatric TBI are similar to those used in adults, there are unique anatomic, physiologic, and pathophysiologic features of children with TBI worth recognizing.

KEY POINTS

- TBI is the leading cause of death in children older than 1 year.
- Fifty percent of children with spinal cord injury have associated TBI.
- Diffuse injury is the most common TBI pattern, and cerebral edema is the most common finding on CT of the head.
- Impaired cerebral autoregulation, hypotension, and CBF mismatched to cerebral metabolism contribute to secondary TBI.
- Children with either a GCS score lower than 9 or a decreasing level of consciousness need tracheal intubation for airway protection and management of increased ICP. The cervical spine must be immobilized.
- Intravenous cerebral vasoconstrictors and muscle relaxants should be used for induction, and volatile anesthetic agents less than 1 MAC, opioid boluses, and muscle relaxants should be used for maintenance of general anesthesia.
- In addition to standard monitors, an arterial cannula and two large peripheral intravenous catheters are placed.
- Hypotension (systolic blood pressure less than the 5th percentile) is treated vigorously after TBI by restoring euvolemia with volume and with vasopressors thereafter.
- Mild or prophylactic hyperventilation ($Paco_2$ <35 mm Hg) should be avoided unless evidence of brain herniation is present.
- Secondary brain injury caused by hyperglycemia, hyperthermia, hypoxia, or coagulopathy should be prevented or aggressively treated.

Acknowledgment

The authors would like to thank Ms. Domonique Calhoun for her assistance in preparation of this manuscript. Funding was provided by NIH//K23 HD044632-04.

FURTHER READING

Adelson PD, Bratton SL, Carney NA, et al: Guidelines for the acute medical management of severe traumatic brain injury in infants, children, and adolescents. Resuscitation of blood pressure and oxygenation and prehospital brain-specific therapies for the severe pediatric traumatic brain injury patient. Pediatr Crit Care Med 2003; 4(3 Suppl):S12-S18.

Adelson PD, Bratton SL, Carney NA, et al: Guidelines for the acute medical management of severe traumatic brain injury in infants, children, and adolescents. Surgical treatment of pediatric intracranial hypertension. Pediatr Crit Care Med 2003; 4(3 Suppl):S56-S59.

Adelson PD, Bratton SL, Carney NA, et al: Guidelines for the acute medical management of severe traumatic brain injury in infants, children, and adolescents. Critical pathway for the treatment of established intracranial hypertension in pediatric traumatic brain injury. Pediatr Crit Care Med 2003; 4(3 Suppl): S65-S67.

Bullock MR, Chesnut R, Ghajar J, et al: Surgical management of acute epidural hematomas. Neurosurgery 2006; 58(3 Suppl):S7-S15.

Bullock MR, Chesnut R, Ghajar J, et al: Surgical management of acute subdural hematomas. Neurosurgery 2006; 58(3 Suppl):S16-S24.

Crosby ET: Airway management in adults after cervical spine trauma. Anesthesiology 2006; 104:1293-1318.

Gausche M, Lewis RJ, Stratton SJ, et al: Effect of out-of-hospital pediatric endotracheal intubation on survival and neurological outcome: A controlled clinical trial. JAMA 2000; 283:783-790.

Pediatric Trauma in Advanced Trauma Life Support Course for Physicians. American College of Surgeons, 1993, pp 261-281.

Skippen P, Seear M, Poskitt K, et al: Effect of hyperventilation on regional blood flow in head injured children. Crit Care Med 1997; 25:1402-1409.

Vavilala MS. Impaired cerebral autoregulation and poor 6 month outcome after severe pediatric traumatic brain injury. Dev Neurosci 2006; 28:348-353.

30

Chapter 31

Postanesthesia Care Unit

Daniel M. Wong • Pirjo H. Manninen

General Considerations

Monitoring
Airway and Ventilation
Fluids and Electrolytes
Laboratory Parameters
Position
Temperature
Imaging

Complications

Airway and Respiratory
Cardiovascular

Neurologic
Pain
Postoperative Nausea and Vomiting
Shivering
Urinary Retention
Thromboembolism
Other

Discharge Criteria

The immediate recovery of neurosurgical patients may take place in an intensive care unit (ICU), neurosurgical ICU, or postanesthesia care unit (PACU), depending on institutional resources, individual patient factors, and the type of procedure. Complications are common in the immediate postoperative period and require close monitoring geared toward detection of neurologic deterioration and optimization of any physiologic parameters that may influence the neurologic outcome.

GENERAL CONSIDERATIONS

Monitoring

On arrival in the PACU or any location designated for recovery, the airway, oxygenation, and hemodynamics should be assessed immediately, along with a neurologic examination. Regular and frequent (every 15 minutes) assessment of the following should also take place:

- Respiratory (oxygen saturation, respiratory rate)
- Cardiovascular (heart rate and rhythm, blood pressure via noninvasive and invasive means if present)
- Neurologic (Glasgow Coma Scale, pupil size and symmetry, sensory and motor function of the upper and lower extremities)
- Temperature
- Fluid balance and urine output
- Pain scores (verbal or visual)
- Presence of nausea and vomiting (PONV)

Table 31-1   Indications for Postoperative Ventilation

Airway concerns	Likelihood of upper airway obstruction (airway edema, macroglossia)
	Failure to regain consciousness or return of airway reflexes
Oxygenation concerns	Concurrent severe respiratory disease
Cardiovascular instability	Poor cardiac function, hypovolemia, major blood loss
Neurologic concerns	Decreased level of consciousness
	Neurologic deficit
	Raised intracranial pressure
	Brainstem injury or cranial nerve dysfunction (lack of gag reflex)
Physiologic disturbances	Hypothermia, acid-base abnormities

Additional neurologic monitoring may include ICP monitoring, which may be routine after certain procedures and is sometimes indicated in patients who are comatose or have deteriorating neurologic status. Advanced monitoring techniques such as electrophysiologic monitoring, transcranial Doppler ultrasonography, and jugular bulb venous oximetry may sometimes be beneficial.

Airway and Ventilation

Extubation of an awake patient is appropriate for the majority of patients before arriving in the PACU, and early extubation is preferred over elective postoperative ventilation to facilitate early neurologic examination and avoid increases in catecholamines because of stress and other ventilator-associated challenges.

Assessment of the gag reflex is essential after posterior fossa surgery because brainstem and cranial nerve function may be altered.

It is important to remember that airway edema may occur after prolonged prone cases, cervical spine surgery, carotid endarterectomy, and procedures involving large fluid shifts.

Postoperative ventilation may be required, the indications for which are presented in Table 31-1.

Fluids and Electrolytes

The perioperative fluid goals for neurosurgical patients should be

- Maintenance of normovolemia
- Avoidance of a reduction in serum osmolarity, hyperglycemia, and hyponatremia

These objectives are achieved with the use of 0.9% saline or physiologic salt solutions (e.g., lactated Ringer's solution) and avoidance of dextrose-containing solutions. Crystalloids or colloids should be used for fluid replacement.

Laboratory Parameters

Correction of changes in plasma biochemistry and rheology may need to commence in the PACU. Changes in plasma sodium are described in Chapter 37.

Blood glucose should be maintained at 80 to 150 mg/dL (4.4 to 8.3 mmol/L) because levels outside the normal range may lead to a worse neurologic outcome.

Modest hyperglycemia at 175 to 250 mg/dL (9.7 to 13.9 mmol/L) may not require intervention, but higher levels should be actively treated with insulin and ongoing blood sugar monitoring. Steroids (dexamethasone, methylprednisolone) may lead to hyperglycemia. Any acid-base imbalance should be investigated.

A hematocrit of 30% gives the optimal combination of viscosity and O_2-carrying capacity. Blood transfusions should be given if appropriate, and any coagulopathy should be rapidly corrected.

Position

A head-up, approximately 30-degree tilt will help improve ventilation; reduce facial, neck, and airway edema; and facilitate cerebral venous and cerebrospinal fluid (CSF) drainage. Patients should lie flat after endovascular procedures requiring femoral artery cannulation.

Temperature

Normothermia should be maintained (use warming blankets if necessary).

Imaging

A chest radiograph should be performed to check central line placement. Patients should be transported to the radiology suite with appropriate monitoring and supplemental oxygen if advanced imaging (computed tomography [CT], CT angiography, magnetic resonance imaging [MRI], MR angiography) is required after major surgery or after any deterioration in neurologic function.

COMPLICATIONS

Airway and Respiratory

Deterioration in the conscious state is an indication for airway management (reintubation) because these patients are at risk for airway obstruction and aspiration and are vulnerable to the effects of hypoxia and hypercapnia on the brain.

After neck surgery (carotid endarterectomy, cervical spine surgery), close monitoring of the airway is required because of the effects of edema and possible hematoma. Measuring neck circumference may be helpful.

Macroglossia is a potentially serious cause of airway obstruction in neurosurgical patients. Intraoperative neck flexion, chin compression, use of an oral airway, and lack of a bite block in prone patients are predisposing factors.

Cardiovascular

Maintenance of stable hemodynamics and cerebral perfusion pressure is important. Both hypertension and hypotension may independently lead to adverse neurologic outcomes. Hypovolemia may accelerate ischemia caused by cerebral vasospasm.

The target blood pressure should be discussed with the surgeon. A compromise may need to be made between maintaining high blood pressure (for cerebral perfusion) and maintaining lower blood pressure (to avoid bleeding). After surgery for arteriovenous malformations, avoidance of hypertension may be critical to prevent postoperative bleeding or hyperperfusion syndrome. Pharmacologic control of blood pressure is often required.

IV

Neurologic causes of cardiovascular instability include raised ICP, brainstem injury, involvement of T1-T4 sympathetic nerves, spinal shock, and autonomic hyperreflexia after spinal injury. Cardiac dysfunction and neurogenic pulmonary edema may be secondary to significant sympathetic activation after subarachnoid hemorrhage. Cardiac and respiratory support with inotropes, invasive hemodynamic monitoring, and ventilation may be indicated.

Neurologic

Any deterioration in the conscious state of the patient requires immediate attention to the airway, oxygenation, and optimization of hemodynamics and cerebral perfusion pressure, followed in most cases by prompt diagnosis via imaging (CT, MRI) or anticipation of surgical intervention, or both.

The possibility of pharmacologic causes (overuse of opioids or sedation) and physiologic abnormalities (airway, oxygenation, hemodynamics, temperature, acid-base status, electrolytes, osmolality, blood glucose) should always be considered.

Focal neurologic deficits should be investigated by imaging and may require early surgical intervention.

Treatment of increased ICP includes attention to the airway or reduction of airway pressure if intubated, head-up position, treatment of hypoxia and hypercapnia, optimization of hemodynamics and cerebral perfusion pressure, administration of mannitol/diuretics, CSF drainage if a ventricular drain is present, surgical management, or any combination of these measures.

Seizures require immediate attention to the airway, protection of the patient, and pharmacologic treatment with benzodiazepines initially, followed by phenytoin or possibly barbiturates.

Pain

Pain should be assessed with a scoring system (verbal or visual) to help guide treatment. Postcraniotomy pain remains challenging and controversial. Measures to decrease postcraniotomy pain include a scalp block; *acetaminophen* alone may be inadequate but should be used as an adjunct with regular dosing and opioids.

Although codeine still remains the most popular first-line agent, disadvantages include administration problems (intramuscular injection) and its poor efficacy in some patients. Traditionally, potent opioids such as morphine were avoided as first-line agents because of concern for hypercapnia, miosis, and sedation (interferes with neurologic monitoring), as well as nausea. However, modest intravenous doses are generally believed to be safe.

Tramadol is associated with less respiratory depression and sedation than morphine is, although its role after craniotomy has not been fully established and its analgesic efficacy may be inferior to that of codeine. Disadvantages include a higher incidence of nausea and vomiting and an increased susceptibility to seizures.

The use of nonsteroidal anti-inflammatory drugs remains controversial. They may contribute to bleeding and postoperative renal failure, although regular postoperative dosing may be effective in pediatric craniectomy patients.

Analgesia for Spine Surgery Patients

Surgery on the lower part of the spine is generally associated with greater analgesic requirements than surgery on the cervical spine is. Patients usually require patient-controlled analgesia or infusion of morphine or an equivalent (or both) after major lumbar and thoracic surgery. If intrathecal morphine or epidural

31

Table 31-2 Antiemetic Treatment Options

Class of Drug	Examples (Intravenous Doses)	Important Side Effects
5-HT$_3$ antagonists	Ondansetron (4 mg), tropisetron (2 mg), granisetron (1 mg), dolasetron (12.5 mg)	Headaches
Antihistamines	Dimenhydrinate (25 mg), promethazine (12.5 mg)	Drowsiness
Anticholinergics	Scopolamine (transdermal patch)	Drowsiness, mydriasis
Antidopaminergics	Droperidol (0.625-1 mg), metoclopramide (10-20 mg)	Extrapyramidal symptoms
Steroids	Dexamethasone (8 mg)	Hyperglycemia

analgesia was administered preoperatively or intraoperatively, extra monitoring requirements may be necessary postoperatively. The use of additional opioids therefore requires great caution. A range of adjuvants (ketamine, gabapentin) should be considered, including regular doses of acetaminophen.

Postoperative Nausea and Vomiting

The incidence of PONV is high after both craniotomy and spine surgery. Prophylactic antiemetics are often administered intraoperatively and in conjunction with postoperative analgesia. Antiemetic prophylaxis with serotonin 5-HT$_3$ antagonists has been shown to be effective in decreasing PONV after both supratentorial and infratentorial surgery.

Options for treatment are presented in Table 31-2.

Shivering

Shivering is treated by rewarming and pharmacologic agents, including meperidine (12.5 to 25 mg intravenously [IV]), clonidine (75 µg IV), and magnesium sulfate (30 mg/kg IV).

Urinary Retention

Transient urinary retention is common, especially after routine neurosurgical spine procedures.

Thromboembolism

The prevalence of deep venous thrombosis is high in the neurosurgical population. Whether to routinely use prophylaxis is controversial. Antiembolic or pneumatic compression stockings are recommended but not always practical. Heparinization of patients requires that the risk of each patient be assessed individually.

Other

Some procedures are associated with specific postoperative concerns, such as endoscopic transsphenoidal hypophysectomy (aspiration of blood in the pharynx), neuroendoscopy (delayed arousal, hyperkalemia, diabetes insipidus, and hypothalamic dysfunction), and deep brain stimulation (movement disorder symptoms).

DISCHARGE CRITERIA

Neurosurgical patients in the PACU may be discharged to an ICU, neurointensive care unit, an intermediate care unit, the ward, and in rare cases, home. Some minor procedures (lumbar microdiscectomy) are suitable for outpatient surgery. Practice guidelines of the American Society of Anesthesiologists allow individual departments to approve their own discharge criteria for PACU patients. The criteria used for general PACU patients (modified Aldrete score) do not sufficiently address the postoperative risks specific to the neurosurgical population. The possibility of rapid neurologic deterioration justifies the observation of neurosurgical patients for a longer fixed amount of time in the PACU before transfer to the ward. Alternatively, it may be appropriate to discharge patients from the PACU earlier to an intermediate care unit equipped for frequent neurologic assessments.

In general, the following principles apply before discharge from the PACU:

- No airway or respiratory problems
- Stable hemodynamics
- No major neurologic problems (awake/alert/oriented, no major sensory or motor blockade)
- Other physiologic parameters within the normal range (temperature, acid-base status, blood sugar level)
- Adequate pain control and minimal PONV

KEY POINTS

- The potential for rapid neurologic deterioration in the immediate postoperative period in the PACU requires regular and frequent monitoring.
- Aggressive management of airway, oxygenation, and ventilation problems is important in view of the detrimental effects of hypoxia and hypercapnia.
- Hypotension and hypertension should be avoided because they may lead to adverse neurologic outcomes.
- Rapid diagnosis of neurologic deterioration with imaging and surgical consultation is essential. Pharmacologic and physiologic causes should also be considered.
- Physiologic parameters such as intravascular volume, osmolality, blood glucose, temperature, cerebral perfusion pressure, and ICP should be kept within the normal range.
- If used carefully, potent opioids such as morphine are appropriate analgesics as an alternative to codeine.
- 5-HT$_3$ antagonists are suitable antiemetics.
- Discharge from the PACU to a suitable location should take place when the patient is stable and discharge criteria have been met.

FURTHER READING

Beauregard CL, Friedman WA: Routine use of postoperative ICU care for elective craniotomy: A cost-benefit analysis. Surg Neurol 2003; 60:483-489.
Bruder N, Ravussin P: Recovery from anesthesia and postoperative extubation of neurosurgical patients: A review. J Neurosurg Anesthesiol 1999; 11:282-293.
de Gray LC, Matta BF: Acute and chronic pain following craniotomy: A review. Anaesthesia 2005; 60:693-704.
Kelly DF: Neurosurgical postoperative care. Neurosurg Clin N Am 1994; 5:789-810.

Leslie K, Williams DL: Postoperative pain, nausea and vomiting in neurosurgical patients. Curr Opin Anaesthesiol 2005; 18:461-465.

Lukins MB, Manninen PH: Hyperglycemia in patients administered dexamethasone for craniotomy. Anesth Analg 2005; 100:1129-1133.

Manninen PH, Raman SK, Boyle K, et al: Early postoperative complications following neurosurgical procedures. Can J Anaesth 1999; 46:7-14.

Niskanen M, Koivisto T, Rinne J, et al: Complications and postoperative care in patients undergoing treatment for unruptured intracranial aneurysms. J Neurosurg Anesthesiol 2005; 17:100-105.

Schubert A, Deogaonkar A, Lotto M, et al: Anesthesia for minimally invasive cranial and spinal surgery. J Neurosurg Anesthesiol 2006; 18:47-56.

Sinha A, Agarwal A, Gaur A, et al: Oropharyngeal swelling and macroglossia after cervical spine surgery in the prone position. J Neurosurg Anesthesiol 2001; 13:237-239.

IV

Section V
Neurointensive Care

Chapter 32

Spinal Cord Injury

Katharine Hunt • Rodney Laing

PATHOPHYSIOLOGY

The pathophysiology of spinal cord injury (SCI) can be divided into primary and secondary components. Primary injury may be caused by stretching of the spinal cord secondary to hyperextension or hyperflexion of the spinal column. If the force is great enough, tearing of the spinal cord can result. The cord may become compromised as a result of compression from fractured and disrupted bony structures and may occasionally be damaged by a direct, penetrating injury. Primary injury leads to disruption of neural tissues, as well as interruption of the vascular supply with hemorrhage, vasospasm, and local ischemia.

Whatever the mechanism of primary injury, the pattern of the ongoing or secondary injury is similar in all cases and involves a complex cascade of events, including release of cytokines and amino acids from injured tissue that generate an inflammatory cascade ultimately leading to free radical formation, cellular edema, and cellular apoptosis. These events may be compounded by systemic hypotension and hypoxia, as well as local cord edema, and result in the destruction of axons nerve cell bodies and the supporting glia.

SCI not only results in neurologic dysfunction but also causes important disturbances in the body's other systems.

Nervous System

Damage to the spinal cord causes an interruption in both somatic and visceral sensation that results in absent somatic and autonomic reflexes and flaccid paralysis. This phenomenon is often termed "spinal shock." Spinal shock may last for up to 6 weeks, but in most cases it resolves within 24 hours of the initial injury. As spinal shock

211

resolves, the initial neurologic findings are replaced by progressive spasticity of the affected segments below the level of injury.

Respiratory System

The degree of airway and respiratory compromise depends on the level of the SCI, as well as the presence of concomitant injuries. In cervical cord injuries, the level of spinal cord edema and hence dysfunction may ascend and make respiratory support necessary. In addition, injuries below the fifth cervical vertebra (C5) affect the intercostal muscles, which may decrease alveolar ventilation and also limit the effectiveness and strength of cough. In unstable thoracic spine injuries, particularly those associated with rib fractures and lung contusions, there is a high risk for the development of respiratory complications.

In lesions at the C4/C5 level, voluntary respiration is maintained but vital capacity is reduced by as much as 20% to 25%. These patients often require ventilatory support. In any lesion above C4, accessory, diaphragmatic, and intercostal muscle function may be lost and require total ventilatory support.

Cardiovascular System

Although patients are often hypertensive at the moment of injury, they quickly become hypotensive because of interruption of sympathetic pathways. Compensatory reflexes are lost, particularly if the lesion is above T1, and a profound bradycardia may occur as a result of unopposed parasympathetic activity.

Gastrointestinal and Genitourinary Systems

Both bladder and bowel atony may occur and are manifested as paralytic ileus, gastric distention, and urinary retention.

Temperature

The ability to control body temperature is lost because of an inability to initiate sweating, coupled with profound cutaneous vasodilation.

DIAGNOSIS AND MANAGEMENT IN THE INTENSIVE THERAPY UNIT

Assessment of Spinal Cord Injury

The initial clinical examination should begin with assessment of airway, breathing, and circulatory status. The neck should be immobilized in a rigid cervical collar, and during transport the patient should be immobilized on a spinal board. The spinal board should be removed as soon as possible once the patient is in the hospital and under specialist supervision. The skin over the spine must be inspected and palpated for deformity and tenderness. Sensory and motor function and tendon reflexes should be examined and documented via the American Spinal Injury Association (ASIA) chart as soon as possible.

Radiographs are taken to screen the vertebral column, but any area of suspected injury should be scanned with computed tomography (CT). CT also allows proper imaging of the cervicothoracic (C7-T1) junction, where injury is common and can be missed with standard radiographs. Imaging should be reviewed by radiologists and by a spinal surgeon to assess the clinical implications of any abnormality.

It is possible for a patient with negative findings on plain radiographs or CT scans to have a soft tissue or ligamentous injury. If despite negative radiologic findings a patient experiences pain or tenderness, particularly with movement, flexion-extension views of the neck or magnetic resonance imaging should be considered. Uncooperative patients should undergo CT scanning of the whole spine.

Associated Injury

Twenty percent to 50% of patients have other systemic injuries, the most common being traumatic brain or major chest injuries. Traumatic brain injury occurs in up to 50% of patients with SCI and is more likely after a motor vehicle accident.

The possibility of other injuries may present several problems. First, other major injuries may cause hypoxia and hypotension, which can result in considerable secondary injury to the spinal cord. Second, the presence of a spinal injury makes secondary injuries harder to diagnose and treat. The airway may also be more difficult to secure because fear of exacerbating a cord injury in the presence of an unstable spine may hinder proper assessment and resuscitation.

Immobilization

During initial transport from the scene to the hospital, patients are commonly immobilized in a rigid cervical collar and placed on a spinal board. Once in an intensive care unit, the neck may be immobilized by continuation of rigid cervical collar support or the use of two sandbags secured on either side of the head. Patients should not be kept on a spinal board in intensive care because of the risk for the development of pressure sores, particularly in areas with diminished or absent sensation. Patients can be log-rolled to allow examination and relief of pressure areas. Immobilization can in itself cause complications, including pressure sores, pain, and atelectasis. Rigid cervical collars are associated with raised intracranial pressure; airway compromise, which can lead to pulmonary aspiration; and pressure necrosis of the underlying skin. Assessment of the stability of the vertebral column and permitted range of movement should be done as soon as possible by experienced clinicians so that immobilization can be discontinued.

32

Airway and Respiratory Support

It is common for patients with spinal injury to require intubation. Indications for intubation in SCI are

- Pa_{O_2} <10 kPa (75 mm Hg)
- Pa_{CO_2} >6.5 kPa (50 mm Hg)
- Vital capacity <20 mL/kg
- Pulmonary edema
- Pulmonary aspiration
- Chest or lung injuries

To minimize movement of the cervical cord, manual in-line stabilization should be used during laryngoscopy and endotracheal intubation. If the patient is awake and cooperative, awake fiberoptic intubation may be considered. In the acute phase of injury (<24 hours), succinylcholine may be administered safely without concern for triggering hyperkalemia.

Cardiovascular Support

Hypotension coupled with bradycardia secondary to loss of cardiac accelerator function and unopposed parasympathetic activity is common after high SCI but can occur after injury at any level. Hypotension may be compounded by active hemorrhage from other associated injuries. Hypotension and hypovolemia should be initially managed with volume replacement guided by central venous pressure measurements. Pulmonary edema commonly occurs after SCI, and although it is probably sympathetically mediated and occurs independently of fluid overload, care must still be taken when optimizing fluid balance. If perfusion remains inadequate despite fluid resuscitation, treatment with vasoconstrictors or inotropes should be commenced and a pulmonary artery catheter inserted. The bradycardia seen in spinal injury responds to atropine.

Other

Bladder and bowel atony is managed by urinary catheterization and insertion of a nasogastric tube, respectively. Prophylaxis against deep venous thrombosis should be given once patients are stabilized and all sources of hemorrhage have been controlled, provided that surgical intervention to decompress the cord or stabilize the spine (or both) is not imminent.

EARLY STEROID INTERVENTION

Corticosteroids have been extensively investigated in both animals and humans. Although their precise mechanism of action is unknown, effects may include stabilization of membrane structures, reduction of vasogenic edema, free radical scavenging, enhancement of spinal cord blood flow, and limitation of the inflammatory response.

The largest human trials, the National Acute Spinal Cord Injury Studies (NASCIS I, II, and III), concluded that early steroid intervention improves neurologic outcome in SCI patients. The NASCIS II study recommended the use of methylprednisolone given as an initial bolus of 30 mg/kg followed by an infusion at 5.4 mg/kg over the next 23-hour period. The NASCIS studies have, however, been criticized on several levels, the most important being that the conclusions of the trial were driven by results taken from subpopulations of patients rather than from the patient study group as a whole. The results have also not been reproducible in any subsequent studies using the same drug and dosage regimens, and the improvement seen in the neurologic level of injury in the NASCIS trials did not equate with an improvement in survival or quality of life.

These criticisms, coupled with the potential side effects associated with high-dose steroid therapy, have led several neurosurgical organizations to suggest that steroid therapy should be used only as an *option* in SCI treatment with the full knowledge that the risks of administration may outweigh the potential benefits of its actions.

AUTONOMIC DYSREFLEXIA

Autonomic dysreflexia is a phenomenon seen after SCI. It typically occurs weeks and months after the initial insult and is characterized by a massive autonomic response to stimuli below the level of the spinal cord lesion.

Pathophysiology

Autonomic dysreflexia is seen in 60% to 80% of patients with complete SCI above T6 (splanchnic outflow), but it may occur in up to 90% of patients with higher thoracic or cervical cord lesions. The response is rarely seen in those with complete injuries below T10. The widespread inappropriate sympathetic response causes profound vasoconstriction. Increased sensitivity to endogenous catecholamines may also develop.

Many stimuli can trigger autonomic dysreflexia, the most common of which is pelvic visceral stimulation. Bladder distention, fecal impaction, uterine contractions, urinary tract infections, long-bone fractures, deep venous thrombosis, pressure sores, and even tight clothing can initiate the reaction. Surgical stimuli can also induce the reflex.

Signs and Symptoms

The most concerning clinical feature of autonomic dysreflexia is paroxysmal hypertension. Blood pressure can reach systolic levels of greater than 260 mm Hg and diastolic pressure ranging from 170 to 220 mm Hg. The rise in blood pressure is commonly accompanied by headache, profuse sweating, and flushing or pallor above the level of the spinal cord lesion. Cardiac function may be disturbed by arrhythmias (especially bradycardia), myocardial ischemia, and in severe cases, congestive cardiac failure. Other features include nausea and vomiting, pupillary changes, nasal obstruction, Horner's syndrome, paresthesias, and anxiety. If left untreated, the precipitous rise in blood pressure may lead to cerebral, retinal, or subarachnoid hemorrhage, seizures, coma, myocardial infarction, and death.

Treatment

The most important aspect in the management of autonomic dysreflexia is awareness and recognition of the phenomenon. Initial treatment involves identifying and removing the precipitating stimulus, loosening all tight clothing and shoes, and when safe, sitting the patient upright. These measures alone may reduce the blood pressure. If an episode occurs under anesthesia, deepening the anesthesia or providing extra analgesia may alleviate the problem. A rapid-onset, short-acting vasodilator is the next drug of choice. Sublingual nifedipine and sublingual, intravenous, or dermal patch glyceryl trinitrate are the most commonly used agents. Intravenous phentolamine and hydralazine have also been used in the acute treatment of this disorder.

Long-term therapy with other antihypertensive agents can be considered. Prazosin, guanethidine, clonidine, and calcium channel blockers have all been used with some success in preventing episodes of the condition from occurring.

Anesthesia

Surgery is a potent stimulus for autonomic dysreflexia, even in patients with no previous history of this disorder. It is generally thought that spinal anesthesia is superior to epidural or general anesthesia in reducing occurrences during surgery.

Before a decision about the type of anesthesia is made, a thorough assessment of renal, cardiac, and respiratory (forced expiratory volume in 1 second [FEV_1]/forced vital capacity [FVC] ratio) function should be undertaken to enable planning of both intraoperative and postoperative care. It is also common to premedicate patients who may be at risk for autonomic dysreflexia with antihypertensives. It is common practice to preload patients with up to a liter of crystalloid before anesthesia to reduce the likelihood of severe hypotension.

32

Careful monitoring of patient temperature should take place in all but the shortest of procedures because patients with SCI are unable to generate heat and are therefore at much higher risk for hypothermia.

General Anesthesia

Propofol is the induction agent of choice, and a short-acting, nondepolarizing muscle relaxant can be administered to aid tracheal intubation. Succinylcholine is known to produce hyperkalemia in SCI patients, which if severe may lead to cardiac arrest. Its use should, when possible, be avoided for 72 hours to 9 months after injury.

Local Anesthesia

Regional techniques may be used alone or in conjunction with general anesthesia. As well as preventing episodes of autonomic dysreflexia, spinal anesthesia maintains good overall cardiovascular stability in these patients and has therefore become the anesthetic of choice, especially for urologic surgery.

In addition to instilling standard local anesthetic agents into the epidural space, opioids can be used. Meperidine, in particular, may prevent autonomic dysreflexia by producing selective blockade of spinal opioid receptors and hence blocking the nociceptive reflexes below the level of cord injury.

Postoperative Care

Autonomic dysreflexia may occur for the first time in the postoperative period. Careful monitoring for this, as well as respiratory function and temperature, is therefore essential. It is wise to allow an extended time for recovery and provide postoperative high-dependency care for these patients.

KEY POINTS

- Initial management of SCI should begin with assessment of the airway, breathing, and circulation.
- Patients should be immobilized until vertebral column injury and stability have been assessed.
- Up to 50% of patients have other associated injuries.
- High-dose corticosteroid therapy is not routinely indicated in early management.
- Autonomic dysreflexia may occur in both the acute and late stages of SCI.

FURTHER READING

Guidelines of the American Association of Neurologic Surgeons and the Congress of Neurologic Surgeons. Pharmacological therapy after cervical spinal cord injury. Neurosurgery 2002; 50(Suppl):63-72.
Hambly PR, Martin B: Anaesthesia for chronic spinal cord lesions. Anaesthesia 1998; 3:273-289.
Smith M, Hunt K: Neurosurgery. In Emergencies in Anaesthesia. London, Oxford University Press, 2005.
Stevens RD, Bhardwaj A, Kirsch JR, Mirski MA: Critical care and perioperative management in traumatic spinal cord injury. J Neurosurg Anesthesiol 2003; 15:215-229.

Chapter 33

Head Injury: Initial Resuscitation and Transfer

Jane E. Risdall

Initial Resuscitation

Airway and Breathing
Circulation and Fluid Resuscitation
Neurologic Status

Transfer of Head-Injured Patients

Head (or brain) injury occurs after a blow to the head in which neurons and intracranial blood vessels are subjected to flexion, extension, and shearing forces as the brain moves within the cranium, as well as the direct effects of the impact.

Primary injury describes the damage that occurs at the time of initial impact. This damage is not generally treatable, and the magnitude of the primary injury is the principal factor that differentiates a viable from a nonviable injury.

Secondary injury is the subsequent insult imposed on neurologic tissue as a consequence of the primary impact. The focus of treatment of patients with severe head injury should be to prevent secondary injury. Providing adequate oxygenation and maintaining sufficient blood pressure to perfuse the brain are the most important means of limiting secondary brain damage and therefore improving outcome.

INITIAL RESUSCITATION

Airway and Breathing

Maintaining a patent airway and adequate oxygenation is of paramount importance. If there is any question about the patient's ability to maintain the airway or achieve adequate gas exchange (Pao_2 <13 kPa [100 mm Hg], $Paco_2$ >6 kPa [45 mm Hg]), if the patient is in coma (i.e., Glasgow Coma Scale [GCS] score <9), if there is a suspicion that intracranial pressure (ICP) is raised acutely (unequal or nonreactive pupils), or if the patient is having seizures, endotracheal intubation is required (Table 33-1).

Because a full stomach is assumed in all trauma patients, endotracheal intubation will require a conventional rapid-sequence induction. Preoxygenation, followed by careful administration of an adequate dose of an intravenous induction agent and succinylcholine, 1 mg/kg, should be the norm. Apart from ketamine, which may adversely affect ICP if used without another hypnotic, the choice of induction agent is not crucial, provided that it is administered carefully to avoid periods of sustained hypotension or hypertension. The risk from the transient rise in ICP associated with the use of succinylcholine is far outweighed by the risks of hypoxemia and hypercapnia.

Table 33-1	Indications for Intubation and Ventilation after Head Injury*

Immediate

Coma/GCS score <9 (not obeying commands, not speaking, no eye opening)
Loss of protective laryngeal reflexes
Inadequate ventilation as judged by arterial blood gas analysis:
Hypoxemia, Pao_2 <13 kPa (100 mm Hg)
Spontaneous hyperventilation causing $Paco_2$ <3.5 kPa (26 mm Hg)
Abnormal respiratory pattern
Uncontrolled seizures

Before Transfer

Deteriorating level of consciousness (drop of 2 points in the GCS score even if not in coma)
Bilateral mandibular fractures
Bleeding into the mouth or airway
Seizures

---

*Intubated patients *must* be ventilated to maintain PaO_2 at greater than 13 kPa (100 mm Hg) and $Paco_2$ at 4.0 to 4.5 kPa (30 to 34 mm Hg).
GCS, Glasgow Coma Scale.

It is important to remember that a significant proportion of severe head injuries are associated with injuries to the cervical spine, so manual in-line immobilization of the cervical spine will be required during induction and endotracheal intubation.

Once the airway is secured, the patient should be ventilated to achieve a Pao_2 higher than 13 kPa (100 mm Hg) and a $Paco_2$ of 4.0 to 4.5 kPa (30 to 34 mm Hg) as checked on arterial blood gas analysis. The patient should be adequately sedated with an intravenous hypnotic (midazolam or propofol), together with an intravenous opioid and, if necessary, a neuromuscular blocking agent to prevent coughing or straining on the tube. Excessive hyperventilation ($Paco_2$ <4 kPa [30 mm Hg]) should be avoided because it has been associated with worsening of cerebral ischemia secondary to excessive cerebral vasoconstriction. Oxygenation should be optimized by increasing the inspired oxygen fraction and judiciously applying positive end-expiratory pressure (no more than 10 mm Hg). Peak inspiratory pressure should be limited to 35 mm Hg to minimize interference with cerebral venous drainage.

Circulation and Fluid Resuscitation

Except for young children, in whom blood loss from a scalp wound is sufficient to cause circulatory shock, hypotension should prompt immediate examination for other sites of blood loss, with urgent laparotomy or thoracotomy performed as indicated. The importance of maintaining systemic perfusion has been confirmed by results from the American National Trauma Coma Data Bank, which demonstrated that systolic blood pressure lower than 80 mm Hg is a significant independent factor contributing to a poor outcome in brain-injured patients. The combination of raised ICP and systemic hypotension is a potent cause of secondary brain injury.

Patients with acutely raised ICP, mass lesions (subdural or extradural hematomas), or subarachnoid hemorrhage may have intense sympathetic activity causing increased systemic vascular resistance. This may mask an inadequate circulating volume. Monitoring of central venous pressure (CVP) is often very useful to ensure adequate fluid resuscitation, particularly since the use of mannitol also removes

V

urine output as a meaningful guide to the adequacy of intravascular volume. A pulmonary artery catheter may be required to guide fluid replacement and inotrope therapy, especially in those with heart disease. Mean arterial pressure above 130 mm Hg or systolic pressure above 180 mm Hg, or both, may need to be controlled, but otherwise a lesser degree of systemic hypertension can be tolerated, thereby ensuring adequate CPP, even in the presence of a degree of intracranial hypertension.

Adequate fluid resuscitation in patients with severe head injury is mandatory. The choice of fluid used for resuscitation is less important than the amount given, although the use of glucose-containing fluids should be avoided unless hypoglycemia is present. Hyperglycemia (with or without lactic acidosis) correlates with poor outcome after head injury. Blood glucose levels should be monitored and rigorously controlled by infusion of insulin if necessary. Blood should be transfused to maintain the hemoglobin level above 8.0 g/dL, and disordered clotting should be corrected aggressively.

Neurologic Status

The GCS score and pupillary light response should be recorded early in the resuscitation process and repeated at intervals. It is important to obtain the GCS score and check pupil reactivity before sedating and paralyzing the patient.

Seizure activity is associated with an increased cerebral metabolic requirement for oxygen ($CMRO_2$) and should be controlled. Initial treatment should be a bolus dose of intravenous benzodiazepine, followed by a loading dose of phenytoin if necessary. If this fails to control the seizures (i.e., the patient is in status epilepticus), consider using an intravenous anesthetic agent such as propofol or thiopental as a temporary measure until effective anticonvulsant therapy can be established. Such patients will need to be intubated and ventilated, but it should be remembered that muscle relaxation will mask (but not prevent) subsequent seizures. Cessation of seizure activity can be confirmed only by electroencephalographic monitoring in paralyzed patients.

Although the incidence of post-traumatic seizures after serious head injuries (GCS score <10 after resuscitation) is up to 18% within the first 24 hours after injury and as high as 48% at 1 week, there is no evidence to support the use of prophylactic anticonvulsant therapy and it is not recommended in the Brain Trauma Foundation guidelines. If in doubt and the opportunity exists, take advice from the duty neurosurgeon at the local/receiving neurosurgical unit.

All patients who have suffered a witnessed seizure or are reported as having done so at or around the time of injury should be loaded with and maintained on anticonvulsants, at least until their neurologic status is stable enough to be assessed.

TRANSFER OF HEAD-INJURED PATIENTS

Moving a patient from one location to another, regardless of the distance involved, is hazardous. The process must be approached with the same attention to detail as the resuscitation that has just been performed, and this applies equally to the move to the computed tomography scanner as to the transfer to a regional neurosurgical center.

Successful and safe transfer involves

- Good communication between the referring and receiving centers or departments
- Adequate resuscitation and stabilization of the patient before transfer

33

- Adequate monitoring of the patient during transfer, with appropriate resuscitative drugs and equipment being available
- An escorting physician with sufficient training, skills, and experience in head injury management to be able to intervene effectively in the event that the patient deteriorates
- A clear, comprehensive handover of the patient to the receiving team, including a verbal briefing to medical and nursing staff, as well as written records of the treatment to date, radiographs, scans, laboratory results, and so forth

Any severe head injury should be discussed with the regional neurosurgical center at an early stage so that treatment priorities can be established and the requirement for transfer identified in timely fashion. The minimum initial information required is listed in Table 33-2.

The fundamental physiologic requirements during transfer are to ensure adequate delivery of oxygen to tissues and maintain cerebral perfusion. Any patient with a significant alteration in consciousness should be sedated, intubated, and ventilated for transfer, and persistent hypotension should be identified and treated before the patient is moved. Treatment of hypotension should include adequate resuscitation of circulating volume with surgical control of bleeding if necessary before recourse to inotropes and vasopressors. Monitoring during transfer should meet standards appropriate to a patient in intensive care, including invasive arterial blood pressure monitoring, central venous pressure monitoring if indicated, and capnography.

Transfers are most likely to be accomplished by road or air (helicopter). Both vehicles offer only confined space with little access to the patient. Lines, tubes, and

---

Table 33-2 Information Required for Neurosurgical Referral

Patient's name, age, and past medical history (if known)
History of the injury
   Time of the injury
   Cause and mechanism (impact velocity, ejection from vehicle, height of fall)
Neurologic status
   Talked or not after injury
   Consciousness level (GCS score) at the scene
   Consciousness level on arrival at the emergency department
   Trends in the GCS score
   Pupillary and limb responses
Cardiorespiratory status
   Blood pressure and pulse rate
   Arterial blood gas results, respiratory rate and pattern
Injuries
   Skull fracture
   Extracranial injuries
   Secondary survey completed or not
Findings on imaging
   Hematoma
   Swelling
   Midline shift
   Images being sent by hard copy or electronically
Management
   Airway protection, ventilatory support
   Circulatory status, fluid therapy, mannitol
   Treatment of associated injuries (emergency surgery, surgical referral)
   Monitoring
   Drugs received and timing

V

drains must all be secured thoroughly because replacing them in transit will not be easy. Estimates of journey times are frequently unreliable and do not usually include the time taken to transfer the patient to the ambulance, load and unload the patient and equipment, and transfer the patient to the unit at the destination. It is therefore important to take a relative oversupply of drugs, fluids, portable gases, and power (in the form of backup batteries) to cover every eventuality. Road and air ambulances will have dedicated fittings for securing the transfer stretcher or trolley.

In more rugged environments where nonambulance helicopters are likely to be used, consideration will need to be given to the means by which and the position in which the stretcher is secured. In general, positioning across the body of an aircraft is preferable to positioning along the longitudinal axis to avoid the variable pitch effects during takeoff (nose down) and landing (tail down). When a nonambulance aircraft is used, it is also important to ensure that the medical equipment traveling with the patient does not interfere with the aircraft systems. A detailed consideration of the logistics and physiologic challenges of airborne transfer of the critically ill is beyond the scope of this chapter, but interested readers are referred to the reading list.

KEY POINTS

- Avoid hypoxia and hypotension at all times because they are the two major contributors to secondary brain injury.
- Assume that the cervical spine is unstable and maintain appropriate immobilization until it has been cleared.
- Resuscitate and stabilize a head-injured patient before transfer.
- Communicate early with the receiving neurosurgical center.
- Ensure that appropriate personnel, monitoring equipment, and records accompany the patient when transferred.

FURTHER READING

American College of Surgeons Committee on Trauma: Advanced Trauma Life Support Course Manual, 7th ed. Chicago, ACS, 2004.

Association of Anaesthetists of Great Britain and Ireland: Recommendations for the transfer of patients with acute head injuries to neurosurgical units. London, AAGBI, 1996.

Brain Trauma Foundation, American Association of Neurological Surgeons, Joint Section on Neurotrauma and Critical Care: Guidelines for cerebral perfusion pressure. J Neurotrauma 2000; 17:507-511.

Gentleman D, Dearden M, Midgely S, Maclean D: Guidelines for the resuscitation and transfer of patients with serious head injury. BMJ 1993; 307:547-552.

Rainford D, Gradwell D (eds): Aviation Medicine, 4th ed. Hoddes Arnold, London, 2006.

33

Chapter 34

Intensive Care Management of Acute Head Injury

Virginia Newcombe • David K. Menon

PRINCIPLES OF MANAGEMENT

Mortality in patients who require intensive care treatment after acute head injury is high, with a rate of 23.5% reported in a recent series of more than 11,000 admissions. A major contributor to outcome is secondary neuronal injury. It is prevention of this secondary damage by avoidance, detection, and treatment of physiologic derangements that is a major focus of the intensive care management of neurotrauma.

Hypotension (systolic blood pressure <90 mm Hg) and hypoxemia (Pao_2 <60 mm Hg or 8 kPa) during the acute to subacute phases of brain injury are associated with a worse outcome. Other factors that have been found to adversely affect outcome include intracranial hypertension, hyperglycemia, hyperthermia, and cerebral perfusion pressure (CPP) less than 50 mm Hg.

MONITORING IN ACUTE NEUROTRAUMA

A multimodal approach to monitoring helps optimize physiology. It allows cross-validation and rejection of artifacts, as well as a better understanding of the pathophysiology and the potential to target therapy individually. Continuous pulse oximetry, regular arterial blood gas analysis, invasive blood pressure monitoring, blood glucose levels, and core temperature monitoring are all important.

Intracranial Pressure Monitoring

Because the clinical signs of intracranial hypertension are often unreliable, may occur late, and are nonspecific, intracranial pressure (ICP) monitoring is needed. Levels higher than 20 mm Hg are an appropriate threshold for commencement of therapy. Intraventricular devices to monitor ICP are regarded as the "gold standard" and have the added advantage that intracranial fluid may be removed to control intracranial hypertension. Intraparenchymal monitors or fiberoptic probes are often preferentially used because of a lower risk of infection and hemorrhage, as well as ease of insertion. Ventricular and subdural transducers may also be used.

In addition to static increases in ICP, phasic increases may also occur and be triggered by a fall in CPP. "A waves" tend to occur in those with high baseline pressure. The increase in pressure can be extreme (50 to 100 mm Hg) and may last several minutes; it is often terminated by a marked rise in mean arterial pressure (MAP). Vasogenic "B waves" are shorter fluctuations lasting approximately 1 minute. Increasing MAP can reduce the occurrence of these waves of intracranial hypertension by preventing vasodilation. Further details regarding ICP monitoring and interpretation can be found in Chapter 40.

Jugular Venous Oximetry

Jugular venous oximetry may be used to aid assessment of cerebral blood flow (CBF) in neurotrauma (see Chapter 41). Jugular venous oxygen saturation ($Sjvo_2$) values below 50% have been associated with a worse outcome. However, this technique may miss focal areas of ischemia because it is a global hemispheric measure of oxygen extraction by the brain. Indeed, positron emission tomography (PET) has been used to show that the ischemic burden required for $Sjvo_2$ to fall below 50% is high, with approximately 13% of the brain needing to be critically ischemic. Marked elevations in $Sjvo_2$ (>85%) may be secondary to cerebral hyperemia or inadequate neuronal metabolism.

Transcranial Doppler Ultrasonography

Elevated flow velocity may indicate vasospasm or hyperemia. Cerebral autoregulation may be assessed with transcranial Doppler ultrasound either by changing MAP or by carotid compression (the transient hyperemic response test) (see Chapter 46).

Other Monitoring Methods

Microdialysis, brain tissue oxygen pressure, near-infrared spectroscopy, and bispectral index (BIS) monitoring have been used at some centers. Although they are still used mainly for research, they can be useful adjuncts to more traditional monitoring methods, and methods such as microdialysis may allow individualization of patient therapy. Further details can be found in the respective chapters in this book.

34

THERAPY

Achieving Adequate Cerebral Perfusion Pressure

Several studies suggest that it is important to ensure that CPP, calculated as the difference between MAP and intracranial pressure, is maintained rather than focusing solely on ICP as a target. The Brain Trauma Foundation guidelines currently recommend a target CPP of greater than 60 mm Hg. In neurotrauma, cerebrovascular autoregulation, if preserved, is at higher blood pressure levels than normal (a rightward shift of the autoregulatory curve), with maintenance of CBF usually at a CPP of greater than 60 to 70 mm Hg. The exact CPP value to target is controversial, and indeed it may need to be higher in some patients with evidence of regional or global ischemia. Targets may be achieved by either decreasing ICP, using techniques mentioned later in this chapter, or increasing MAP via volume expansion, inotropes, and vasopressors.

The correlation between arterial blood pressure and ICP waves can be used to create a pressure reactivity index (PRx) that may reflect cerebrovascular autoregulation in response to changes in blood pressure. A PRx of less than 0.3 is thought to reflect an intact cerebrovascular response, whereas a PRx higher than 0.3 indicates an impaired response (i.e., ICP follows MAP in a linear fashion) and has been associated with a poorer clinical outcome (see Chapter 40).

Ventilatory Support and the Use of Hypocapnia for Intracranial Pressure Reduction

A Glasgow Coma Scale (GCS) score of 8 or less, ventilatory failure, central neurogenic hyperventilation, and recurrent seizures are all indications for intubation and ventilation. Reasonable targets include a Pao_2 higher than 75 mm Hg (10 kPa) and a $Paco_2$ of 36 to 40 mm Hg (4.5 to 5.0 kPa).

Hyperventilation has been shown to increase the volume of hypoperfused tissue in a severely injured brain. Therefore, although it is effective in rapidly reducing ICP, prolonged or profound hyperventilation may further stress the traumatized brain and lead to secondary neuronal damage.

Fluid Therapy

Fluid management aimed at restoring euvolemia and preventing hypotension is important in acute head trauma. However, it may be complicated by hemorrhage, concealed or continuing, from associated extracranial trauma. Clinical and laboratory assessment of fluid status should guide fluid replacement, which usually involves administration of maintenance fluids at 30 to 40 mL/kg daily.

Nutrition

By the seventh day after trauma, these patients require 140% of resting metabolic expenditure, with 15% of these calories being supplied as protein. Early feeding may be associated with a trend toward improved survival and decreased disability. If enteral feeding cannot be achieved, parenteral feeding with gastric stress ulcer prophylaxis and good glycemic control should be considered.

Thromboprophylaxis

Neurotrauma patients, particularly those with extracranial injuries, are at increased risk for the development of venous thromboembolism. Although the evidence is limited, it is generally agreed that therapeutic doses of anticoagulants should be avoided until improvement of the intracranial pathology/hemorrhage is seen on computed tomography (CT). Prophylactic doses of heparin may be safe from the second to third day after injury. Reasonable but unproven alternatives include the nonpharmacologic methods of elastic stockings or pneumatic compression devices.

Hyperosmolar Therapy

Hyperosmolar therapy is an effective means of elevating plasma osmolarity and decreasing cerebral edema. Hypertonic saline has been shown to produce better ICP control than mannitol does, but no significant difference in either neurologic outcome or mortality has been demonstrated. To avoid side effects, these fluids should be discontinued when ICP no longer responds significantly. Care should be taken to monitor intravascular volume status, not allow plasma osmolality to rise above 320 mOsm/L, and keep plasma sodium below 155 mmol/L.

Sedation and Suppression of Cerebral Metabolism

Intravenous anesthetic agents cause a dose-dependent reduction in both the cerebral metabolic rate of oxygen ($CMRO_2$) and CBF. However, this flow-metabolism coupling may be impaired in neurotrauma, and thus the reduction in CBF may be greater than that in $CMRO_2$, which leads to widening of the cerebral arteriovenous oxygen content difference.

Although agents such as propofol are preferred over barbiturates because of their better pharmacokinetic profiles, propofol may induce both hypotension and a decrease in CPP, especially in volume-depleted patients. Midazolam is an alternative, but its accumulation means that propofol is often preferable if rapid emergence is required. Intravenous barbiturates are effective in reducing ICP. However, their side effect profile, which includes cardiovascular depression, longer intensive care stay, and increased respiratory infections, means that they are generally reserved for use in intracranial hypertension refractory to other treatments.

Analgesia

Effective analgesia for these patients, who often have multiple injuries, is important to reduce the autonomic responses to stimulation. Opioids have minimal effect on cerebral metabolism, blood flow, and ICP, as long as ventilation and normotension are preserved.

Neuromuscular Blockade

Prophylactic neuromuscular blockade is associated with longer intensive care unit stay, a higher incidence of respiratory complications, and with some agents, neuromyopathy without a concomitant improvement in outcome. However, these drugs can help prevent rises in ICP produced by coughing and straining on the endotracheal tube. Atracurium is often used because it does not accumulate and has not been associated with myopathy.

34

Seizure Prophylaxis

Risk factors for the development of post-traumatic seizures include GCS scores lower than 10, cortical contusion, intracranial hematoma, depressed skull fracture, or a penetrating injury. There is some evidence to support prophylaxis in these patients to prevent early (within 7 days of injury) seizures, but anticonvulsants appear to be less useful in preventing the occurrence of late seizures.

Hypothermia

Hypothermia reduces cerebral metabolism with a concurrent reduction in ICP. However, apart from one clinical trial[10] indicating that a subgroup of patients with GCS scores of 5 to 6 may benefit, there has been little evidence that hypothermia improves outcome. Other questions, including the optimal timing and degree of hypothermia required for neuroprotection, are yet to be answered. Caution is advised because of the known side effects of cooling, which include suppression of innate immunity. Hyperthermia should certainly be avoided because it has been shown to worsen outcome after brain injury.

Steroids

The routine use of corticosteroids in head injury to reduce edema is not currently recommended. A randomized placebo-controlled trial (Corticosteroid Randomization after Significant Head Injury [CRASH]) assessing the use of intravenous corticosteroids showed that at both 2 weeks and 6 months the risk for death or poor neurologic outcome was higher in the group given methylprednisolone.

Decompressive Craniectomy

Surgical treatment of brain edema via decompressive craniectomy allows the injured brain space to swell thus lowering ICP and improving CPP, either early, with removal bone flap when a mass lesion is evacuated (primary craniectomy), or later when other measures of ICP control have been or are nearly exhausted. While this technique has been shown to be effective in lowering ICP there is currently no level I evidence that it improves functional outcome. To address this question there are currently two multicentre prospective randomized controlled trials being performed; RESCUEicp (Randomised Evaluation of Surgery with Craniectomy for Uncontrollable Elevation of Intra-Cranial Pressure, www.rescueicp.com) and the DECRA Trial (Early Decompressive Craniectomy in Patients with Severe Traumatic Brain Injury, http://clinicaltrials.gov/show/NCT00155987).

HEAD INJURY MANAGEMENT PROTOCOLS

Many therapeutic options are available for neurotrauma, the efficacy of which has often not yet been tested. When combined with the heterogeneous nature of the pathophysiology, it can be difficult to devise appropriate treatment plans to encompass all patients and all scenarios. Nonetheless, protocol-driven therapy has been shown to improve outcomes in the specialist setting. Thus, many centers have devised protocols for the management of patients with neurotrauma; these protocols tend to involve a stepwise escalation of treatment with the choice of intervention guided by clinical and physiologic parameters. Figure 34-1 illustrates the ICP/CPP management

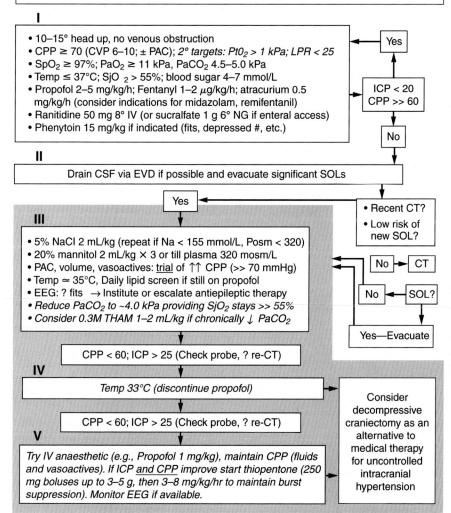

Figure 34-1 Addenbrooke's NCCU ICP/CPP management algorithm. CPP, cerebral perfusion pressure; CSF, cerebrospinal fluid; CVP, central venous pressure; EEG, electroencephalogram; EVD, external ventricular drain; ICP, intracranial pressure; LPR, lactate-pyruvate ratio; NCCU, neurosciences critical care unit; NG, nasogastric tube; PAC, pulmonary artery catheter; $Paco_2$, arterial carbon dioxide partial pressure; Pao_2, arterial oxygen partial pressure; Pto_2, brain tissue oxygen partial pressure; Rt, right; Rx, therapy; Sjo_2, jugular bulb oxygen saturation; SOLs, space-occupying lesions; THAM, tris(hydroxymethyl)aminomethane.

protocol used in the neurosciences critical care unit (NCCU) at Addenbrooke's Hospital, University of Cambridge in the United Kingdom.

KEY POINTS

- The main aim of management is to prevent secondary brain injury, particularly by avoiding hypoxia and hypotension.
- The use of multimodal monitoring can help facilitate the early identification and treatment of secondary insults.
- ICP should be kept below 20 to 25 mm Hg.
- A CPP higher than 60 mm Hg is currently recommended by the Brain Trauma Foundation.
- After injury there is regional heterogeneity in CBF and metabolism that may not be identified by common monitoring methods.

FURTHER READING

Hyam JA, Welch CA, Harrison DA, Menon DK: Case mix, outcomes and comparison of risk prediction models for admissions to adult, general and specialist critical care units for head injury: A secondary analysis of the ICNARC Case Mix Programme Database. Crit Care 2006; 10(Suppl 2):S2.

The Brain Trauma Foundation: Management and prognosis of severe traumatic brain injury. 2000, last updated 2003. http://www.braintrauma.org

Adamides AA, Winter CD, Lewis PM, et al: Current controversies in the management of patients with severe traumatic brain injury. Aust N Z J Surg 2006; 76:163-174.

Nortje J, Menon DK: Traumatic brain injury: Physiology, mechanisms, and outcome. Curr Opin Neurol 2004; 17:711-718.

Coles JP, Fryer TD, Smielewski P, et al: Incidence and mechanisms of cerebral ischemia in early clinical head injury. J Cereb Blood Flow Metab 2004; 24:202-211.

Lang EW, Lagopoulos J, Griffith J, et al: Cerebral vasomotor reactivity testing in head injury: The link between pressure and flow. J Neurol Neurosurg Psychiatry 2003; 74:1053-1059.

Perel P, Yanagawa T, Bunn F, et al: Nutritional support for head-injured patients. Cochrane Database Syst Rev 2006; 4. CD001530.

Denson K, Morgan D, Cunningham R, et al: Incidence of venous thromboembolism in patients with traumatic brain injury. Am J Surg 2007; 193:380-383; discussion 383-384.

Vialet R, Albanese J, Thomachet L, et al: Isovolume hypertonic solutes (sodium chloride or mannitol) in the treatment of refractory posttraumatic intracranial hypertension: 2 mL/kg 7.5% saline is more effective than 2 mL/kg 20% mannitol. Crit Care Med 2003; 31:1683-1687.

Polderman KH, Tjong Tjin Joe R, Peerdeman SM, Vandertop WP, Girbes AR: Effects of therapeutic hypothermia on intracranial pressure and outcome in patients with severe head injury, Intensive Care Med 28 (2002) 1563-1573.

Edwards P, Arango M, Balica L, et al: Final results of MRC CRASH, a randomised placebo-controlled trial of intravenous corticosteroid in adults with head injury—outcomes at 6 months. Lancet 2005; 365:1957-1959.

V

Chapter 35

Intracranial Hemorrhage: Intensive Care Management

Susan Ryan • Alexander Kopelnik • Jonathan Zaroff

Common causes of intracranial hemorrhage include subarachnoid hemorrhage (SAH) from an aneurysm, bleeding from an arteriovenous malformation (AVM) (see Chapter 17), or intracerebral bleed. The latter is commonly associated with hypertension, anticoagulation therapy or other coagulopathy, drug and alcohol abuse, neoplasia, or amyloid angiopathy. This chapter focuses on the intensive care management of SAH.

CLINICAL FINDINGS AND DIAGNOSIS

Patients with intracranial hemorrhage typically have a sudden onset of a severe headache accompanied by nausea, vomiting, neck stiffness, photophobia, and sometimes loss of consciousness. On examination, patients may have altered consciousness, meningismus, focal neurologic deficits, or retinal hemorrhage. Patients are commonly hypertensive and may have dysrhythmias and electrocardiographic (ECG) abnormalities.

Non–contrast-enhanced head computed tomography (CT) is the first step, followed by a lumbar puncture (LP) if the CT scan is nondiagnostic. If either the CT scan or LP suggests intracranial hemorrhage, further characterization of the vascular abnormality should be obtained with cerebral angiography or CT angiography.

INITIAL MANAGEMENT

Rupture of an aneurysm allows blood to flow into the subarachnoid space with the rapid development of multiple sequelae. SAH induces catecholamine surges with resulting hypertension, dysrhythmias, and possible cardiac damage. Hemorrhage may result in elevated intracranial pressure (ICP) from the volume of blood alone, as well as from surrounding edema or impaired ventricular drainage. Neurologic

35

dysfunction ranges from headache to coma. Initial management focuses on (1) management of hemodynamic and cardiac issues, (2) airway and ventilatory management in the setting of neurologic dysfunction, and (3) evaluation of neurologic function and the need for ICP monitoring or ventricular drainage, or both.

Hemodynamic Control

Most patients with intracranial hemorrhage have some degree of hypertension. Because hypertension may contribute to rebleeding, blood pressure should be maintained within a normotensive range until the aneurysm or AVM is treated. "Normotensive" may refer to the individual's baseline blood pressure, but typically a target mean arterial pressure (MAP) of less than 100 mm Hg is recommended. Although higher blood pressure may be desirable in patients with elevated ICP or vasospasm, the risk of rebleeding and the benefits of relative hypertension must be considered on an individual basis.

Initial antihypertensive therapy should include short-acting agents. Antihypertensives that are not significant vasodilators, such as β-blockers and labetalol, are preferred over hydralazine and calcium channel blockers because vasodilation could worsen elevated ICP. However, elevated ICP is often much less of an issue in patients with an external ventricular drain in place. With persistent hypertension, an intravenous infusion of labetalol or nicardipine will provide more consistent control. Headaches should be treated with the judicious use of analgesics, which may also improve hypertension. Patients with SAH are normally commenced on therapy with the calcium channel blocker nimodipine, which in theory acts as a neuroprotectant agent (despite the concern for vasodilation) and may also decrease blood pressure, particularly when administered intravenously. There is no evidence to suggest that nimodipine is of any benefit for intracranial hemorrhage not resulting from SAH.

A smaller group of patients may have hypotension that may be due to myocardial dysfunction, usually caused by SAH. Myocardial infarction secondary to coronary artery disease in addition to subendocardial ischemia associated with catecholamine surges after SAH must also be considered.

Subarachnoid Hemorrhage–Related Cardiac Abnormalities

Cardiac abnormalities after SAH can be divided into ECG abnormalities, cardiac arrhythmias, myocardial injury, and ventricular dysfunction. All patients with SAH should have a 12-lead electrocardiogram performed regardless of age at admission.

Electrocardiographic Abnormalities

Forty percent to 70% of SAH patients exhibit ECG abnormalities. QT prolongation is the most common (70%) ECG abnormality, followed by inverted or flat T waves (55%), ST-segment changes (28%), and new U waves (15%). ECG changes do not require specific treatment. Cardiovascular monitoring and appropriate testing should be pursued to identify causes or contributors in addition to SAH.

Cardiac Arrhythmias

Arrhythmias may contribute to mortality, and most occur within the first week. They are seen in 35% to 100% of patients and include bradycardia, supraventricular tachycardia, atrial flutter, atrial fibrillation, ectopic beats, ventricular tachycardia, torsades de pointes, and ventricular fibrillation. Up to 5% may suffer a life-threatening ventricular arrhythmia. Arrhythmias should be managed immediately according to advanced cardiac life support guidelines, and hypokalemia, hypomagnesemia, and acidosis must be corrected. Drugs that prolong the QT interval should be discontinued.

Myocardial Injury and Dysfunction

SAH may induce neurocardiogenic injury. Catecholamine-induced subendocardial lesions typically occur in the vicinity of the cardiac nerves and not in the distribution seen in patients with coronary disease. SAH may produce a functional cardiac denervation that is associated with release of troponin and regional wall motion abnormalities on echocardiography.

Cardiac enzyme elevations, indicative of myocardial necrosis, are common in SAH. Elevated creatine kinase (CK) levels are seen in 45% of patients, and there is good correlation between elevation in CK-MB and ECG changes or cardiac arrhythmias. Cardiac troponin I elevations have been described in 25% of patients. Global or regional left ventricular systolic dysfunction has been described in 10% to 28% of SAH patients. Diastolic dysfunction is also common and is associated with the severity of neurologic injury and may be the cause of pulmonary edema. Left ventricular dysfunction occurs early in the course of SAH and may normalize over time.

Neurocardiogenic injury has implications beyond straightforward cardiac morbidity and mortality. An association exists between myocardial injury or dysfunction and adverse neurologic outcomes. In some SAH patients, reduction of cardiac output from normally elevated levels may increase their risk for cerebral ischemia related to vasospasm. Troponin elevation after SAH is associated with an increased risk for cardiopulmonary complications, delayed cerebral ischemia, and death or poor functional outcome at discharge. An elevated brain natriuretic peptide level is independently associated with delayed ischemic neurologic deficits, predicts the 2-week Glasgow Coma Scale score, and is an independent and strong predictor of inpatient mortality after SAH.

The current focus of treatment should be on the underlying neurologic injury because the cause of cardiac injury is neurogenic and the degree of cardiac injury is related to the severity of SAH. In the majority of cases, treatment of the cardiac injury should be supportive. β-Blockers may provide cardioprotection but to date have no proven mortality benefit.

Pulmonary/Airway Management

Patients with intracranial hemorrhage are at risk for pulmonary complications, most commonly pneumonia, pulmonary edema, and aspiration, which may require intubation and mechanical ventilation.

If a patient requires intubation, hypertension should be avoided during laryngoscopy. Mechanical ventilation should provide adequate oxygenation and ventilation with a normal Po_2, Pco_2, and pH. In addition, patients with neurologic injury often generate high minute ventilation (above the ventilator settings) with resulting alkalemia. Only if this produces dangerous or symptomatic extremes of alkalemia or hypocapnia should sedation be increased to decrease ventilation and normalize blood gas values.

Sedation

Sedation is usually necessary to reduce agitation, provide comfort, and allow better synchrony with the ventilator, all of which will permit better hemodynamic control and enable management of ICP and cerebral perfusion pressure. Propofol provides sedation with the best pharmacokinetic/dynamic profile, and the addition of an opioid such as fentanyl, sufentanil, or remifentanil helps reduce the total dose of propofol used. For patients requiring longer-term sedation (>48 hours), midazolam can be used as a substitute for propofol. Neuromuscular blockade may be used as an adjunct to sedative agents if necessary to assist with ventilator synchrony and to control ICP. Atracurium and cisatracurium are the most commonly used agents because they are noncumulative. However, many neuromuscular blocking agents, including atracurium, have been associated with myopathy; they should be used only when necessary and terminated as quickly as possible.

Seizure Prophylaxis

The risk of seizures in SAH is relatively low. About 10% of patients will experience seizures within several weeks of the initial hemorrhage. There is no evidence to support seizure prophylaxis.

Detection and Treatment of Vasospasm

Patients are at risk for vasospasm from approximately day 4 to day 16, with the peak incidence occurring on days 5 to 10 after SAH. Subarachnoid blood and blood breakdown products such as hemosiderin incite inflammation and leukocyte infiltration into adjacent blood vessels, which then become thickened and potentially spastic. About two thirds of patients demonstrate angiographic vasospasm, whereas 30% to 50% become symptomatic. Focal or global neurologic dysfunction can develop as a result of vasospasm-induced cerebral ischemia. In patients in whom vasospasm develops, the risk of stroke or death is 20%.

Neuroangiography is currently the diagnostic "gold standard" for vasospasm; however, this is not a practical daily diagnostic solution. Transcranial Doppler ultrasonography is currently the most frequently used noninvasive technique to diagnose vasospasm, but its sensitivity varies by vessel and it is subject to operator-dependent results. Promising methods that more directly detect shifts in cerebral blood flow and ischemia include perfusion-sensitive CT and magnetic resonance imaging.

Hemodynamic augmentation of cerebral perfusion has become a well-accepted medical therapy for symptomatic vasospasm. This therapy is commonly referred to as HHH, or "triple-H" therapy, because of the three simultaneous goals of hypertension, hypervolemia, and hemodilution. A hypertensive blood pressure is targeted and volume is augmented with crystalloid (0.9% NaCl) or colloid (albumin) solutions. If the degree of hypertension is inadequate for the target cerebral perfusion pressure and neurologic deficits persist, pressors, inotropes, or both are used. Dopamine, phenylephrine, and norepinephrine are all acceptable drugs for increasing blood pressure.

In general, MAP between 110 and 120 mm Hg should be targeted in patients whose aneurysms have been secured. In those who have unsecured aneurysms, the target MAP should be 90 to 100 mm Hg. Blood flow characteristics are best at a hemoglobin value of 10, and patients do not generally receive transfusions above this value. Even though no prospective, double-blind, controlled trials of triple-H therapy exist at this point, this therapy is commonly used and considered effective. The benefit of prophylactic triple-H therapy in asymptomatic patients, however, remains more controversial.

Although the majority of patients tolerates triple-H therapy, cardiopulmonary and neurologic complications can occur. Complications identified include congestive heart failure, myocardial ischemia and infarction, noncardiogenic pulmonary edema, and cerebral edema. A recent study found that phenylephrine is relatively ineffective in increasing blood pressure in patients with a low left ventricular ejection fraction. In this setting, additional inotropic therapy with dobutamine or milrinone may be effective. Norepinephrine offers an alternative that combines inotropy and increased vascular tone. Central monitoring that includes cardiac output will help guide inotropic therapy.

Endovascular Treatment of Vasospasm

Endovascular treatment of symptomatic vasospasm includes several effective and well-validated therapeutic strategies. They are most often used when medical management (some degree of triple-H therapy) has failed. An angiographically guided endovascular catheter first identifies the cerebral vessel or vessels in spasm. Balloon angioplasty (for larger vessels) or vasodilatory agents such as papaverine are selectively used to relieve the spasm. Complications of endovascular therapy include femoral vessel dissection and hemorrhage, cerebral vessel dissection or rupture, thrombosis leading to ischemia or stroke, and reperfusion cerebral edema. Triple-H therapy is typically continued after endovascular therapy for vasospasm.

Electrolyte Disturbances

The most commonly observed electrolyte disturbances include hyponatremia, hypomagnesemia, hypokalemia, and hypocalcemia. Hypomagnesemia is found in more than 50% of patients during their hospital stay. Early hypomagnesemia correlates with the extent of hemorrhage; later, it is also related to the occurrence of delayed cerebral ischemia and poor outcome at 3 months. Hypokalemia and hypocalcemia are also common in the early course of SAH and should be treated as needed. Although electrolyte abnormalities are associated with ECG abnormalities, the electrolyte values—not the ECG abnormalities—should guide replacement therapy.

Hyponatremia develops in 30% to 40% of patients. It is most often related to one of two distinct disorders: the syndrome of inappropriate antidiuretic hormone secretion (SIADH) and cerebral salt-wasting syndrome (CSWS). Patients with neurologic disease, as well as a variety of non-neurologic diseases, are at risk for SIADH. CSWS, on the other hand, results specifically from neurologic intracranial disease and is associated with increased levels of natriuretic peptides. It is critical to distinguish between these two entities because their therapeutic interventions are diametrically opposed (see Chapter 37).

GENERAL INTENSIVE CARE MANAGEMENT ISSUES

Patients with intracranial hemorrhage usually require management in an intensive care unit (ICU) for longer than 2 weeks. During this stay, patients are vulnerable to the usual ICU complications, as well as those specific to SAH. Current recommendations are briefly reviewed in Table 35-1.

DEFINITIVE TREATMENT

Definitive management of aneurysmal SAH and AVM is described in Chapter 17. Patients who have primary intracerebral bleeding with no evidence of aneurysm or AVM will require the primary cause to be treated, which may include control of hypertension or correction of coagulopathy. Evidence from the International

35

Table 35-1 Critical Care Issues for Patients with Intracranial Hemorrhage

General Issues	Diagnosis/Management Recommendations
Cardiovascular	Close blood pressure and volume monitoring and maintenance of euvolemia and normal blood pressure before aneurysm treatment; continue euvolemia but allow hypertension afterward; 12-lead ECG for all patients
Pulmonary	Aspiration precautions, head of the bed at 30 degrees or higher, VAP prevention protocols
Pain	Treat with simple analgesics or IV or PO narcotics with close monitoring; avoid NSAIDs
Activity	Ensure a quiet environment and bed rest before aneurysm treatment
Gastrointestinal	Prophylaxis with an H_2 blocker or PPI in all patients, stool softener to avoid constipation
Seizures	Treat with antiseizure medication; prophylaxis in the absence of seizure is controversial
Blood glucose	Treat hyperglycemia (above 120 mg/dL [10 mmol]) with IV insulin infusion
DVT prophylaxis	Provide stockings and sequential compression devices before aneurysm treatment; continue the same or consider SC heparin afterward
Fever	Treat with acetaminophen and active cooling if necessary; culture as indicated
Sedation	For patients who are mechanically ventilated, sedation with propofol or midazolam for amnesia, supplemented with intravenous short-acting opioid infusion, helps with ICP/CPP control and tube tolerance; neuromuscular blockade may be required
Condition (Complications)	
Myocardial Injury	Obtain an echocardiogram; monitor troponins, BNP; consider inotropic agents and pulmonary catheter monitoring for cardiac output
Arrhythmias	ACLS protocol and antiarrhythmics, correct electrolyte abnormalities, discontinue contributory medications
Vasospasm	Monitor by transcranial Doppler sonography and angiography, as well as examination. Medical treatment: triple-H therapy. Procedural intervention: endovascular cerebral angioplasty or vasodilation
Electrolytes	Correct abnormal electrolytes; for hyponatremia, distinguish between SIADH and CSWS for appropriate treatment
Pulmonary edema	Consider an echocardiogram as well as CXR to distinguish between cardiogenic and noncardiogenic edema; provide oxygen, ventilatory support
Pneumonia	Follow CXR and cultures; provide antibiotics, oxygen/ventilatory support as needed
Elevated ICP	CT for diagnosis; extraventricular drainage for cerebral edema, hydrocephalus, and intraventricular hemorrhage; surgery for decompression of hemorrhage or refractory edema

ACLS, advanced cardiac life support; BNP, brain natriuretic peptide; CPP, cerebral perfusion pressure; CSWS, cerebral salt-wasting syndrome; CT, computed tomography; CXR, chest x-ray; DVT, deep venous thrombosis; ECG, electrocardiogram; ICP, intracranial pressure; NSAIDs, nonsteroidal anti-inflammatory drugs; PPI, proton pump inhibitor; SIADH, syndrome of inappropriate antidiuretic hormone secretion; VAT, ventilator-associated pneumonia.

Surgical Trial in Intracerebral Haemorrhage (STICH) suggests that conservative medical management with surgery for clot removal if initial medical management fails has an outcome comparable to that of early surgery.

RESOLUTION OF INTENSIVE CARE UNIT ISSUES

Improvement in neurologic function and objective indicators of resolution of vasospasm should guide the length of triple-H therapy and the need for close ICU observation. Once triple-H therapy is terminated, patients should be carefully observed for possible recurrence of symptoms. Nimodipine is usually administered for 21 days, and because hypertension is a common comorbidity, continued antihypertensive therapy may be indicated. The degree of persistent neurologic impairment after the period of susceptibility to vasospasm will begin to determine the level of support required by a patient in a number of areas. Tracheostomy should be considered for ventilator-dependent patients. Patients requiring nutrition by feeding tube may benefit from gastrostomy or jejunostomy tube placement. Longer-term deep venous thrombosis prophylaxis should also be considered in relatively immobile patients. For the majority of patients with intracranial hemorrhage, physical and occupational therapy may be the next step.

KEY POINTS

- Major sources of morbidity & mortality include: Neurologic (ischemia from vasospasm and elevated ICP); Cardiopulmonary (arrhythmias, myocardial injury, pulmonary edema) and Electrolyte abnormalities (hypomagnesemia, hypokalemia, and hyponatremia).
- Initial management focuses on: appropriate cerebral perfusion pressure to prevent ischemia or rerupture and treatment of elevated ICP; correction of electrolyte abnormalities; stabilization of cardiopulmonary status.
- Sedation and pain management consistent with neurologic status and monitoring are key components for comfort, improved ICP and hypertension, and, if intubated, synchrony with the ventilator.
- Definitive treatment of the aneurysm should be provided early. Both surgical clipping and endovascular coiling are acceptable treatments.
- Vasospasm occurs from days to weeks following SAH. All patients should receive nimodipine. Symptomatic vasospasm should be treated expeditiously.
- Symptomatic vasospasm is first treated medically with HHH therapy (hypertension, hemodilution, hypervolemia). Persistent symptomatic vasospasm can be treated by selective intracerebral arterial angioplasty and intra-arterial vasodilators.

35

FURTHER READING

Hoh BL, Ogilvy CS: Endovascular treatment of cerebral vasospasm: Transluminal balloon angioplasty, intra-arterial papaverine, and intra-arterial nicardipine. Neurosurg Clin N Am 2005; 16:vi, 501-516.

Mayer S, Lin J, Homma S, et al: Myocardial injury and left ventricular performance after subarachnoid hemorrhage. Stroke 1999; 30:780-786.

McGirt MJ, Blessing R, Nimjee SM, et al: Correlation of serum brain natriuretic peptide with hyponatremia and delayed ischemic neurological deficits after subarachnoid hemorrhage. Neurosurgery 2004; 54:1369-1373; discussion 1373-1364.

Mendelow AD, Gregson BA, Fernandes HM, et al: Early surgery versus initial conservative treatment in patients with spontaneous supratentorial intracerebral haematomas in the International Surgical Trial in Intracerebral Haemorrhage (STICH): A randomised trial. Lancet 2005; 365:387-397.

Naidech AM, Kreiter KT, Janjua N, et al: Cardiac troponin elevation, cardiovascular morbidity, and outcome after subarachnoid hemorrhage. Circulation 2005; 112:2851-2856.

Naval NS, Stevens RD, Mirski MA, Bhardwaj A: Controversies in the management of aneurysmal subarachnoid hemorrhage. Crit Care Med 2006; 34:511-524.

Suarez JI, Tarr RW, Selman WR: Aneurysmal subarachnoid hemorrhage. N Engl J Med 2006; 354: 387-396.

Tisdall M, Crocker M, Watkins J, Smith M: Disturbances of sodium in critically ill adult neurologic patients: A clinical review. J Neurosurg Anesthesiol 2006; 18:57-63.

Treggiari MM, Walder B, Suter PM, Romand JA: Systematic review of the prevention of delayed ischemic neurological deficits with hypertension, hypervolemia, and hemodilution therapy following subarachnoid hemorrhage. J Neurosurg 2003; 98:978-984.

Tung P, Kopelnik A, Banki N, et al: Predictors of neurocardiogenic injury after subarachnoid hemorrhage. Stroke 2004; 35:548-551.

V

Chapter 36

Fluid Management

David Zygun

Indications for Administration of Fluid and Resuscitation End Points

Monitoring Fluid Status

Fluid Administration in Neurologically Injured Patients

Hyperosmolar Therapy

Fluid management strategies need to be individualized and guided by an understanding of the underlying pathophysiologic mechanisms because there is a paucity of clinical outcome evidence. This chapter reviews the common indications for fluid administration, fluid resuscitation end points, and types of fluids and discusses issues pertinent to neurologically injured patients.

INDICATIONS FOR ADMINISTRATION OF FLUID AND RESUSCITATION END POINTS

Routine maintenance fluid is perhaps the most common indication for administration of fluid in hospitalized patients. The "4-2-1 rule" provides an approximation of hourly water requirements (4 mL/kg for each kilogram of body weight up to 10 kg + 2 mL/kg for body weight of 11 to 20 kg + 1 mL/kg for each kilogram of body weight over 20 kg). The daily sodium requirement (1.5 mEq/kg/day or mmol/kg/day) is dissolved in the daily fluid requirement. The daily potassium requirement (1 mEq/kg/day) is commonly included in the daily fluid requirement, although this may be limited because of chemical irritation when delivered through a peripheral vein. Fluid management of perioperative patients must also take into account the vasodilation and cardiac depression caused by anesthesia and sedation, unreplaced preoperative deficits, ongoing losses, and redistribution of third-space losses.

MONITORING FLUID STATUS

The traditional markers of the adequacy of fluid resuscitation, including heart rate, blood pressure, and urine output, remain essential indicators of successful resuscitation. However, despite normalization of these markers, a considerable proportion of patients will have evidence of inadequate tissue oxygenation. Level 1 recommendations include use of the initial base deficit, lactate level, or gastric intramucosal pH (pHi) to stratify patients with regard to the need for ongoing fluid resuscitation and the risk for multiple organ dysfunction syndrome and death.

36

The use of central venous pressure (CVP) and pulmonary artery occlusion pressure (PAOP) as a measure of intravascular filling is relatively common. In clinical practice, the relationship between intravascular volume and filling pressure cannot be assumed to be linear and most certainly is dynamic over short periods of time. Furthermore, the response to fluids is not reliably predicted from any given level of filling pressure. Pulse pressure variability ($\%PPV = [PPmax - PPmin]/[\{PPmax + PPmin\}/2] \times 100\%$) and systolic pressure variability ($\%SPV = [SBPmax - SBPmin]/[\{SBPmax + SBPmin\}/2] \times 100\%$) have been shown to be better predictors of response to fluid management than PAOP and CVP are. Thus, although the trends are clinically useful, the use of absolute values of PAOP or CVP as predictors of fluid responsiveness is not advised.

There is a paucity of studies regarding optimal transfusion practice in the neuro-critical care population. Animal studies have suggested that a hematocrit of 30% to 33% may optimize the balance of viscosity and oxygen-carrying capacity whereas a hematocrit of 42% to 45% maximizes oxygen delivery in normal humans. However, recent evidence suggests that although transfusion in patients with brain injury may improve cerebral tissue oxygenation, a significant effect on cellular metabolism was not observed. Thus, definitive transfusion practice recommendations in patients with neurologic injury cannot be made at this time.

FLUID ADMINISTRATION IN NEUROLOGICALLY INJURED PATIENTS

Lactated Ringer's solution and normal saline distribute evenly throughout the extracellular space and are essentially isotonic with human plasma. Sodium is the primary osmotically active particle. Only a fifth to a quarter of the infused volume remains in the intravascular space 1 hour after infusion. Colloid solutions contain albumin or synthetic molecules that are relatively impermeable to the vascular membrane. Albumin is responsible for 80% of plasma colloid oncotic pressure. This protein distributes throughout the extracellular space, and it stays in the intravascular compartment longer than crystalloids do (half-life, 16 hours). Synthetic colloids include hydroxyethyl starch, modified gelatin, and dextran. However, optimal use of crystalloids and colloids in fluid management continues to be a matter of debate. Survey data suggest that no clear consensus exists among clinicians and that strategies vary widely across clinical situations.

A multicenter, randomized, double-blind trial published in 2004 compared the effect of resuscitation with albumin or saline on mortality in a heterogeneous population of nearly 7000 patients in the intensive care unit (ICU) (the SAFE study). There were no significant differences between groups in the mean numbers of days spent in the ICU, days spent in the hospital, days of mechanical ventilation, or days of renal replacement therapy. A trend toward improved survival was observed in patients with severe sepsis who were randomized to the albumin group. However, there was also a worse outcome in the traumatic brain-injured patients randomized to albumin. These results are congruent with findings by Neff and colleagues, who performed a prospective, randomized, controlled trial of the safety of large doses of medium-molecular-weight hydroxyethyl starch in patients with traumatic brain injury. The control group, which received a different starch and albumin as an add-on colloid, had a significantly higher incidence of intracranial pressure (ICP) peaks above 30 mm Hg and more cumulative hours of elevated ICP. This suggests that the type of colloid may not simply be interchangeable.

Although negative fluid balance during the first 96 hours has been associated with detrimental outcomes in patients with traumatic brain injury and the use of colloids may facilitate the clinician's ability to control this parameter, one cannot ignore the potential negative effect of albumin on outcome in patients with traumatic brain injury, nor the detrimental effects of crystalloids in some experimental studies. In particular, hypo-osmolar solutions such as 5% dextrose in water reduce serum sodium and increase brain water and ICP and should be strictly avoided in patients with neurologic injury. Moreover, dextrose-containing solutions contribute to hyperglycemia. After neurologic injury, hyperglycemia has been associated with increased areas of contusion, enhanced neutrophil accumulation experimentally, and poor neurologic outcome.

Overall, unfortunately, there is insufficient evidence to make definitive recommendations regarding the optimal use of crystalloids or colloids in terms of patient outcome in the neurocritical care population.

HYPEROSMOLAR THERAPY

Hyperosmolar therapy is used for the treatment of patients with cerebral edema and intracranial hypertension. These solutions are thought to treat intracranial hypertension through plasma expansion with optimization of blood hematocrit, blood viscosity, and cerebral blood volume. In addition, creation of an osmotic gradient may draw fluid from brain tissue into the vasculature and thereby reduce total brain volume.

Mannitol (0.25 to 1 g/kg) has been used for decades and has a well-recognized side effect profile. Its main mechanisms of action include osmotic removal of water from the brain, especially when the blood-brain barrier is intact. In addition, mannitol improves blood rheology, which increases cerebral blood flow and results in autoregulation-mediated vasoconstriction, as well as helps reduce ICP. It may also act as a free radical scavenger and inhibit programmed cell death. Its main side effect is an osmotic-mediated diuresis that can result in intravascular volume depletion. Volume depletion commonly results in hypotension, an important secondary insult to the brain and strongly associated with poor neurologic outcome. Mannitol may cross a damaged blood-brain barrier and consequently worsen cerebral edema and ICP. There is also debatable concern regarding the maximum safe osmolarity (commonly cited as 320 mOsm/L). Hyperosmolality has been shown to have little association with mortality until it exceeds approximately 340 mOsm/L.

Hypertonic saline solutions may be more effective in reducing ICP and have a longer duration of action than mannitol does. In addition, hypertonic saline may provide blood-brain barrier protection and beneficially modulate the inflammatory response to injury. Similar to mannitol, hypertonic saline is a volume-expanding agent, but its use is not accompanied by subsequent osmotic diuresis. Disadvantages of hypertonic saline include non–anion gap metabolic acidosis, unknown safe maximum serum concentration (serum sodium concentrations >160 mmol/L have been independently associated with a poor outcome), and unknown optimal dosing (use of 3%, 5%, 7.5%, and 23% solutions has been reported).

KEY POINTS

- The most common indications for fluid therapy include maintenance fluid and treatment of intravascular volume depletion.
- Fluid resuscitation end points include heart rate, blood pressure, urine output, base deficit, gastric pHi, lactate, pulse pressure variability, and systolic pressure variability.

- There is little convincing evidence that the choice of colloid or crystalloid has a differential effect on patient outcome. However, hypo-osmolar and glucose-containing solutions should be avoided in those with neurologic injury.
- Albumin solutions may be beneficial in focal cerebral ischemia, including patients with subarachnoid hemorrhage, but current evidence associates albumin with worsened outcomes in traumatic brain injury. Isotonic crystalloid should be considered first line in the resuscitation of patients with traumatic injuries.
- Hypertonic solutions may be used in the management of intracranial hypertension. Plasma osmolality (<320 mOsm/L or osmotic gap <20), sodium concentration (<160 mmol/L), and renal function need to be carefully monitored during administration of hypertonic fluid.

FURTHER READING

Clifton GL, Miller ER, Choi SC, Levin HS: Fluid thresholds and outcome from severe brain injury. Crit Care Med 2002; 30:739-745.

Finfer S, Bellomo R, Boyce N, French J, Myburgh J, Norton R; SAFE Study Investigators. A comparison of albumin and saline for fluid resuscitation in the intensive care unit. N Engl J Med. 2004 May 27;350(22): 2247-56.

Finfer S, Bellomo R, Boyce N, et al: A comparison of albumin and saline for fluid resuscitation in the intensive care unit. N Engl J Med 2004; 350:2247-2256.

Kramer A, Zygun D, Hawes H, et al: Pulse pressure variation predicts fluid responsiveness following coronary artery bypass surgery. Chest 2004; 126:1563-1568.

Neff TA, Doelberg M, Jungheinrich C, et al: Repetitive large-dose infusion of the novel hydroxyethyl starch 130/0.4 in patients with severe head injury. Anesth Analg 2003; 96:1453-1459.

Pendem S, Rana S, Manno EM, Gajic O: A review of red cell transfusion in the neurological intensive care unit. Neurocrit Care 2006; 4:63-67.

Suarez JI, Shannon L, Zaidat OO, et al: Effect of human albumin administration on clinical outcome and hospital cost in patients with subarachnoid hemorrhage. J Neurosurg 2004; 100:585-590.

Tisherman SA, Barie P, Bokhari F, et al: Clinical practice guideline: Endpoints of resuscitation. J Trauma 2004; 57:898-912.

V

Chapter 37

Electrolyte Disorders

Adam Peets • David Zygun

Sodium Disorders	**Magnesium Disorders**
Hyponatremia	Hypomagnesemia
Hypernatremia	**Phosphate Disorders**
Potassium Disorders	Hypophosphatemia
Hypokalemia	
Hyperkalemia	

An electrolyte disorder is an imbalance of ionized salts in the blood. A complete review of all electrolyte disturbances is beyond the scope of this chapter. Common electrolyte disorders encountered in clinical practice include hyponatremia, hypernatremia, hypokalemia, hyperkalemia, hypophosphatemia, and hypomagnesemia. This chapter reviews the manifestations and management of these disorders with a specific focus on patients with neurologic disorders.

SODIUM DISORDERS

Sodium is the primary cation in extracellular fluid. It is a crucial component of the electrochemical gradient responsible for nerve conduction and cellular function. Sodium is the major osmole in blood and therefore determines extracellular fluid volume.

Hyponatremia

Hyponatremia is present when the serum sodium concentration is less than 136 mmol/L. Symptoms of hyponatremia include headache, nausea, vomiting, muscle cramps, lethargy, and seizures. Severe acute hyponatremia may result in cerebral edema and subsequent coma and respiratory arrest. A general approach to the causes of hyponatremia is presented in Figure 37-1. The syndrome of inappropriate antidiuretic hormone secretion (SIADH) and cerebral salt wasting (CSW) are two potential causes of hyponatremia in patients with disorders of the central nervous system.

Syndrome of Inappropriate Antidiuretic Hormone Secretion

This hypotonic hyponatremia is due to excessive release of arginine vasopressin (ADH) with subsequent water reabsorption. Patients with SIADH are in a water-expanded state but do not usually display signs of intravascular volume expansion

37

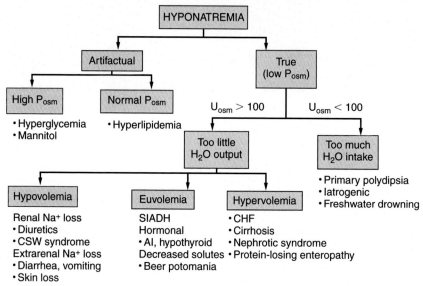

Figure 37-1 Approach to hyponatremia. AI, adrenal insufficiency; CHF, congestive heart failure; CSW, cerebral salt wasting; P_{osm}, plasma osmolarity; SIADH, syndrome of inappropriate antidiuretic hormone secretion; U_{osm}, urine osmolarity.

because two thirds of the total retained water remains in the intracellular compartment. A diagnosis of SIADH requires hyponatremia, hypo-osmolality, inappropriately high urine osmolality, and exclusion of hypoadrenalism and hypothyroidism. Neurologic conditions commonly associated with SIADH include central nervous system infection, intracranial hemorrhage, traumatic brain injury, brain neoplasm, and cerebral vasculitis or thrombosis. Certain drugs, most commonly narcotics, can also induce the release of ADH. Physiologic stimuli of ADH should also be considered, including pain, nausea, hypovolemia, and stress.

Cerebral Salt Wasting

CSW is a primary natriuresis observed in those with neurologic injury. It results in negative sodium balance and volume depletion. The cause probably relates to circulating natriuretic factors or decreased sympathetic input to the kidney, or both. Clinical assessment of extracellular fluid volume is an important discriminatory element to differentiate SIADH and CSW syndrome (Table 37-1).

Management

Treatment of hyponatremia depends on the underlying cause. Disorders of increased water intake, SIADH, and hypervolemic states generally require free water restriction, whereas other disorders such as CSW require sodium replacement. The rapidity of correction of hyponatremia must take into account the rate of its development and associated symptoms. In general, a 0.5-mmol/L increase in serum sodium per hour with a maximum total increase in 24 hours of 10 to 12 mmol/L is recommended. If the patient is seizing or has acute hyponatremia-related cerebral edema, hypertonic saline is administered for 2 to 4 hours with the goal of a 1.5- to 2.0-mmol/L/hr increase in sodium concentration. Because intravascular volume depletion must be avoided in those with neurologic injury, hypertonic saline infusions may be necessary. However, this therapy is not without risk and must be provided only in

Table 37-1   Differentiating the Syndromes of Inappropriate Antidiuretic Hormone Secretion and Cerebral Salt Wasting

	SIADH	CSW
Extracellular fluid volume	↔ or slightly ↑	↓
Serum [Na⁺]	↓	↓
Urine osmolarity	↑	↑
Urine [Na⁺]	↑	↑↑
Urine volume	↔ or ↓	↑ or ↑↑
Serum urate	↓	↔ or ↓
Hematocrit	↔	↑
[Albumin]	↔	↑
Blood urea nitrogen/creatinine	↔ or ↓	↑
Serum [K⁺]	↔	↔ or ↑

specialized units with frequent monitoring by experienced personnel. If the sodium concentration is corrected too quickly, central pontine myelinolysis can occur and result in dysarthria, dysphagia, paresis, coma, and death. In patients with chronic refractory SIADH, demeclocycline, 150 to 300 mg twice daily, can be used because it interferes with action of ADH at renal collecting ducts; fludrocortisone has also been used.

Hypernatremia

Clinical manifestations of hypernatremia include lethargy, weakness, irritability, seizures, and coma. It results from insufficient water intake, hypotonic fluid loss, or solute excess. Insufficient water intake may be due to unavailability of water, hypodipsia secondary to osmoreceptor dysfunction, or neurologic deficits. Hypotonic fluid loss may be due to diabetes insipidus (DI), osmotic diuresis, diuretic drugs, or the diuretic phase of acute tubular necrosis (ATN). In addition, hypotonic fluids may be lost as a result of vomiting, diarrhea, nasogastric suction, sweating, burns, or hyperventilation. Iatrogenic solute excess resulting from infusions of sodium chloride or sodium bicarbonate may also be a factor.

Central Diabetes Insipidus

Central DI is a failure of ADH homeostasis related to dysfunction of the hypothalamopituitary axis. Characteristics of central DI include polyuria (>3 L/day), inappropriately dilute urine (<350 mmol/kg), and a rise in plasma osmolarity (>305 mmol/kg) and serum sodium (>145 mmol/L). A urine specific gravity of less than 1.005 with increasing serum sodium suggests DI. Not uncommonly, it is seen in the intensive care unit after pituitary surgery, traumatic brain injury, subarachnoid hemorrhage, and brain death. Management consists of free water replacement and parenteral or intranasal vasopressin. Free water replacement should be titrated to the sodium concentration with the aim of reducing the serum sodium concentration 1 to 2 mmol/hr if the change in sodium concentration is acute, the patient is symptomatic (seizures), or the sodium concentration is greater than 160 mmol/L. Sodium should be corrected more slowly (0.5 mmol/hr) if the hypernatremia is chronic and the patient is asymptomatic. DDAVP (desmopressin), a two–amino acid substitute of ADH, reduces urine output and simplifies fluid therapy. DDAVP is given in doses of 0.4 to 1 µg intravenously, and its duration of action is 8 to 12 hours.

37

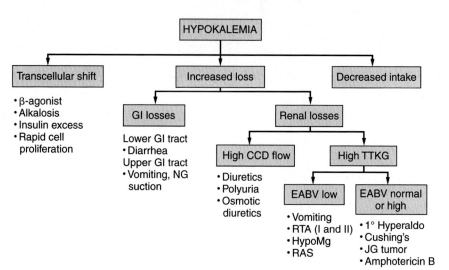

Figure 37-2 Approach to hypokalemia. CCD, cortical collecting duct; EABV, effective arterial blood volume; Hyperaldo, hyperaldosteronism; RTA, renal tubular acidosis; TTKG, transtubular potassium gradient = (urine [K+]/serum [K+])/(urine osmolarity/serum osmolarity).

POTASSIUM DISORDERS

Potassium is the major intracellular cation (total body stores ≈3500 mmol in an average patient). It is reabsorbed in the proximal convoluted tubule (passive) and ascending loop (active). Secretion into the collecting duct is dependent on tubular flow, the aldosterone concentration, and the sodium concentration.

Hypokalemia

Hypokalemia can result in severe muscle weakness, paralysis, rhabdomyolysis, cardiac arrhythmias, and nephrogenic DI. A general approach is presented in Figure 37-2. Electrocardiographic (ECG) changes include ST depression, T-wave flattening, and U waves. In addition to treating the underlying cause, oral or intravenous potassium replacement is required. Because of the irritant effects on peripheral veins, a maximum of 10 mmol/hr may be given via a peripheral line. Central venous access allows 20-mmol/hr replacement. For life-threatening arrhythmia, a maximum of 40 mmol/hr may be given via a central line with cardiac monitoring. It is important to note that a drop in serum potassium of 1 mmol/L equates to a total body potassium store deficit of 200 to 400 mEq and that adequate serum magnesium levels are required for reabsorption of potassium in the kidney.

Hyperkalemia

A general approach to hyperkalemia is presented in Figure 37-3. Clinical manifestations of hyperkalemia do not usually become apparent until serum levels are greater than 7 mmol/L or levels increase rapidly. Symptoms can include muscle weakness or paralysis. Hyperkalemia can result in severe ECG conduction abnormalities, including peaked T waves, prolonged PR and QRS intervals, sine waves, ventricular fibrillation, and asystole. Treatment of hyperkalemia-induced cardiac toxicity includes

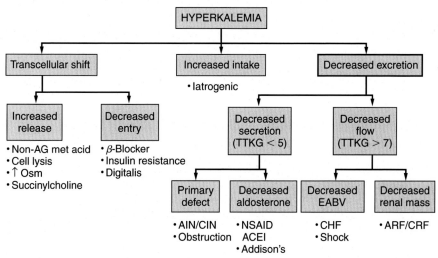

Figure 37-3 Approach to hyperkalemia. ACEI, angiotensin-converting enzyme inhibitor; AIN/ CIN, acute/chronic interstitial nephritis; ARF/CRF, acute/chronic renal failure; CHF, congestive heart failure; EABV, effective arterial blood volume; met acid, metabolic acidosis; Non-AG, non–anion gap; NSAID, non-steroidal anti-inflammatory drug; Osm, osmolarity; TTKG, transtubular potassium gradient = (urine [K+]/serum [K+])/(urine osmolarity/serum osmolarity).

intravenous calcium gluconate or chloride to stabilize cardiac myocytes, insulin and glucose, bicarbonate, salbutamol or albuterol to induce transcellular shifts, and resins, furosemide, or dialysis to increase excretion.

MAGNESIUM DISORDERS

Magnesium is essential for all reactions that require adenosine triphosphate, replication and transcription of DNA, cellular energy metabolism, cell membrane stabilization, nerve conduction, and calcium channel activity.

Hypomagnesemia

Hypomagnesemia is common in patients admitted to intensive care and has been associated with increased mortality. Clinical manifestations include weakness, anorexia, dysrhythmias (torsades de pointes, ventricular tachycardia), muscular dysfunction (fasciculation, cramps, tremor, tetany, respiratory muscle weakness), and seizures. Hypomagnesemia is due to decreased intake, increased loss, or redistribution. Decreased intake as a result of malnutrition and alcoholism is not infrequent. Magnesium may be lost through the gastrointestinal tract (vomiting, diarrhea, fistula, pancreatitis, malabsorption) or via renal mechanisms (diuretics, hypercalcemia, post-ATN status, hypothermia-induced polyuria). Redistribution may occur in association with hypoparathyroidism, correction of metabolic acidosis, or the refeeding syndrome. Treatment of hypomagnesemia includes correction of the underlying cause and magnesium replacement orally or intravenously. For life-threatening arrhythmia, 1 to 2 g of magnesium sulfate solution may be given intravenously over a 5-minute period. Otherwise, replacement should be given via infusion over a period of several hours or orally.

PHOSPHATE DISORDERS

Phosphate is the most common intracellular anion and is essential for membrane structure, energy storage, DNA and RNA production, and bone production.

Hypophosphatemia

Clinical manifestations of hypophosphatemia generally occur at serum values of less than 0.3 mmol/L and include weakness, dysphagia, ileus, rhabdomyolysis, respiratory muscle failure, decreased myocardial contractility, impaired phagocytosis/chemotaxis, thrombocytopenia, and decreased oxygen delivery related to reduced 2,3-diphosphoglycerate (2,3-DPG). Hypophosphatemia is due to decreased intake, increased loss, or transcellular shift. Decreased intake may be related to malnutrition (especially when phosphate-binding antacids are consumed), vomiting, or severe diarrhea. Increased loss is observed in hyperparathyroidism, vitamin D deficiency, diuretic use, and Fanconi's syndrome. Hypophosphatemia related to transcellular shift can be seen in recovery from malnutrition and diabetic ketoacidosis, respiratory alkalosis, and rapid cell proliferation. Hormone administration (insulin, epinephrine, dopamine, steroids, and glucagon) can also cause a transcellular shift. Treatment is directed at the underlying cause, and replacement of phosphate can be accomplished enterally or parenterally in the form of sodium or potassium phosphate.

KEY POINTS

- Although multiple causes of hyponatremia are possible, SIADH and CSW are most common in patients with neurologic disease.
- Diagnosis of SIADH requires hyponatremia, hypo-osmolarity, inappropriately high urine osmolarity, and exclusion of hypoadrenalism and hypothyroidism.
- CSW is a primary natriuresis observed in those with neurologic injury. It results in negative sodium balance and volume depletion.
- Characteristics of central DI include polyuria (>3 L/day), inappropriately dilute urine (<350 mmol/kg), and a rise in plasma osmolarity (>305 mmol/kg) and serum sodium (>145 mmol/L). A urine specific gravity of less than 1.005 in the setting of increasing serum sodium suggests DI.

FURTHER READING

Adler SM, Verbalis JG: Disorders of body water homeostasis in critical illness. Endocrinol Metab Clin North Am 2006; 35:xi, 873-894.
Rabinstein AA, Wijdicks EF: Hyponatremia in critically ill neurological patients. Neurologist 2003; 9:290-300.
Tisdall M, Crocker M, Watkiss J, Smith M: Disturbances of sodium in critically ill adult neurologic patients: A clinical review. J Neurosurg Anesthesiol 2006; 18:57-63.

Chapter 38

Status Epilepticus

John M. Taylor

Epidemiology	**Treatment**
Risk Factors	First-Line Treatment
Complications of Status Epilepticus	Second-Line Treatment
	Additional Treatment Options
Diagnosis	Refractory Status Epilepticus

Status epilepticus (SE) is a medical emergency that is associated with high morbidity and mortality. Early recognition and appropriate treatment are paramount for meaningful outcomes.

A seizure is a nonspecific term defined as a suddenly occurring change in mental status or behavior that is usually transient. An epileptic seizure is a manifestation of hypersynchronous neuronal activity in the brain resulting in involuntary disturbances in consciousness, behavior, or emotion. These seizures may or may not be associated with tonic or clonic activity (or both). Of note, a pseudoseizure is a misnomer; it is a psychogenic nonepileptic seizure and does not result in SE.

In 1993, the Epilepsy Foundation of America convened a work group that established a definition of SE. Patients who experience two or more consecutive seizures without return to their baseline mental status or those who have continuous seizure activity for 30 or more minutes fulfill the diagnostic criteria for SE. A more practical definition defines SE as a seizure of more than 5 minutes' duration or two consecutive seizures without return to baseline mental status.

SE may be convulsive or nonconvulsive. Convulsive SE may be generalized (arising from both hemispheres) or partial (arising from a specific region), overt or subtle, and symmetric or asymmetric, with tonic or clonic movements (or both). Nonconvulsive status epilepticus (NCSE) is most commonly manifested as altered mental status with no other apparent etiology. Patients afflicted with NCSE appear alert, although they have alterations in affect. When other causes of altered mental status have been excluded, neurologic evaluation for NCSE must be performed.

Several methods can be used to classify SE, although no single approach has been widely accepted. Even though discussion of the classification of SE is beyond the scope of this review, it is important to identify seizure activity as SE to institute appropriate treatment in a timely manner.

EPIDEMIOLOGY

SE occurs in approximately 150,000 people in the United States each year and results in approximately 42,000 deaths annually. Mortality, defined as death within 30 days of SE, ranges from 22% to 26%. Data from one study showed a mortality rate of 38% in the elderly. Mortality in children is low, ranging from 3% to 8%. Mortality is most often due to precipitating factors rather than SE alone.

An epidemiologic study conducted in Richmond, Virginia, found that partial SE accounts for 69% of adult SE and 64% of pediatric SE. SE occurs most frequently in people younger than 1 year or older than 60 years. A follow-up prospective single-center study found NCSE in 8% of patients with coma and no signs of seizure activity.

RISK FACTORS

SE may occur in patients with epilepsy or in those with no previous history of neurologic disorder. The most common cause of SE is an inadequate serum level of antiepileptic drugs (AEDs). Other causes include hyponatremia, fever, central nervous system infection, intracranial mass, subarachnoid hemorrhage, head trauma, stroke, hypoglycemia, uremia, hypoxemia, hyperglycemia, alcohol or benzodiazepine withdrawal, and local anesthetic toxicity.

In children, infection with fever is the leading cause of SE and accounts for 50% or more of cases. In the elderly, stroke (either acute or remote) and inadequate AED levels are the most common causes of SE.

COMPLICATIONS OF STATUS EPILEPTICUS

Convulsive SE results in hypoglycemia, hypoxemia, lactic acidosis, hyperthermia, or hypotension and can result in brain damage. Neuronal necrosis and apoptosis occur as a result of the excitotoxic neurotransmitter release (N-methyl-D-aspartate [NMDA] receptor stimulation) that occurs in SE. In addition, convulsive disorders cause massive release of catecholamines. Catecholamine release may result in hypertension, increased oxygen consumption, and arrhythmias. Other complications include aspiration, rhabdomyolysis, and secondary injury.

The primary factors that determine outcome after SE are age, duration of the seizure, and cause of the SE. Patients with SE secondary to cerebral anoxia and stroke have very high mortality, whereas those with SE secondary to subtherapeutic AED levels or alcohol withdrawal have very low mortality. The likelihood of SE becoming refractory is dependent on the duration of SE and the rapidity of treatment.

DIAGNOSIS

The clinical diagnosis of SE is often not straightforward. Patients with SE may exhibit hypertension, tachycardia, hypoventilation, hypoxemia, hypercapnia, aspiration, alterations in behavior, altered mental status, tonic or clonic movements (or both), or unresponsiveness.

In addition to a complete physical examination, all patients with SE should undergo brain-imaging studies, except pediatric patients with febrile SE. Patients should also have a neurology consultation, and electroencephalographic (EEG) studies should be performed. EEG monitoring is necessary because of the high percentage of patients with electrographic evidence of seizure activity despite cessation of clonic-tonic movements.

TREATMENT

First-Line Treatment

As with all medical emergencies, initial management should concentrate on airway management, maintenance of oxygenation and ventilation, treatment of hemodynamic instability, establishment of vascular access, and appropriate pharmacologic therapy. Hemodynamic monitoring is essential during treatment of SE because almost all pharmacologic therapies can result in hypotension or myocardial depression. Although algorithms have been established for the treatment of SE, it is important to note that clinical care must be case specific. Figure 38-1 outlines an approach to treatment of SE.

Benzodiazepines are the most effective first-line medications for the treatment of SE. Lorazepam, diazepam, and midazolam have all been used in the treatment of SE. Several studies have demonstrated that lorazepam is the most efficacious pharmacologic treatment of SE. Lorazepam and diazepam result in rapid cessation of seizure activity, but lorazepam has a more favorable pharmacokinetic profile. Patients treated with lorazepam are less likely to have recurrent seizures and require fewer additional doses of medication to stop seizure activity.

When compared with diazepam, lorazepam is less lipid soluble and exerts a much longer duration of action. Lorazepam has a smaller volume of distribution and binds more avidly to the γ-aminobutyric acid A ($GABA_A$) receptor. The typical loading dose of lorazepam is 0.1 mg/kg up to a maximum of 4 mg administered intravenously. The onset of action of lorazepam is 2 to 4 minutes, and it has a half-life of 12 to 14 hours.

Diazepam is highly lipid soluble and has a short onset of action; however, it redistributes rapidly to fatty tissues. The usual intravenous loading dose for diazepam is 0.15 mg/kg (typical maximum adult dose 10 mg), which provides anticonvulsant activity for 20 to 30 minutes.

Midazolam has a short duration of action because of a unique imidazole ring that allows it to be water and lipid soluble, depending on pH. The water solubility allows intranasal, intramuscular, and sublingual administration if vascular access is not established. Use of single-dose midazolam results in more frequent seizure recurrence as a result of rapid serum clearance of the drug.

A large clinical trial established that prehospital treatment of SE with lorazepam or diazepam is safe and effective for early termination of SE. Effective doses of lorazepam are 2 to 4 mg intravenously and equivalent doses of diazepam are 5 to 10 mg intravenously.

Side effects of benzodiazepines include respiratory depression, decreased level of consciousness, alteration in mental status, and hypotension.

Second-Line Treatment

The next group of medications used in the treatment of SE consists of the hydantoins *phenytoin* and *fosphenytoin*. These barbiturate-like drugs slow the rate of recovery of voltage-gated sodium channels, thus reducing the number of action potentials and controlling seizure activity. Both phenytoin and fosphenytoin have a 15-minute onset of action, which makes these drugs less desirable in the acute treatment of SE.

Phenytoin has poor water solubility. The loading dose of phenytoin used for SE is 10-20 mg/kg administered at 50 mg/min; for adults, a 1-g loading dose is typical. Phenytoin has several undesirable side effects: hypotension, QT prolongation, dysrhythmias, and local ischemia associated with extravasation. Phenytoin is highly protein bound and has multiple drug interactions.

Fosphenytoin is the water-soluble prodrug of phenytoin. After administration, fosphenytoin has 100% bioavailability. Plasma phosphatases convert the phosphate

38

249

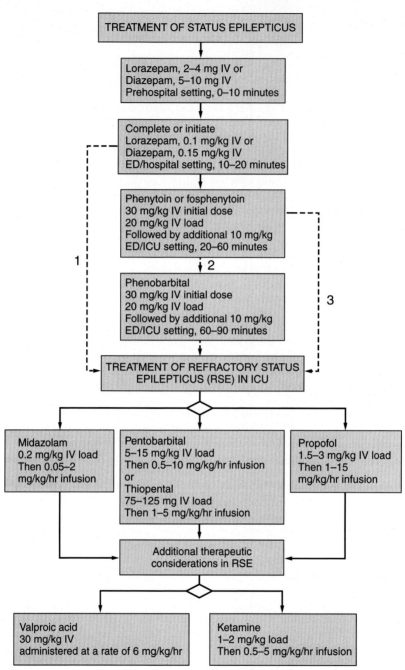

Figure 38-1 Treatment algorithm for status epilepticus and refractory status epilepticus. Times are approximate. Pathway 1: If seizure activity continues after benzodiazepine administration, continue with RSE treatment. Pathway 2: Phenobarbital is the third-line therapeutic option, after benzodiazepines and hydantoins. Pathway 3: Second-line treatment after benzodiazepines and before treatment of RSE. ED, emergency department; ICU, intensive care unit. (Adapted from Manno EM: New management strategies in the treatment of status epilepticus. Mayo Clinic Proc 2003; 78:508-518.)

ester fosphenytoin to phenytoin. This conversion takes about 15 minutes to occur. The advantage of fosphenytoin relates to its water solubility, which allows more rapid administration with a higher safety profile if extravasation occurs. A 1.5-mg dose of fosphenytoin is equivalent to 1 mg of phenytoin. The cost of fosphenytoin is significantly greater than that of phenytoin. Hypotension and myocardial depression are still present in the side effect profile.

Phenobarbital is a barbiturate. Like benzodiazepines, phenobarbital increases chloride ion influx, thereby resulting in hyperpolarization and increased inhibition of neuronal activity. The typical loading dose of phenobarbital is 20 to 30 mg/kg given over a period of 30 minutes. Because phenobarbital is solubilized in propylene glycol, rapid infusion may cause myocardial depression, peripheral vasodilation, acute renal failure, respiratory depression, or seizures. Phenobarbital has a duration of action of up to 100 hours. It is not considered a first-line treatment because the mechanism of action of phenobarbital is similar to that of benzodiazepines and treatment after a fast-acting benzodiazepine is unlikely stop seizure activity.

Additional Treatment Options

Valproic acid (VPA) is an anticonvulsant medication with an unclear mechanism of action. There is some evidence that VPA acts through GABA receptors. At this time VPA has not been approved by the Food and Drug Administration for the treatment of SE because of infusion rate limitations. One trial has reported effective treatment of SE with intravenous VPA, 15-30 mg/kg at a rate of 6 mg/kg/min. Intravenous VPA has side effects that include hypertension, hypotension, tachycardia, hepatotoxicity, and gastrointestinal distress.

Ketamine is a noncompetitive NMDA-glutamate receptor antagonist. It has a serum half-life of 2 to 3 hours with hepatic metabolism via the P-450 system. Metabolism of ketamine produces an active metabolite, norketamine. Animal models suggest that ketamine may exert neuroprotective effects through anticonvulsant activity and by blocking excitatory neurotransmitter activity at NMDA receptors. Ketamine has been used for the treatment of SE in doses ranging from 0.5 to 5 mg/kg/hr. Broad acceptance of ketamine for SE has been limited by its side effect profile and lack of clinical studies for use in SE. Side effects include hypertension, increased intracranial pressure, cardiac arrhythmias, increased metabolic rate, and myocardial depression.

Small recent studies have shown the efficacy of using levetiracetam (Keppra) and topiramate (Topamax) for the treatment of refractory SE (RSE). The mechanism of action is unknown. Levetiracetam and topiramate can be considered second-line drugs for the treatment of RSE; they have minimal interactions with other AEDs and a minimal side effect profile. At present, both medications are available only in enteral formulations.

Carbamazepine (Tegretol) and lamotrigine (Lamictal) have also been used with some success as second- or third-line agents in the treatment of RSE.

Refractory Status Epilepticus

Seizure activity that is refractory to standard treatment algorithms is termed *refractory status epilepticus*. RSE occurs in approximately 30% of patients with SE. Treatment of RSE involves anesthetic doses of medications. Medications commonly used are midazolam infusion, propofol infusion, and short-acting barbiturates.

A typical loading dose of midazolam is 0.1 to 0.2 mg/kg, followed by an infusion of 0.05 to 0.2 mg/kg/hr. Metabolism is hepatic and may be enhanced by the administration of other AEDs. Rapid tachyphylaxis may develop and necessitate adjunctive pharmacologic treatment. The dose range for propofol induction is 1.5 to 3.0 mg/kg,

38

with maintenance infusion rates of 50 to 200 μg/kg/min. Side effects include hypotension, myocardial depression, and hypertriglyceridemia. Patients should have frequent monitoring of serum triglycerides.

The short-acting barbiturates pentobarbital and thiopental are also used in RSE. These medications are highly protein bound, have a large volume of distribution, and readily redistribute to adipose tissue, thus accounting for prolonged clinical activity after cessation of infusion. The typical loading dose for pentobarbital is 5 to 10 mg/kg administered over a 30- to 60-minute period, followed by infusion at 0.5 to 10 mg/kg/hr. Thiopental is typically used for rapid control of RSE; loading doses are 0.5 to 2 mg/kg given over a period of several minutes.

Ideally, the dosage of these agents for RSE should be tailored to maintain burst suppression on EEG monitoring.

Isoflurane and other volatile anesthetics have been used for severe intractable RSE, but their use is complicated by the need for exhaled gas–scavenging equipment and monitoring of end-tidal concentrations of volatile anesthetics. Failure of multiple simultaneous intravenous agents typically precedes consideration of the use of volatile anesthetics.

Debate continues over the need for persistent neuromuscular blockade (NMB) in the treatment of RSE. Certainly, NMB facilitates endotracheal intubation and securing the patient airway. It also allows ventilation at lower peak airway pressure and may reduce oxygen consumption, as well as intracranial pressure, if elevated. Continuing NMB necessitates mechanical ventilation and predisposes patients to complications, including ventilator-associated pneumonia, as well as myopathy and neuropathy associated with protracted NMB. EEG monitoring is necessary if NMB is used because seizure activity may be masked by NMB.

KEY POINTS

- SE is defined as two or more consecutive seizures without return to baseline mental status or as continuous seizure activity for 30 or more minutes.
- SE may be generalized or partial, convulsive or nonconvulsive, and symmetric or asymmetric.
- Mortality is approximately 20% and primarily determined by age, duration of seizure, and cause of the SE.
- Lorazepam is the most effective first-line treatment of SE.
- Refractory SE occurs in approximately 30% of patients with SE.
- Other treatments of SE include midazolam, barbiturate, and propofol infusion.

FURTHER READING

Bassin S, Smith TL, Bleck TP: Clinical review: Status epilepticus. Crit Care 2002; 6:137-142.
Bleck TP: Refractory status epilepticus. Curr Opin Crit Care 2005; 11:117-120.
Borris DJ, Bertram EH, Kapur J: Ketamine controls prolonged status epilepticus. Epilepsy Res 2000; 42:117-122.
Claassen J, Hirsch LJ, Emerson RG, Mayers SA: Treatment of refractory status epilepticus with pentobarbital, propofol, or midazolam: A systematic review. Epilepsia 2002; 43:146-153.
DeLorenzo: A prospective, population-based epidemiologic study of status epilepticus in Richmond, Virginia. Neurology 1996; 46:1029-1035.
Epilepsy Foundation of America Work Group on SE. JAMA 1993; 270:854.
Ulvi H, Yoldas T, Müngen B, Yigiter R: Continuous infusion of midazolam in the treatment of refractory generalized convulsive status epilepticus. Neurol Sci 2002; 23:177-182.
Walker MC, Howard RS, Smith SJ, et al: Diagnosis and treatment of status epilepticus on a neurological intensive care unit. Q J Med 1996; 89:913-920.
Walker MC: Diagnosis and treatment of nonconvulsive status epilepticus. CNS Drugs 2001; 15:931-939.
Wasterlain CG, Treiman DM (eds): Status Epilepticus: Mechanisms and Management. Massachusetts Institute of Technology, Cambridge, MA, 2006.

Chapter 39

Brain Death

Peter M. Schulman

HISTORICAL PERSPECTIVE

Determination of death must be made by qualified professionals in accordance with conventional medical standards and practices. Historically, this was straightforward because death was defined as permanent cessation of circulatory and respiratory function.

However, in 1968 a committee at Harvard Medical School decided that it was important to redefine death by using "irreversible coma" as a new criterion. This had become necessary because advancements in techniques of cardiopulmonary resuscitation and the widespread use of mechanical ventilators resulted in a growing number of patients who could be kept temporarily "alive" even though they had suffered devastating and irreversible neurologic injury. The committee members were also concerned that the then emerging field of organ transplantation would be unduly hindered by "obsolete criteria" for determining death. Consequently, the landmark Harvard criteria were developed and have formed the basis for all brain death guidelines that followed.

BRAINSTEM DEATH VERSUS WHOLE-BRAIN DEATH

There are significant differences in how brain death is defined and diagnosed throughout the world. In many countries, including the United States and the majority of Europe, neurologic death has been defined as irreversible cessation of function of the entire brain, including the brainstem. Because clinical examination alone is insufficient to diagnose whole-brain death, confirmatory tests to demonstrate the absence of cerebral blood flow, electroencephalography (EEG), or both are frequently used.

In the United Kingdom, the brain death guidelines initially published in 1976 were revised in 1995 to replace the concept of whole-brain death with that of brainstem death. This new definition represented a substantive change in thinking because it affirmed that confirmatory tests were not required (i.e., appropriate clinical examination in addition to a clear diagnosis of severe brain injury is adequate).

39

Criteria for diagnosing brain death vary widely from country to country, and practice standards in most instances have not yet been legally mandated. It is therefore advisable to first determine the guidelines or requirements that are specific to the particular region or institution.

THE CLINICAL EXAMINATION PROCESS

The primary purpose of the clinical examination is to demonstrate the absence of brainstem function. Although widespread differences exist in examination requirements, such as the number of observers, the specialty and the number of years since qualification of the assessing physician, the duration of observation, and the use of confirmatory testing, the examination should always include several key elements.

Evaluation of Coma

The patient must be totally unresponsive and ventilator dependent. Total unresponsiveness includes absence of seizures and limb movement, except for spinal reflexes. Furthermore, the underlying cause of the comatose state should be determined. This is generally easier in cases of head injury or intracranial bleeding, but it may be significantly more difficult when hypoxic arrest has occurred. A computed tomography scan and full neurologic examination (as outlined later) are essential to definitively establish the diagnosis of brain death.

Search for Reversible Causes and Confounding Conditions

A core temperature higher than 35° C is required because brainstem responses are blunted when core temperature is lower than 32° C. A core temperature lower than 27° C can mimic brain death.

Many drugs cause central nervous system depression and can mimic brain death. Drug-induced central nervous system depression is associated with complete but reversible loss of brainstem reflexes, an isoelectric EEG, or both. Examples include barbiturates, tricyclic antidepressants, opiates, benzodiazepines, and high concentrations of volatile anesthetic agents. It is also important to determine whether any neuromuscular blocking agents have recently been administered and whether their effects are still present. Both drugs that depress the central nervous system and neuromuscular blocking agents must be allowed time to wear off or their effects reversed. A toxicology screen should be performed if drug ingestion is suspected.

Severe electrolyte abnormalities or acid-base disturbances may impair cerebral function or alter the neurologic assessment.

Other conditions such as Guillain-Barré or the locked-in syndrome may mimic brain death and must be excluded.

Clinical Examination of the Brainstem

Sensory input to the upper part of the face (cranial nerve V) and motor response (grimace) to pain (cranial nerve VII) should be tested by applying a painful stimulus to the supraorbital nerve, temporomandibular joint, or finger nail bed.

The following brainstem reflexes should be tested: corneal reflex (cranial nerves V and VII), pupillary response to light (cranial nerves II and III), oculovestibular response (cranial nerves VII, III, and VI), and cough (IX and X). Of note, although the pupil is usually midposition in brain death, pupillary size is considered irrelevant in establishing the diagnosis of brain death.

Finally, an apnea test should be conducted to assess for the presence or absence of spontaneous breathing. The patient should first be adequately preoxygenated with an FiO_2 of 1.0 for about 10 minutes. With a PaO_2 of 200 mm Hg or greater and a $PaCO_2$ of 40 mm Hg or greater, the patient can then be disconnected from the ventilator. Supplemental oxygen is administered via T piece or suction catheter while the physician monitors for respirations and ensures that the patient remains hemodynamically stable. Apnea is confirmed if the $PaCO_2$ is 60 mm Hg or greater or there is an increase of more than 20 mm Hg from the normal baseline value without any attempted respiratory effort.

ADJUNCTIVE AND CONFIRMATORY TESTS

Because clinical examination alone cannot distinguish brainstem death from whole-brain death, this distinction must be based on the cause of the brain injury, neuroimaging, or electrophysiology (or any combination). Therefore, adjunctive or confirmatory testing is used frequently in the United States but only rarely in the United Kingdom. Confirmatory testing is generally recommended in all cases for children younger than 1 year and is mandated by law for patients of all ages in several European, Central and South American, and Asian countries.

Adjunctive tests used to support the clinical diagnosis of brain death include EEG, evoked potentials, and intracranial pressure measurement. Although EEG is probably the best validated, it is not in itself sufficient to establish whole-brain death because patients may have absent cortical function with an isoelectric recording yet may still retain brainstem function.

Confirmatory tests include transcranial Doppler ultrasonography, single-photon emission computed tomography (SPECT), and angiography. These tests prove that brain death has occurred because they evaluate cerebral blood flow. The absence of perfusion means that the brain is not viable. Angiography is considered the "gold standard"; however, it is invasive. Doppler ultrasonography is quick but operator dependent and is considered less reliable than angiography. SPECT is noninvasive but is not considered a definitive test.

PATHOPHYSIOLOGY OF BRAIN DEATH
AND MANAGEMENT OF ORGAN DONORS

Brain death is commonly associated with a catastrophic rise in intracranial pressure. As this occurs, massive amounts of catecholamine stores are released and lead to increased systemic arterial blood pressure, sometimes associated with concomitant reflex bradycardia, bradyarrhythmia, or both. Decreased cardiac output, pulmonary edema, and cardiac ischemia are other clinical conditions that may be encountered while brain death is evolving.

Once total brain infarction has occurred, catecholamines are abruptly depleted and sympathetic nervous system output is lost. This results in peripheral vasodilation and systemic hypotension. Other common problems occurring soon after brain death that can threaten organ viability include diabetes insipidus, hypothermia, electrolyte disturbances such as hypokalemia and hypernatremia, acidosis, pulmonary edema, and cardiac arrest.

Consent from family for organ donation can be obtained after the diagnosis of brain death is established. Once an organ donor is identified, vigilant medical care

39

is needed to ensure that the greatest number of organs can be recovered in the best possible condition. The primary goal is to preserve organ viability. This is best accomplished by ensuring oxygenation and ventilation, maintaining homodynamic stability, and correcting electrolyte problems and acid-base abnormalities.

Ventilatory support should be adjusted to provide adequate arterial oxygen saturation while minimizing toxicity associated with high F_{IO_2}. High airway pressure should be avoided to prevent lung injury. In addition, acid-base status should be normalized.

Hypotension is generally managed by volume expansion and vasopressors if necessary. Therapy should be guided by central venous pressure monitoring, fluid replacement should be judicious to prevent pulmonary edema, but the use of vasopressors should be minimized to prevent end-organ damage from vasoconstriction and hypoperfusion.

Treatment of diabetes insipidus may require hormone replacement, volume expansion, and correction of hypernatremia and potassium and magnesium losses.

KEY POINTS

- There are significant differences in how brain death is defined throughout the world. The United States and other countries use whole-brain death, whereas the United Kingdom has accepted the concept of brainstem death.
- Criteria for diagnosing brain death are highly variable, so it is advisable to determine the guidelines or requirements specific to the particular region or institution.
- A comprehensive clinical examination is required to diagnose brain death. The primary purpose of the examination is to demonstrate the absence of brainstem function.
- Adjunctive or confirmatory tests (or both) are often used to diagnose whole-brain death. Adjunctive tests can be used to support the diagnosis, whereas confirmatory tests can be used to prove that brain death has occurred.
- Brain death is often accompanied by severe hemodynamic instability, diabetes insipidus, and other acute medical problems.
- Vigilant care of a brain-dead organ donor is required to preserve organ viability.

FURTHER READING

Darby JM: Care of the organ donor. In O'Donnell JM, Nacul FE (eds): Surgical Intensive Care Medicine, Boston, Kluwer, 2002, pp 795-803.

Diringer MN, Wijdicks EFM: Brain death in historical perspective. In Wijdicks EFM (ed): Brain Death. Philadelphia, Lippincott Williams & Wilkins, 2001, pp 5-27.

Doig CJ, Burgess E: Brain death: Resolving inconsistencies in the ethical declaration of death. Can J Anaesth 2003; 50:725-731.

Larson MD, Gray AT: The diagnosis of brain death [letter]. N Engl J Med 2001; 345:616-618.

Munari M, Zucchetta P, Carollo C, et al: Confirmatory tests in the diagnosis of brain death: Comparison between SPECT and contrast angiography. Crit Care Med 2005; 33:2068-2073.

Powner DJ, Hernandez MS, Rives TE: Variability among hospital policies for determining brain death in adults. Crit Care Med 2004; 32:1284-1288.

Shemie SD: Must the entire brain be dead to diagnose brain death [reply of letter to the editor]? Can J Anaesth 2006; 53:1061-1062.

Sutcliffe AJ: Current issues in the diagnosis of brain stem death. Scand J Trauma Resusc Emerg Med 2005; 13:89-92.

Wijdicks EFM: The diagnosis of brain death. N Engl J Med 2001; 344:1215-1221.

Wijdicks EFM: Brain death worldwide: Accepted fact but no global consensus in diagnostic criteria. Neurology 2002; 58:20-25.

Wood KE, Becker BN, McCartney JG, et al: Care of the potential organ donor. New Engl J Med 2004; 351:2730-2739.

Section VI
Monitoring

Chapter 40

Intracranial Pressure Monitoring

Marek Czosnyka

Methods of Measurement	Optimal Cerebral Perfusion Pressure
Microtransducers	Pulse Waveform Analysis of Intracranial
Intraventricular Drains	Pressure
Other Sensors	Noninvasive Intracranial Pressure
Typical Events and Trends Seen	**Measurement**
in Intracranial Monitoring	**Intracranial Pressure and Outcome**
Cerebrovascular Pressure Reactivity	**after Severe Head Injury**

Intracranial pressure (ICP) is an essential modality in most brain-monitoring systems and requires the use of an invasive sensor. Attempts to monitor ICP noninvasively, though promising, are still in a phase of technical refinement.

Measurement of ICP allows estimation of cerebral perfusion pressure (CPP):

$$\text{Mean CPP} = \text{Mean arterial blood pressure (ABP)} - \text{Mean ICP}$$

ICP also provides information regarding autoregulation of cerebral blood flow, pressure reactivity, and compliance of the cerebrospinal system.

ICP is more than a number. Its instant value based on a single measurement (which is what we can see on most bedside monitors) is not clinically as relevant as its long-term average, variability in time, presence of waveforms, and correlation with other variables in brain monitoring (Fig. 40-1).

METHODS OF MEASUREMENT

Microtransducers

Modern ventricular, subdural, or intraparenchymal microtransducers reduce infection rates and have demonstrated excellent metrologic properties during bench tests. Intraparenchymal systems may be inserted through an airtight support bolt (e.g., Codman or Camino systems) or tunneled subcutaneously from a bur hole either at the bedside or after craniotomy (Codman system). With the most common intraparenchymal arrangement, the measured pressure may be local and not necessarily representative of ventricular cerebrospinal fluid (CSF) pressure. Microtransducers cannot generally be recalibrated after insertion, and zero drift may occur with long-term monitoring.

Intraventricular Drains

An external pressure transducer connected to a catheter ending in the ventricular system that allows direct pressure measurement is still considered the "gold standard" for measurement of ICP. Additional advantages include the capability of periodic

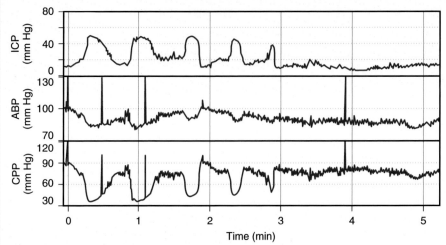

Figure 40-1 Example of unstable intracranial pressure (ICP) leading to repetitive decreases in cerebral perfusion pressure (CPP). Notably, intracranial hypertension after head injury is frequently of a temporary nature. In this particular case, ICP finally stabilized at a satisfactory level of 12 mm Hg. However, the reverse situation often takes place, and the onset of sudden refractory hypertension may lead to fatal complication. Therefore, in intensive care, ICP should be monitored continuously! ABP, arterial blood pressure.

external calibration and CSF drainage. However, insertion of a ventricular catheter may be difficult or impossible in patients with advanced brain swelling, and the risk of infection is increased significantly after 3 days of monitoring. When measurement is performed by open extraventricular drainage (EVD), care should be taken to not interpret ICP readings as valid while the EVD is open (Fig. 40-2). EVD should be closed for measurement (for at least 15 minutes), or an independent intraparenchymal transducer should be used.

Other Sensors

The least invasive systems use epidural probes, but there is still uncertainty regarding the precise relationship between ICP and extradural pressure. Contemporary epidural sensors are much more reliable than those 10 years ago. Manometric lumbar CSF pressure measurement should not be considered a reliable method in neurointensive care.

TYPICAL EVENTS AND TRENDS SEEN IN INTRACRANIAL MONITORING

Specific patterns of the ICP waveform can be identified when mean ICP is monitored continuously. Patients with a low and stable ICP (<20 mm Hg) characteristically have no ICP vasogenic waves, with the exception of a phasic response of ICP to rapid variations in ABP. This pattern is specific for uncomplicated patients after head injury or during the initial hours after trauma before ICP increases.

The most common picture after head injury consists of high and stable ICP (>20 mm Hg) with vasogenic waves of limited amplitude. Vasogenic B waves, plateau waves, or waves related to changes in arterial pressure and hyperemic events are common in postinjury intensive care.

VI

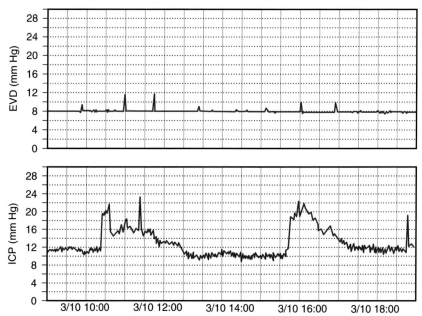

Figure 40-2 Time course of intracranial pressure (ICP) in a patient measured with a ventricular catheter (extraventricular drainage [EVD]) and an intraparenchymal transducer, respectively. With ventricular drainage opened, periods of increased ICP were recorded while EVD remained constant.

CEREBROVASCULAR PRESSURE REACTIVITY

The correlation between spontaneous waves in ABP and ICP is dependent on the ability of cerebral vessels to autoregulate. With intact autoregulation, a rise in ABP produces vasoconstriction, a decrease in cerebral blood volume, and a fall in ICP. With disturbed autoregulation, changes in ABP are transmitted to the intracranial compartment and result in a passive pressure effect.

The correlation coefficient between slow changes in mean ABP and ICP (termed the pressure reactivity index [PRx]) is negative when cerebral vessels are pressure reactive. A positive correlation coefficient indicates disturbed cerebrovascular pressure reactivity (Fig. 40-3). This index may fluctuate with time as ICP and CPP vary (Fig. 40-4), but on average it expresses most of the phenomena related to cerebral hemodynamics and volume expansion processes.

OPTIMAL CEREBRAL PERFUSION PRESSURE

In adults with head trauma, PRx plotted against CPP gives a "U-shaped" curve that indicates, for the majority of patients, a value of CPP for which pressure reactivity is optimal (Fig. 40-5). This optimal pressure can be estimated by plotting and analyzing the PRx-CPP curve in sequential 6-hour periods; the greater the distance between the current and the "optimal" CPP, the more likely that the outcome will be poor. This potentially useful methodology attempts to refine our current approach to CPP-oriented therapy: both too low (ischemia) and too high (hyperemia and secondary increase in ICP) a CPP are detrimental. It has been suggested that CPP in adults should be optimized to maintain CPP in the most globally favorable state. Probably,

40

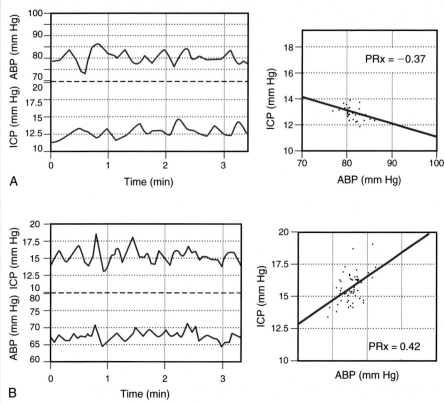

Figure 40-3 Examples of a negative pressure reactivity index (PRx) (**A,** good pressure reactivity) and a positive PRx (**B,** disturbed pressure reactivity). PRx is calculated as a moving correlation coefficient between slow waves of intracranial pressure (ICP) and arterial blood pressure (ABP) with a period of 4 to 6 minutes. Slow waves may be detected by low-pass filtering or a simple moving average with a period of 6 to 8 seconds.

such a strategy could help in reaching a consensus between "CPP therapy" and a "Lund concept" on an individual basis.

PULSE WAVEFORM ANALYSIS OF INTRACRANIAL PRESSURE

To adequately identify potentially harmful intracranial hypertension in individual patients, an analysis of the amplitude of ICP waveforms can be performed. The pulse waveform of ICP provides information about the transmission of arterial pulse pressure through the arterial walls to the CSF space. As CPP decreases, the wall tension in reactive brain vessels decreases. This in turn increases transmission of the arterial pulse to ICP. Therefore, when cerebral vessels are normally reactive, a decrease in CPP should provoke an increase in ABP-to-ICP pulse transmission. If this relationship is disturbed, the cerebral vessels are no longer pressure reactive.

A moving linear correlation coefficient between mean ICP and ICP pulse amplitude values (termed the RAP index: R, symbol of correlation; A, amplitude; P, pressure) calculated over a 3-to 5-minute time window is used for continuous detection of the amplitude-pressure relationship (Fig. 40-6). The advantage is that the coefficient

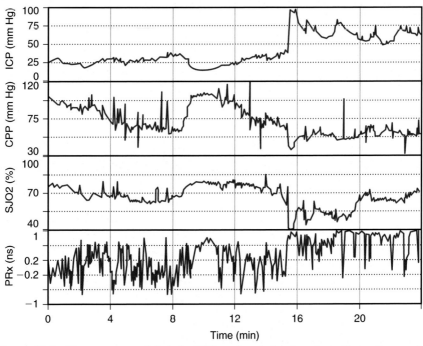

Figure 40-4 The pressure reactivity index (PRx) can be calculated continuously as a time-varying index. It is quite noisy but on average reflects time-related variations in brain perfusion, intracranial hypertension, or inadequate cerebral perfusion pressure. CPP, cerebral perfusion pressure ICP, intracranial pressure.

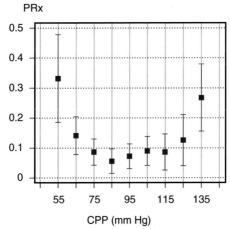

Figure 40-5 Plotting the pressure reactivity index (PRx) against cerebral perfusion pressure (CPP) results in a "U-shaped" curve (results averaged from around 250 head-injured patients). With too low a CPP, pressure reactivity is disturbed, but it is disturbed equally for too high a CPP. "Optimal CPP" occurs around 70 to 90 mm Hg and ensures the best reactivity. This optimal CPP can be traced in individual cases and may vary over time. Following the "optimal CPP" allegedly increases the chance of achieving a better outcome after head trauma.

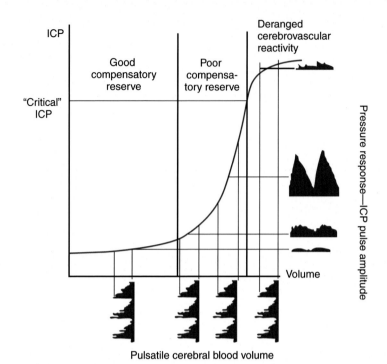

Pulsatile cerebral blood volume

Figure 40-6 In a simple model, the extraventricular drainage pulse amplitude of intracranial pressure (ICP) (expressed along the y-axis on the right side of the panel) results from pulsatile changes in cerebral blood volume (expressed along the x-axis) transformed by the pressure-volume curve. This curve has three zones: a flat zone that expresses good compensatory reserve, an exponential zone that depicts poor compensatory reserve, and a flat zone again seen at very high ICP (above the "critical" ICP) that depicts derangement of normal cerebrovascular responses. The pulse amplitude of ICP is low and does not depend on mean ICP in the first zone, thereby resulting in RAP values close to 0. The pulse amplitude increases linearly with mean ICP in the zone of poor compensatory reserve, thereby resulting in RAP values close to +1. In the third zone, the pulse amplitude starts to decrease with rising ICP, thus making RAP theoretically negative. (Adapted from Löfgren J,Von Essen C, Zwetnow NN, The pressure-volume curve of the cerebrospinal fluid space in dogs. Acta Neurol Scand 1973; 49:557-574; and Avezaat CJ, Van Eijndhoven JH, Wyper DJ. et al: cerebrospinal fluid pulse pressure and Intracranial volume-pressure relationships. J Neurol Neurosurg Psychiatry 1979; 42:687-700.)

has a normalized value from −1 to +1 and thus allows comparison between patients. In a pooled analysis of patients with head injury, the value of RAP was close to +1. This is expected in head-injured patients with moderately raised ICP (>15 mm Hg) and CPP (>50 mm Hg) and indicates decreased compensatory reserve with preserved cerebrovascular reactivity. A decrease in RAP to 0 or negative values, found with very high ICP and very low CPP, indicates loss of cerebrovascular reactivity with a risk of brain ischemia and is also predictive of a poor outcome.

NONINVASIVE INTRACRANIAL PRESSURE MEASUREMENT

It would be very helpful to measure ICP or CPP without invasive transducers. To this end, transcranial Doppler examination, tympanic membrane displacement, and ultrasound "time-of-flight" techniques have been suggested. The description of transcranial Doppler sonography by Aaslid and colleagues in 1982 permitted bedside monitoring of one index of cerebral blood flow noninvasively, repeatedly, and even continuously. The

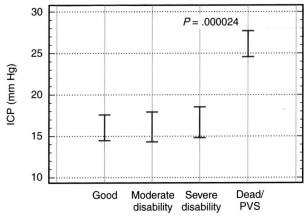

Figure 40-7 Averaged intracranial pressure (ICP) in nearly 500 patients after traumatic brain injury monitored in a specialized neuroscience center, with a breakdown of different outcome groups. PVS, persistent vegetative state.

problem has been that it is a "big tube technique" that measures flow velocity in branches of the circle of Willis, most commonly the middle cerebral artery (MCA). Compliant branches of the MCA can be compared with two physiologic pressure transducers. The pattern of blood flow within these tubes is certainly modulated by transmural pressure—that is, CPP and distal vascular resistance (also modulated by CPP). However, what is the calibration factor and how should we compensate for unknown nonlinear distortion?

There is reasonable correlation between the pulsatility index of MCA velocity and CPP after head injury, but absolute measurements of CPP cannot be extrapolated. Others have suggested that "critical closing pressure" derived from flow velocity and arterial pressure waveform analysis approximates the value of ICP. The accuracy of this method, however, has never been satisfactory. Aaslid and colleagues suggested that an index of CPP could be derived from the ratio of the amplitudes of the first harmonics of ABP and MCA velocity (detected by transcranial Doppler sonography) multiplied by mean flow velocity. Recently, a method for noninvasive assessment of CPP has been reported: mean ABP multiplied by the ratio of diastolic to mean flow velocity. This estimator can predict actual CPP—in the adult range (60 to 100 mm Hg)—with an error of less than 10 mm Hg for more than 80% of measurements. This is of potential benefit for continuous monitoring of changes in actual CPP over time in situations in which direct measurement of CPP is not readily available. Finally, a more complex method aimed at noninvasive assessment of ICP has been introduced and tested by B. Schmidt and colleagues. The method is based on the presumed transformation between ABP and ICP waveforms.

INTRACRANIAL PRESSURE AND OUTCOME AFTER SEVERE HEAD INJURY

In severe head injury, an average ICP higher than 25 mm Hg is associated with a twofold-increased risk for death. The distribution of mean ICP in patients achieving different outcomes suggests that postinjury intracranial hypertension is really a matter of life and death (Fig. 40-7). In addition, the PRx and RAP indices are strong independent predictors of death. Good vascular reactivity is an important element of brain homeostasis that enables the brain to protect itself against uncontrollable rises in intracerebral volume.

40

KEY POINTS

- Proper continuous measurement of ICP is a key element of brain monitoring after head injury.
- The PRx reflects the autoregulatory reserve of cerebral blood vessels.
- Analysis of the PRx and the ICP pulse waveform gives useful information regarding the adequacy of CPP.
- Noninvasive measurement of ICP and CPP, though of limited accuracy, is possible.

FURTHER READING

Balestreri M, Czosnyka M, Steiner LA, et al: Intracranial hypertension: What additional information can be derived from ICP waveform after head injury? Acta Neurochir (Wien) 2004; 146:131-141.

Banister K, Chambers IR, Siddique MS, et al: Intracranial pressure and clinical status: Assessment of two intracranial pressure transducers. Physiol Meas 2000 Nov 21(4):473-9.

Chambers IR, Jones PA, Lo TY, et al: Critical thresholds of intracranial pressure and cerebral perfusion pressure related to age in paediatric head injury. J Neurol Neurosurg Psychiatry 2006; 77:234-240.

Czosnyka M, Pickard JD: Monitoring and interpretation of intracranial pressure. J Neurol Neurosurg Psychiatry 2004; 75:813-821.

Czosnyka M, Smielewski P, Kirkpatrick P, et al: Continuous assessment of the cerebral vasomotor reactivity in head injury. Neurosurgery 1997; 41:11-19.

Hlatky R, Valadka AB, Robertson CS: Intracranial hypertension and cerebral ischemia after severe traumatic brain injury. Neurosurg Focus 2003; 14(4):e2.

Marmarou A, Signoretti S, Fatouros PP, et al: Predominance of cellular edema in traumatic brain swelling in patients with severe head injuries. J Neurosurg 2006; 104:720-730.

Steiner LA, Czosnyka M, Piechnik SK, et al: Continuous monitoring of cerebrovascular pressure reactivity allows determination of optimal cerebral perfusion pressure in patients with traumatic brain injury. Crit Care Med 2002; 30:733-738.

VI

Chapter 41

Jugular Venous Oximetry

Anuj Bhatia • Arun K.Gupta

Insertion Technique

Methods of Measurement

Factors Affecting Jugular Venous Oximetry

Clinical Applications

Limitations

Jugular venous oximetry (Sjvo$_2$) is a method of estimating *global* cerebral oxygenation and metabolism.

INSERTION TECHNIQUE

A catheter is inserted into the internal jugular vein via the Seldinger technique and advanced cephalad beyond the outlet of the common facial vein into the jugular bulb at the base of the skull (Fig. 41-1). Correct placement is confirmed when the catheter tip is level with the mastoid process above the lower border of C1 on a lateral neck radiograph. To sample the most representative side of the brain, it is common practice to cannulate the dominant internal jugular vein, which is usually on the right side. Contraindications and complications are similar to those for an internal jugular central venous pressure line.

METHODS OF MEASUREMENT

Serial samples can be taken to estimate the arteriovenous oxygen difference (AVDo$_2$), lactate, and glucose, which is technically easy and inexpensive. However, this method will give only a "snapshot" of the state of cerebral oxygenation and metabolism at the time of sampling, and samples may be contaminated by factors such as extracranial venous blood, catheter placement that is too low or against the petrosal veins, or blood sampling that is too rapid.

Insertion of fiberoptic catheters enables continuous monitoring of Sjvo$_2$, with normal values ranging from 55% to 85% (mean, 62%). No blood samples need be taken except for initial calibration. The advantages of a continuous on-line display of Sjvo$_2$ are readily apparent. This technique, however, does have disadvantages. Calibration drift may occur, and frequent in vivo recalibration may be required. Inaccurate readings may be obtained if the sensor is impacted against the vessel wall or if there is a decrease in intensity of the near-infrared light in the fiberoptic sensor, which occurs with thrombus formation on the catheter tip or changes in head position or blood flow characteristics in the vein.

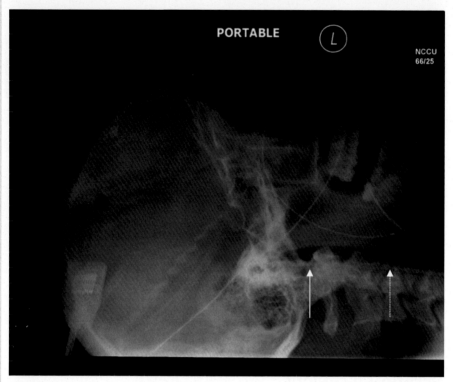

Figure 41-1 Lateral Cervical Spine X ray demonstrating the correct placement of Jugular Bulb Catheter. The dashed arrow indicated the point of insertion, the solid arrow indicates the tip of the catheter.

FACTORS AFFECTING JUGULAR VENOUS OXIMETRY

Although $Sjvo_2$ does not give quantitative information about either cerebral blood flow (CBF) or the cerebral metabolic rate of oxygen ($CMRO_2$), it does reflect the balance between the two variables.

> *Low $Sjvo_2$* values indicate either low oxygen delivery to the brain (low CBF or arterial O_2 content) or high $CMRO_2$ and increased oxygen extraction.
>
> *High $Sjvo_2$* values reflect high oxygen delivery (hyperemia, arteriovenous mixing) or low $CMRO_2$.

The threshold of $Sjvo_2$ below which cerebral ischemia is occurring may vary with the individual and the pathology. The two most common causes of jugular bulb desaturation ($Sjvo_2$ <55%) are

- *Decreased cerebral perfusion pressure* as a result of raised intracranial pressure (ICP) or systemic hypotension.
- *Hypocapnia.* In head-injured patients, $Sjvo_2$ values less than 50% have been shown to increase mortality. In patients undergoing cardiopulmonary bypass for cardiac surgery, cerebral venous desaturation below 50% correlated with worse postoperative cognitive function.

CLINICAL APPLICATIONS

A rise in ICP associated with a normal or low $Sjvo_2$ would suggest that edema is the predominant cause. If ICP and $Sjvo_2$ were both high, hyperemia would be implicated and hyperventilation would be the appropriate therapy. $Sjvo_2$ is a useful technique to guide hyperventilation therapy. Excessive hyperventilation causes profound cerebral vasoconstriction, which results in a reduction in $Sjvo_2$, assuming that brain metabolism remains constant. $Sjvo_2$ should be kept above 55% if hyperventilation is indicated.

There are also benefits in measuring $Sjvo_2$ to assess cerebral hypoperfusion during the intraoperative and postoperative management of patients with subarachnoid hemorrhage.

LIMITATIONS

The main limitation of this form of monitoring is that it is a global measure and a regional change in cerebral oxygenation will not be detected unless it is of sufficient magnitude to affect overall brain saturation. It is, however, the most widely used monitor for cerebral oxygenation in neuroanesthesia and intensive care.

KEY POINTS

- $Sjvo_2$ is a global measure of the balance of cerebral blood flow and metabolism.
- The insertion technique and complications are similar to those of an internal jugular central venous line.
- Measurement can be intermittent or continuous.
- $Sjvo_2$ is particularly useful in monitoring interventions such as hyperventilation therapy.
- Lack of sensitivity to regional changes is a major limitation.

FURTHER READING

41

Bhatia A, Gupta AK. Neuromonitoring in the intensive Care Unit II. Cerebral oxygenation monitoring and microdilalysis. Intensive Care Medicine 2007. 33:1322-1328.

Croughwell ND, White WD, Smith LR, et al: Jugular bulb saturation and mixed venous saturation during cardiopulmonary bypass. J Card Surg 1995; 10:503-508.

Dearden NM, Midgley S: Technical considerations in continuous jugular venous oxygen saturation measurement. Acta Neurochir 1993; 59(Suppl):91-97.

Robertson CS, Cormio M: Cerebral metabolic management. New Horizons 1995; 3:410-422.

Robertson CS, Gopinath SP, Goodman JC, et al: $Sjvo_2$ monitoring in head injured patients. J Neurotrauma 1995; 12:891-896.

Sheinberg M, Kanter MJ, Robertson CS, et al: Continuous monitoring of jugular venous oxygen saturation in head injured patients. J Neurosurg 1992; 76:212-271.

Chapter 42

Tissue Oxygenation

Jurgens Nortje • Arun K.Gupta

Measurement of Brain Tissue Oxygen Tension	Near-Infrared Spectroscopy
Equipment	Principles
Validation and Safety	Equipment
Clinical Applications	Clinical Applications
Therapeutic and Research Applications	Summary
Summary	

Hypoxia and hypotension worsen outcomes after brain injury, and avoidance of cerebral hypoxia may improve outcomes after traumatic brain injury (TBI). Jugular bulb oximetry (see Chapter 41) has been the traditional technique used, but the more reproducible technique of direct intraparenchymal oxygen tension measurement is increasingly being applied. There has also been a resurgence in the use of near infrared spectroscopy (NIR).

MEASUREMENT OF BRAIN TISSUE OXYGEN TENSION

Brain tissue oxygen tension (Pbo_2) is the partial pressure of oxygen in the extracellular fluid of the brain and reflects the availability of oxygen for oxidative energy metabolism (production of adenosine triphosphate). It represents the balance between oxygen delivery and consumption.

Potential benefits include

- Optimization of cerebral oxygen delivery
- Early detection and possible amelioration of secondary cerebral insults
- Monitoring of focal areas of injured brain
- Monitoring of uninjured brain and thus allowing assumptions about global cerebral oxygenation
- Greater assessment of therapeutic interventions such as manipulation of cerebral perfusion pressure (CPP)
- Elucidation of underlying pathophysiology after brain injury

Equipment

The Licox sensor is now the most commonly used sensor although the Neurotrend sensor has also been used in the past.

- The Licox (GMS, Kiel-Mielkendorf, Germany) measures Pbo_2 and temperature. Covering an estimated 15-mm^2 Po_2-sensitive area, the Licox sensor uses a

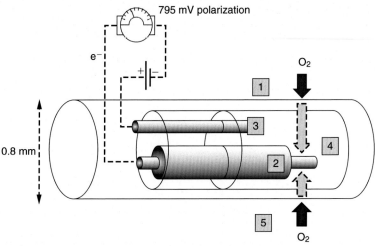

Figure 42-1 The Licox oxygen sensor tip. 1, Polyethylene tube with diffusible membrane; 2, gold polarographic cathode; 3, silver polarographic anode; 4, electrolyte chamber; 5, brain parenchyma. (Adapted from the manufacturer's manual.)

closed polarographic (Clark-type) cell with reversible electrochemical electrodes (Fig. 42-1). After diffusion from brain tissue across a semipermeable membrane, oxygen is reduced by a gold polarographic cathode to produce a flow of electrical current directly proportional to the oxygen concentration. This oxygen-consuming process is temperature dependent.

- The Neurotrend (Codman, Johnson & Johnson, Raynham, MA) measures Pbo_2, $Pbco_2$, pH, and temperature, but its production has been discontinued.

Insertion

Sensors can be inserted either via a cranial access device through a bur hole in the intensive care unit (ICU) or under direct vision at surgery. The Licox has a sensor-specific precalibrated smart card that allows immediate implantation. Exact localization of the sensor tips on computed tomography after insertion is essential for accurate interpretation and use. To exclude insertion-related microhemorrhage or sensor damage, Fio_2 can be increased transiently to confirm appropriate corresponding increases in Pbo_2. An equilibration time of about half an hour after insertion is required before readings are stable.

Validation and Safety

Measurement of Pbo_2 has been significantly correlated with cerebral venous blood Po_2, $Sjvo_2$, regional cerebral blood flow (CBF), positron emission tomography (PET)-derived end-capillary Po_2, and microdialysis glucose and lactate. Despite the invasiveness of these intraparenchymal sensors, there are very few reports of complications, with studies totalling 552 patients reporting no infections and three iatrogenic hematomas. Measurement accuracy with negligible zero drift is also a consistent finding.

Clinical Applications

Though predominantly used for TBI and subarachnoid hemorrhage (SAH) both in the ICU and intraoperatively, Pbo_2 monitoring has also been applied to resection of arteriovenous malformations and brain tumors and determination of the pharmacodynamics of anesthetic agents.

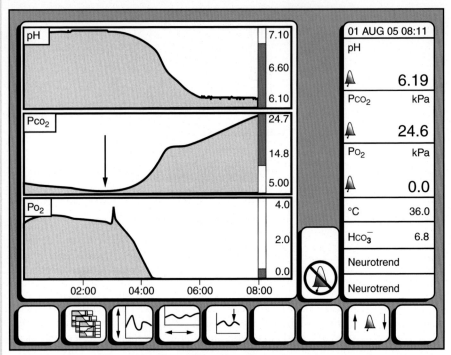

Figure 42-2 Neurotrend trace reflecting changes at the time of fatal intracranial hypertension–induced cerebellar tonsillar herniation *(arrow)* in a patient with traumatic brain injury.

Traumatic Brain Injury

Cerebral ischemia after TBI may be the result of fluctuations in CBF, and this is compounded by cerebral edema and raised intracranial pressure (ICP). Monitoring of Pbo_2 has revealed not only evidence of hypoxia but also differences in normal and abnormal brain tissue. Trends in cerebral oxygenation assist in early detection and treatment of secondary insults, as well as in assessing responses to therapeutic interventions such as hyperventilation. Decreases in Pbo_2 and pH with concomitant increases in $Paco_2$ occur during brain death (Fig. 42-2).

Subarachnoid Hemorrhage

Correctly positioned intraoperative Pbo_2 sensors may allow assessment of the effect and reversibility of temporary aneurysm clipping, as well as correct positioning of the subsequent permanent clip. A Pbo_2 value of less than 8 mm Hg for 30 minutes during temporary clipping is predictive of cerebral infarction. Pbo_2 monitoring during aneurysm clipping also supplements somatosensory evoked potential (SEP) monitoring in identifying ischemia. Though attractive for continuous surveillance and detection of delayed vasospasm-induced ischemia in patients with SAH in the ICU, targeting the relevant tissue with Pbo_2 monitoring has remained a hurdle.

Normal Values

Human measurements have been restricted to "normal" values during neurosurgery and in "normal-appearing" brain after TBI, with Pbo_2 varying from 37 to 48 mm Hg.

Hypoxic Thresholds

Though important, these thresholds need to be considered in the context of probe type, probe site, underlying pathology, and duration of hypoxia. Various Pbo_2 thresholds have been proposed (8.5, 10, 14, 20, and 25 mm Hg), but a level of 10 mm Hg is generally taken as a clinically significant hypoxic threshold.

Pbo_2 Reactivity

Pbo_2 reactivity is the increase in Pbo_2 after an increase in Pao_2 and is thought to be controlled by an oxygen regulatory mechanism that may be disturbed after brain injury. The "brain tissue oxygen response" has been shown to be an independent predictor of an unfavorable outcome (odds ratio, 4.8).

Pbo_2 "Autoregulation"

Pbo_2 autoregulation is the ability of the brain to maintain Pbo_2 despite changes in CPP and has implications for optimal CPP targets.

Therapeutic and Research Applications

Monitoring of Pbo_2 has been used to assess the adequacy of CPP, the dangers of excessive hyperventilation, and optimum brain temperature after injury, as well as controversial interventions such as decompressive craniectomy and normobaric hyperoxia.

Summary

Advantages

- Continuous oxygenation monitor
- Accurate and technically more reliable than jugular venous oximetry
- Calibrated before insertion
- Selective monitoring of "at risk" tissue
- Direct brain temperature measurement
- Increasing data on clinical usefulness

Disadvantages

- Invasive with attendant risks
- Fragile sensors
- Focal monitor, although global assumptions can be made if located in normal tissue

42

NEAR-INFRARED SPECTROSCOPY

NIRS is a noninvasive monitor of regional cerebral oxygenation whereby human cerebral tissue is penetrated by light in the near-infrared band.

Principles

Light in the near-infrared band (700 to 1000 nm) passes through human tissue (including skin and bone) relatively easily. Its resultant absorption and scatter allow assessment of changes in the chromophores oxyhemoglobin (HbO_2), deoxyhemoglobin (Hb), and cytochrome oxidase, each of which has different absorption spectra. The concentrations of these substances depend on their oxygenation status. The isobestic point of HbO_2 and Hb is 810 nm, with greater light absorption by HbO_2 above this point and greater absorption by Hb below this point. Maximal light absorption by cytochrome oxidase occurs at about 830 nm.

The change in concentration of the chromophores is quantified by using a modification of the Beer-Lambert law, so-called differential spectroscopy. Beer's law states that the intensity of transmitted light decreases exponentially as the concentration of the substance increases, whereas Lambert's law states that the intensity of transmitted light decreases exponentially as the distance traveled through the substance increases. The modified law provides the optical attenuation with use of the following equation:

$$A = logI_0/I\alpha CLB + G$$

where

A = optical density
I_0 = incident light intensity
I = detected light intensity
α = absorption coefficient of the chromophore
C = concentration of the chromophore
L = distance between the light entry and exit points
B = light path length factor
G = tissue geometry and type factor (scatter correction)

In neonates, the thin skull allows light transmission from one side and detection on the other (transmission spectroscopy). However, in adults, because of the diameter and thickness of the skull, light transmission is significantly attenuated and reflectance spectroscopy is required. Using spatially resolved reflectance spectroscopy, cerebral oxygenation may be expressed with high sensitivity and specificity as the tissue oxygen index (TOI):

$$TOI = HbO_2/HbO_2 + Hb \times 100$$

Equipment

Although configurations of the clinically available instruments vary, pulsed laser light–emitting diodes deliver near-infrared light of different wavelengths into cerebral tissue, which is then detected by photodiodes placed at specific distances (Fig. 42-3). The optodes are held in a lightproof holder and can be set at a distance of around 4 to 7 cm. A fiberoptic plate detector window allows light to be conducted from the skin surface to the sensors without distorting the spatial distribution. Correct detector orientation relative to the laser diode bundle is essential.

The probes illuminate a volume of up to 10 cc of cerebral tissue, with radial depth depending on the interoptode distance. Placement of the probe on one side of the forehead away from the midline is important to avoid the cerebral venous sinuses and temporalis muscle. A derived algorithm, which is equipment specific, measures changes in attenuation at each wavelength (for each chromophore), and this is then converted to changes in concentrations of HbO_2, Hb, and cytochrome oxidase from a zero baseline. Spatial resolution relies on measurement of the attenuation gradient as a function of source-detector separation.

Clinical Applications

NIRS is well established in neonates and provides brain hemoglobin oxygen saturation, cerebral blood volume (CBV), and cerebrovascular responses to therapeutic interventions. Use in adults has been predominantly in the ICU to

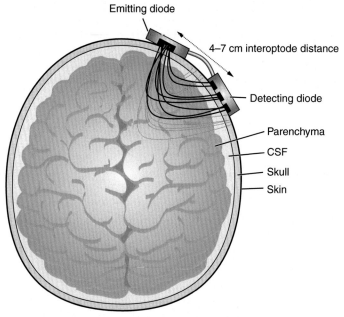

Emitting diode

4–7 cm interoptode distance

Detecting diode

Parenchyma

CSF

Skull

Skin

Figure 42-3 Schematic representation of near-infrared spectroscopy. CSF, cerebrospinal fluid.

monitor patients with TBI and SAH or in the operating room in patients undergoing carotid endarterectomy and other neurovascular procedures.

Traumatic Brain Injury

NIRS allows important estimations of regional cerebral oxygenation, CBF (modified Fick principle with HbO_2 as the tracer), and CBV at the ICU bedside after head injury. The cerebral oxygenation, however, is a mean value for arterial, venous, and capillary oxygenation, in contrast to $Sjvo_2$, for instance.

Carotid Endarterectomy and Neurovascular Procedures

As part of multimodality monitoring in the operating theater, NIRS can detect cerebral desaturation at cross-clamping and identify patients who require intraoperative shunt placement.

Summary

Advantages

- NIRS is a noninvasive monitor, as opposed to Pbo_2 or $Sjvo_2$.
- It is a continuous real-time bedside monitor, as opposed to snapshot methods such as PET, which requires extensive postprocessing.
- Patients are not exposed to ionizing radiation.
- NIRS can provide measures of cerebral oxygenation, as well as CBV and CBF, with newer applications in functional imaging.

Disadvantages

- Readings are restricted to a small region with a variable sample volume.
- NIRS has wide variability in readings without the reproducibility of PET.

42

- The major disadvantage is that extracranial blood flow and oxygenation contaminate readings to a significant and variable degree. Although increasing the interoptode distance reduces this influence, the signal then becomes weaker.
- The complex multilayered human cranium causes variable distorted penetration with optical channels and unpredictable scatter.
- Outside light and head movement distort the readings, and maintaining optode positioning can be difficult.
- Machines have traditionally been bulky.
- The derived algorithms may not be robust under varying clinical conditions.

KEY POINTS

Brain Tissue Oxygen Sensors

- Pbo_2 sensors are accurate with minimal complications and are more reproducible and robust than $SjvO_2$.
- CPP and $Paco_2$ levels can be optimized with Pbo_2 sensors.
- They provide an indication of the efficacy of research interventions.
- Hypoxic thresholds have clear implications for outcome in SAH and TBI, with possible scope for improving outcome with targeted Pbo_2 therapy.

Near-Infrared Spectroscopy

- NIRS is a transcutaneous noninvasive monitor of regional cerebral oxygenation.
- Monitoring is based on the differential absorption of near-infrared light by oxyhemoglobin, deoxyhemoglobin, and cytochrome oxidase.
- Positioning and interoptode distance can influence measurement.
- It can be used in the operating room or in the ICU.
- NIRS is a good trend monitor, but it is beset by reliability issues because of extracranial blood contamination.

FURTHER READING

Al-Rawi PG, Kirkpatrick PJ: Tissue oxygen index: Thresholds for cerebral ischemia using near-infrared spectroscopy. Stroke 2006; 37:2720-2725.

Calderon-Arnulphi M, Alaraj A, Amin-Hanjani S: Detection of cerebral ischemia in neurovascular surgery using quantitative frequency-domain near-infrared spectroscopy. J Neurosurg 2007; 106:283-290.

Clausen T, Scharf A, Menzel M, et al: Influence of moderate and profound hyperventilation on cerebral blood flow, oxygenation and metabolism. Brain Res 2004; 1019:113-123.

Kett-White R, Hutchinson PJ, Al-Rawi PG, et al: Cerebral oxygen and microdialysis monitoring during aneurysm surgery: Effects of blood pressure, cerebrospinal fluid drainage, and temporary clipping on infarction. J Neurosurg 2002; 96:1013-1019.

Madsen PL, Secher NH: Near-infrared oximetry of the brain. Prog Neurobiol 1999; 58:541-560.

Nortje J, Gupta AK: The role of tissue oxygen monitoring in patients with acute brain injury. Br J Anaesth 2006; 97:95-106.

Owen-Reece H, Smith M, Elwell CE, Goldstone JC: Near infrared spectroscopy. Br J Anaesth 1999; 82:418-426.

Stiefel MF, Spiotta A, Gracias VH, et al: Reduced mortality rate in patients with severe traumatic brain injury treated with brain tissue oxygen monitoring. J Neurosurg 2005; 103:805-811.

Strangman G, Franceschini MA, Boas DA: Factors affecting the accuracy of near-infrared spectroscopy concentration calculations for focal changes in oxygenation parameters. Neuroimage 2003; 18:865-879.

Chapter 43

Microdialysis

Ivan Timofeev • Peter Hutchinson

Microdialysis is a monitoring method that allows measurement of extracellular chemistry in living tissue. After its development in the 1970s, it was used predominantly in laboratory research. Since the 1990s microdialysis has been applied in the clinical area and is now used by many specialties. Monitoring cerebral tissue chemistry in neurointensive care remains one of its main applications.

PRINCIPLES

A fine polyurethane catheter (1 mm Ø) is placed into the tissue of interest, where it acts as an artificial "blood capillary" (Fig. 43-1). It consists of outer and inner tubes and contains a semipermeable membrane at the distal end. A small portable pump is used to perfuse the catheter with solution containing Na^+, K^+, Ca^+, Mg^{2+}, and Cl^- at 0.1 to 2.0 μL/min. Once the fluid passes through the inner tube of the catheter and reaches the membrane area, the chemical substances at higher concentration in the extracellular fluid (ECF) passively diffuse into the perfusate driven by the concentration gradient. The membrane pore size defines the maximum weight of molecules that can cross, most commonly 20 or 100 kD clinically, thus allowing sampling of amino acids and small proteins. At a constant rate, fluid flows proximally via the outer tube and accumulates in the microvial. After a predefined period (usually 1 hour), the microvial is changed and the collected dialysate is analyzed. Measurement of common biochemical markers (glucose, lactate, pyruvate, glutamate, glycerol, and urea) can be performed by enzyme assay with colorimetry. Virtually any substance that is small enough to cross the membrane can be measured with an appropriate analytic technique.

Chemical substances can also be added to the perfusion fluid and will diffuse across the membrane into the ECF. This technique is known as retrodialysis and can be used for delivery of pharmacologic and experimental agents directly into tissue.

43

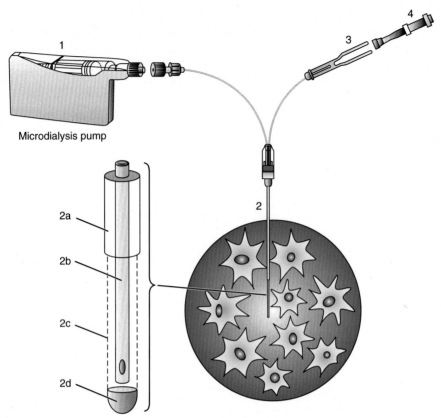

Figure 43-1 Principle of microdialysis. 1, Precision pump. 2, Microdialysis catheter implanted in tissue. The catheter consists of outer (2a) and inner (2b) tubes and a semipermeable membrane at the distal end (2c). The golden tip (2d) facilitates visualization on computed tomography. 3, Microvial holder with a needle that on insertion of the vial penetrates its lid. 4, Microvial for collection of dialysate.

RECOVERY

Constant exchange of perfusion fluid at the membrane helps maintain a concentration gradient but at the same time prevents complete equilibration of concentrations between the ECF and perfusate. Consequently, the concentration of substance detectable in the dialysate, known as "the recovery," represents only a proportion of its true extracellular concentration. Relative recovery defines the concentration of the substance in the dialysate after it leaves the membrane area and is expressed as the percentage of its total ECF concentration. Relative recovery increases with a reduction in the perfusion flow rate because of the longer time available for diffusion; it approaches 100% of the ECF concentration when flow rates approach zero. Catheters with greater membrane area provide higher recovery at the same flow rate as a result of an increased area of diffusion. Unfortunately, the reduction in flow rates limits the amount of dialysate available for analysis, and increasing the membrane area leads to difficulty in catheter implantation. It has been estimated that standard catheters with a membrane size of 10 mm at a flow rate of 0.3 μL/min provide relative recovery of 70% of the true tissue concentration. Other factors that may influence recovery are the charge of the molecule or the membrane, pH, temperature, pressure, and osmolarity of the ECF.

COMMON MICRODIALYSIS MARKERS

The clinical application of microdialysis is based on early detection of changes in tissue biochemistry, which represent impeding or ongoing tissue injury. In some situations, microdialysis may be the only modality to detect unfavorable tissue conditions at an early stage. Changes in bedside microdialysis markers reflect the general pathophysiology of cellular injury and therefore can be applied to many organs. In cerebral tissue they are predominantly used to detect ischemia, impaired mitochondrial function, and excitotoxic and structural damage. The most commonly used bedside microdialysis markers include glucose, lactate, pyruvate, glutamate, and glycerol.

Glucose, Lactate, and Pyruvate

Adequate aerobic production of adenosine triphosphate relies on a constant supply of glucose and oxygen and preserved mitochondrial function. Under normal conditions glucose is metabolized to pyruvate and lactate, and the former is used as substrate for the citric acid cycle. There is normally a relative balance between glucose, lactate, and pyruvate concentrations in ECF. Lack of oxygen or impaired mitochondrial function may lead to failure of oxidative phosphorylation. Pyruvate is then not used to the same extent and is increasingly converted to lactate, thereby leading to accumulation of the latter. The ratio of lactate to pyruvate (L/P ratio) reflects this changing balance and benefits from being independent of absolute values of parameters. The L/P ratio has been proved to be a sensitive marker of impaired energy metabolism and relates to neurologic outcome.

A reduction in cerebral blood flow or increased consumption of glucose may lead to a decrease in its extracellular concentration. Low extracellular glucose levels are associated with poor outcome after traumatic brain injury (TBI) and are indicative of poor perfusion in aneurysmal subarachnoid hemorrhage (SAH). The lactate-to-glucose ratio can also serve as a marker of ischemia or increased glycolysis.

Glutamate

Cerebral extracellular glutamate levels increase in tissue ischemia and hypoxia. This process may be manifested as raised extracellular glutamate in the absence of ischemia despite the fact that the origin of extracellular glutamate is generally extrasynaptic.

Glycerol

One of the manifestations of cellular distress and injury is degradation of the cell membrane, which results in the release of glycerol from phospholipids and leads to a rise in the ECF glycerol concentration, thus making it a marker of brain injury. Although the main source of cerebral glycerol is the cellular membrane, systemic increases in glycerol as a result of peripheral lipolysis or the administration of glycerol-containing drugs may affect its cerebral levels.

The concentrations of microdialysis markers in uninjured brain are summarized in Table 43-1. It needs to be stressed that analysis of trends over time is most useful.

43

Table 43-1   Values of Microdialysis Markers in Normal Brain and in Different Catheter Locations in Relation to Traumatic Contusion (Values Represent Means ± Standard Deviations)

Biochemical Marker	Normal Brain, Awake Patient	Microdialysis Catheter Located in a Minimally Injured Brain Contralateral to the Lesion in TBI	Microdialysis Catheter Located in the Penumbra of the Lesion in TBI
Glucose (mmol/L)	1.7 ± 0.9	3.1 ± 0.1	1.2 ± 0.1
Pyruvate (mmol/L)	166 ± 47	160 ± 50	170 ± 80
Lactate (μmol/L)	2.9 ± 0.9	2.9 ± 0.1	6.3 ± 0.1
Lactate-pyruvate ratio	23 ± 4	20 ± 0.3	45 ± 1
Glutamate (μmol/L)	16 ± 16	17 ± 1	63 ± 2
Glycerol (μmol/L)	35 ± 11	38 ± 1	175 ± 6

TBI, traumatic brain injury.
Data from Engstrom M, Polito A, Reinstrup P, et al: Intracerebral microdialysis in severe brain trauma: The importance of catheter location. J Neurosurg 2005; 102:460-469; and Reinstrup P, Stahl N, Mellergard P, et al: Intracerebral microdialysis in clinical practice: Baseline values for chemical markers during wakefulness, anesthesia, and neurosurgery. Neurosurgery 2000; 47:701-709; discussion 709-710.

CATHETER LOCATION

A cerebral microdialysis catheter monitors only several cubic millimeters of brain tissue, and therefore interpretation of microdialysis data requires knowledge of the catheter's location in relation to pathologic areas in the brain tissue. The tip of the standard microdialysis catheter can be visualized on computed tomography. The values obtained with the catheter located in diffusely injured brain correlate with whole-brain metabolism, whereas a catheter located in the vicinity of contusion or ischemic penumbra provides focal information on the state of this vulnerable tissue (Table 43-1). In many cases the concurrent use of two catheters in different locations is recommended. No catheter should be placed into necrotic tissue.

CLINICAL APPLICATIONS OF MICRODIALYSIS

TBI and SAH remain the main areas of clinical application. In TBI, in conjunction with other methods of multimodality monitoring, microdialysis allows early detection of ischemia, hypoxia, and seizures, all of which may lead to secondary injury (Fig. 43-2). Microdialysis markers can be used to individualize cerebral perfusion pressure management, evaluate the adequacy of tissue perfusion and oxygenation, and assess the physiologic response to therapy (e.g., hyperventilation, sedation, surgical interventions). In SAH, one of the main benefits of monitoring with microdialysis is the possibility of detecting ischemic changes early, before the development of clinical symptoms of delayed ischemic neurologic deficit.

Microdialysis has also been used to monitor stroke (ischemic penumbra or malignant brain edema in major-vessel occlusion), intracranial hemorrhage, epilepsy, tumors, infections, and hepatic encephalopathy. Microdialysis may help evaluate the

VI

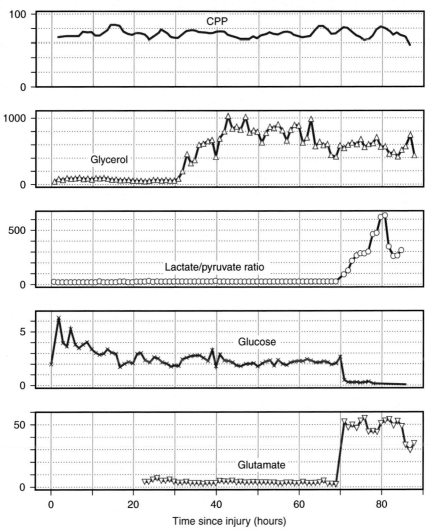

Figure 43-2 Example of clinical microdialysis trends. Significant elevation in the extracellular glycerol concentration is seen on the second day after severe traumatic brain injury, followed by other biochemical markers despite the absence of significant changes in cerebral perfusion pressure. The patient did not survive.

safety of intraoperative manipulations and the duration of hypoperfusion (e.g., during temporary clipping or anastomosis).

RESEARCH APPLICATIONS OF MICRODIALYSIS

Current research applications include evaluating pharmacokinetics and the tissue bioavailability of pharmacologic agents, exploring the pathophysiology of tissue injury, and developing and validating novel biochemical markers. In clinical research, microdialysis markers can be used as surrogate end points to evaluate the physiologic benefits of therapeutic interventions.

LIMITATIONS OF MICRODIALYSIS

Microdialysis provides retrospective measurement of biochemical markers, depending on the rate of vial change, and therefore cannot be considered an on-line technique. Many factors can affect recovery and the tissue concentration of biochemical substances in vivo, and this coupled with invasiveness and dependence on highly trained personnel currently limits its widespread use.

KEY POINTS

- Microdialysis allows in vivo measurement of biochemical substances in extracellular fluid.
- The system consists of a perfusion pump, catheter implanted in the tissue, microvials for collection of the dialysate, and an analyzer.
- Recovery of substances is proportional to their true extracellular concentration.
- Glucose, lactate (L), and pyruvate (P) are bedside markers of energy metabolism.
- The L/P ratio is a sensitive marker of impaired aerobic metabolism.
- Glutamate and glycerol are additional markers of adverse tissue conditions.
- Biochemical trends provide useful clinical information.
- Catheter location in relation to the areas of injured tissue needs to be taken into account when interpreting results.

FURTHER READING

Bellander BM, Cantais E, Enblad P, et al: Consensus meeting on microdialysis in neurointensive care. Intensive Care Med 2004; 30:2166-2169.

Engstrom M, Polito A, Reinstrup P, et al: Intracerebral microdialysis in severe brain trauma: The importance of catheter location. J Neurosurg 2005; 102:460-469.

Hillered L, Vespa PM, Hovda DA: Translational neurochemical research in acute human brain injury: The current status and potential future for cerebral microdialysis. J Neurotrauma 2005; 22:3-41.

Hlatky R, Valadka AB, Goodman JC, et al: Patterns of energy substrates during ischemia measured in the brain by microdialysis. J Neurotrauma 2004; 21:894-906.

Hutchinson PJ, O'Connell MT, Al-Rawi PG, et al: Clinical cerebral microdialysis: A methodological study. J Neurosurg 2000; 93:37-43.

Reinstrup P, Stahl N, Mellergard P, et al: Intracerebral microdialysis in clinical practice: Baseline values for chemical markers during wakefulness, anesthesia, and neurosurgery. Neurosurgery 2000; 47:701-709; discussion 709-710.

Sarrafzadeh A, Haux D, Sakowitz O, et al: Acute focal neurological deficits in aneurysmal subarachnoid hemorrhage: Relation of clinical course, CT findings, and metabolite abnormalities monitored with bedside microdialysis. Stroke 2003; 34:1382-1388.

Vespa P, Bergsneider M, Hattori N, et al: Metabolic crisis without brain ischemia is common after traumatic brain injury: A combined microdialysis and positron emission tomography study. J Cereb Blood Flow Metab 2005; 25:763-774.

VI

Chapter 44

Electromyography and Evoked Potentials

Jeremy A. Lieberman

Electromyography	Somatosensory Evoked Potentials
Anesthetic Considerations	Motor Evoked Potentials
Evoked Potentials	
Visual Evoked Potentials	
Brainstem Auditory Evoked Potentials	

Electromyography and evoked potentials are monitors of neurologic function that are used during some neurosurgical procedures (Table 44-1). Evidence suggests that these techniques can identify reversible changes in neurologic function intraoperatively, thereby allowing intervention and possible prevention of injury. However, no randomized prospective trials have clearly demonstrated that such techniques improve outcome.

ELECTROMYOGRAPHY

Electromyography allows continuous assessment of cranial and peripheral motor nerves by placing needle electrodes into or near specific muscles. If a nerve is touched or stretched during surgery, electromyographic (EMG) activity will occur in the muscle that is innervated by that nerve. Mild nerve irritation leads to transient EMG discharges that resolve rapidly. More serious nerve irritation may produce sustained EMG discharges. Electrocautery and saline irrigation are major sources of interference.

Electromyography is commonly used when trying to preserve the facial nerve (cranial nerve VII) during procedures involving the base of the skull, such as resection of acoustic neuromas. EMG activity may also be recorded from other cranial nerves that innervate muscles, including nerves III, IV, VI, IX, X, XI, and XII.

EMG activity may be recorded from muscles of the upper and lower extremities and be used to detect injury to the spinal cord and spinal nerve roots during spine surgery. Electrodes are placed in muscles deemed most at risk from surgically induced neurologic injury. In addition, vertebral pedicle screws may be stimulated electrically to determine whether they are wholly within the bony pedicle and vertebral body. If there is a breach into the spinal canal, EMG activity will occur with much lower stimulation current.

44

Table 44-1 Lesions for Which Evoked Potential Monitoring or Electromyography Might Be Used

Visual Evoked Potentials	Brainstem Auditory Evoked Potentials	Somatosensory Evoked Potentials	Motor Evoked Potentials	Electromyography
Pituitary or suprasellar lesions	Acoustic neuroma Fifth nerve compression— trigeminal neuralgia	Spinal deformity Spinal cord tumors	Spinal deformity Intramedullary spinal cord tumors	Acoustic neuroma Posterior fossa lesions
Retro-orbital lesions		Spinal cord vascular lesions	Cerebral tumors near the motor cortex	Lumbar spine defects
Lesions near the occipital cortex	Seventh nerve compression— facial spasm	Lesions of the posterior fossa	Cerebrovascular structures near the motor cortex	Cervical spine defects
Neurovascular lesions— posterior circulation	Lesions in the posterior fossa Lesions of the temporal or parietal cortex	Lesions near the thalamus Lesions of the parietal cortex		

Anesthetic Considerations

There are no anesthetic agents that interfere with EMG responses. Muscle relaxants do block the neuromuscular junction and should be avoided during periods of EMG recording.

EVOKED POTENTIALS

As the name implies, this technique of monitoring applies a stimulus to evoke a response. Sensory evoked potentials may be recorded after various types of sensory input: somatosensory (SSEP), visual (VEP), or auditory (brainstem auditory [BAEP]). Motor evoked potentials (MEPs) involve stimulation of the motor cortex to elicit a response in the spinal cord, peripheral nerves, or muscles.

All evoked potential responses are described in terms of latency (the time from the stimulus until the response) and amplitude (the size of the response) (Fig. 44-1). Neurologic injury typically leads to prolonged latency and decreased amplitude. Most sensory evoked potential amplitudes are very small relative to background EEG activity. Therefore, it is necessary to evoke many responses to permit "signal averaging," which filters out this background and yields a more distinct evoked potential waveform.

Visual Evoked Potentials

VEPs monitor the visual pathway from the eye through the optic nerve and chiasm to the visual cortex. The eyes are exposed to a series of bright lights by using special goggles or contact lenses while scalp electrodes record the VEPs. VEPs may be useful in assessing visual pathway integrity for surgery near the optic nerve and chiasm (e.g., pituitary resection). They may also help when resecting tumors in the occipital cortex or correcting neurovascular lesions involving the posterior circulation.

VEPs are technically difficult to obtain and are exquisitely sensitive to most anesthetic agents, so consistent responses are hard to obtain and interpret under general anesthesia. Thus, they are not commonly used in the operating room.

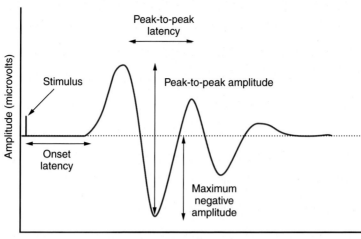

Figure 44-1 Example of an evoked potential response curve depicting latency and amplitude measurements. Note that "onset latency" is the time from the stimulus to the beginning of the response. "Peak-to-peak" or "interpeak" latency is the time between various amplitude peaks. Peak amplitude may be characterized as either the largest voltage deviation in one direction from baseline or as the maximum total voltage spread (maximum positive + maximum negative amplitude).

Brainstem Auditory Evoked Potentials

BAEPs record the integrity of the auditory pathway, starting from the ear (tympanic membrane, ossicles) and including nervous system structures such as hair cells, spiral ganglion, cranial nerve VIII, cochlear nuclei, superior olivary complex, lateral lemniscus, inferior colliculus, and medial geniculate thalamic nuclei.

To generate BAEPs, a transducer is placed in the external auditory canal. The auditory stimulus is typically a series of clicks. Responses are measured across electrodes placed over the scalp. Multiple signals are averaged (≈2000) to yield a series of six or seven positive waves, each given a Roman numeral designation (Fig. 44-2). Each wave was originally believed to arise from a specific structure along the auditory pathway, but subsequent studies have shown that many waves originate from multiple structures. Thus, pathologic lesions or surgical trauma may affect several waves.

Interpretation

To elicit interpretable BAEPs, the patient must have adequate hearing function. With middle ear or cochlear deficits, no waves will be generated. Eighth nerve injury affects all waves after wave I. Cerebellar retraction often causes prolongation of interpeak latency between waves I and V. Transient changes are not predictive of hearing loss, but when complete loss of these later waves occurs, permanent auditory tract damage is more likely.

Typical Procedures

BAEPs are most commonly used during microvascular decompression of cranial nerves V or VII. BAEPs may help reduce hearing loss during resection of acoustic neuromas. Auditory tract injury is due to brainstem compression, direct trauma to the eighth nerve, or ischemia of the nerve. BAEPs are less useful for posterior fossa tumors. They may miss focal brainstem injury because abnormal BAEPs might occur only with global brainstem damage.

44

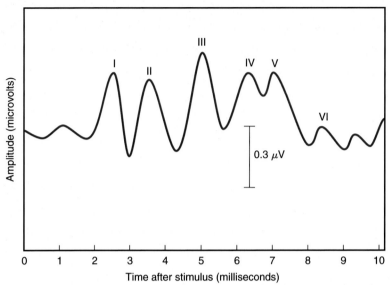

Figure 44-2 Brainstem auditory evoked potential tracing demonstrating multiple waveform peaks after an auditory stimulus. Loss of wave amplitude and prolongation of interpeak latency may suggest injury.

Anesthetic Considerations

BAEPs are very robust and resistant to most anesthetics. Volatile inhalational agents are the most suppressive, but the effects are minimal and signals are easily obtained with any regimen. Muscle relaxants have no effect on BAEPs.

Somatosensory Evoked Potentials

SSEPs monitor the integrity of sensory pathways, including peripheral nerves, the spinal cord, the brainstem, subcortical structures, and the sensory cortex. Disruption along any part of this pathway may disrupt normal SSEP responses. A repetitive electrical stimulus is applied to a peripheral nerve and responses are measured over the cerebral cortex with scalp electrodes. Subcortical responses may be recorded by placing electrodes near the upper cervical spine. A transcutaneous electrical stimulus is applied to a peripheral nerve, typically the median or ulnar nerve of the upper extremity or the posterior tibial nerve of the lower extremity. The main sensory pathways travel up the posterior spinal cord in the dorsal columns. Some sensory tracts from the lower extremities travel along ventral and lateral pathways as well. The fibers cross at the brainstem and proceed up through the thalamus to the postcentral gyrus of the cortex. Scalp electrodes record the evoked potentials. SSEPs have small amplitude, and averaging of more than 1000 responses is needed to produce a clear signal.

Typical Procedures

SSEPs are commonly used during spine surgery when injury to the spinal cord may be due to ischemia secondary to spinal distraction and disruption of perforating radicular vessels. Direct trauma may occur during pedicle screw placement or other instrumentation or while resecting a pathologic lesion that is proximate to the sensory tracts.

SSEPs may be used to ensure adequate perfusion to the cortex during intracranial or extracranial vascular surgery (e.g., aneurysm, carotid endarterectomy). If SSEPs change, inadequate blood flow may be indicated. SSEP responses elicited from posterior tibial nerve stimulation are mediated by cortex supplied by the anterior cerebral artery. In contrast, stimulation of the median nerve evokes responses in the cortex supplied by the middle cerebral artery.

Interpretation of Responses

Loss or decrease of SSEP responses may be due to disruption of any component of the sensory pathway. The common definition of significant change is a 50% drop in amplitude or a 10% increase in latency, or both. Asymmetric changes are also suspicious.

Frequent causes of false-positive changes (i.e., changes but without resulting injury) include anesthetics, hypothermia, acute changes in $Paco_2$, hypotension, hypovolemia, and anemia. Because SSEPs monitor the integrity of sensory tracts, isolated injury to motor tracts might be missed (i.e., a false-negative response).

Anesthetic Considerations

Cortical SSEPs are more sensitive than BAEPs to anesthetic agents. Cortical SSEP responses can be obtained with any anesthetic regimen, but avoidance of rapid changes in anesthetic depth is warranted, especially at critical stages of the operation. Volatile agents and N_2O are the most suppressive agents (Table 44-2). It is difficult to obtain reliable SSEPs when giving more than 0.5 to 1 minimal alveolar concentration (MAC) of these agents. Intravenous anesthetics such as propofol are less suppressive. They are commonly used with opioids, which have minimal effects on SSEPs. Ketamine and etomidate do not depress SSEP responses, nor do muscle relaxants interfere with SSEP responses.

Motor Evoked Potentials

MEPs involve stimulation of the motor cortex to activate the motor pathways and elicit a movement response. MEPs have only recently been used clinically and are still being evaluated for optimal use in detecting and preventing motor injury. For spine surgery, SSEP and EMG monitoring has reduced the need for intraoperative wake-up tests. MEP monitoring also appears to have value in reducing motor deficits during cranial surgery near the motor cortex.

For spine surgery, direct activation of neurons of the motor cortex is performed. Magnetic stimulation is noninvasive and less painful but is more difficult to use in the operating room. Instead, electrical stimulation via electrodes placed into the scalp are preferred. A brief pulse or train of pulses directly depolarize motor neurons, as well as other cortical nerve cells, which then activate the motor neurons. This produces waves of depolarization that travel down the corticospinal tracts of the spinal cord and then summate at the ventral horn. Here, signals synapse with alpha motor neurons, and the resulting compound motor action potential triggers muscle movement.

Alternative stimulation can be performed at the level of the spinal cord, proximal to the surgical site. Responses are recorded as muscle movement (myogenic MEPs) or activity in a peripheral nerve (neurogenic MEP) or the distal spinal cord (epidural). Myogenic is the most prevalent because responses are strong, but more sensitive to anesthetic suppression, especially by volatile agents that have muscle relaxation properties. Epidural recordings are technically challenging, invasive, and hard to reproduce.

44

Table 44-2 Relative Effects of Anesthetic Agents on Somatosensory and Motor Evoked Potentials

| Agent | Cortical SSEPs | | MEPs |
	Latency	Amplitude	Amplitude
Volatile agents*	↑↑↑	↓↓↓	↓↓↓
Nitrous oxide	↑	↓↓	↓
Barbiturates*	↑↑	↓↓↓	↓↓
Propofol*	↑↑	↓↓	↓↓
Benzodiazepines	↑	↓	↓↓
Narcotics/opioids	+/−	+/−	+/−
Ketamine	↑	↑	+/−
Etomidate	↑	↑↑	↑
Muscle relaxants*	0	0	↓↓↓

*The degree of suppression is highly dose dependent.
↑, Mild increase; ↑↑, moderate increase; ↑↑↑, significant increase; ↓, mild decrease; ↓↓, moderate decrease; ↓↓↓, significant decrease.

Interpretation of Responses

A decrease in amplitude and prolonged latency of MEP responses suggest neurologic injury, as do acute increases in the threshold voltage needed to obtain an MEP response. Acute and asymmetric changes are more suggestive of true injury. Changes in the duration or complexity of the morphology of the myogenic response may also predict motor damage. There is still much disagreement about what constitutes a meaningful change, however.

Several physiologic factors depress MEP responses, including hypothermia, hypotension, and hypovolemia. MEP responses may be difficult or impossible to obtain from patients with preexisting muscle weakness (as a result of neuropathy or myopathy). In addition, young children require stronger stimuli to elicit MEP responses, probably because of lack of complete myelinization of immature motor pathways.

Anesthetic Considerations

VI

Myogenic MEPs are highly susceptible to suppression by anesthetics (Table 44-2). Volatile inhalational agents are the most suppressive. Nitrous oxide appears to be less depressing than the MAC equivalent of volatile agents. Intravenous agents such as propofol produce dose-dependent MEP suppression but are less depressing than equivalent amounts of vapor. Ketamine and etomidate are well tolerated, as are narcotics. Gradual decreases in MEP response amplitudes occur over time while under general anesthesia—a process described as "anesthetic fade."

Muscle relaxants clearly weaken myogenic responses but do not affect neurogenic or epidural recordings. It is ideal to avoid any muscle relaxation during critical parts of the operation. However, if required, partial neuromuscular blockade is compatible with myogenic MEP monitoring if constant depth of blockade is carefully maintained.

KEY POINTS

- Electromyography monitors cranial and peripheral nerve integrity.
- Electromyography is not affected by anesthetics, but muscle relaxants should be avoided.

- Evoked potentials use a stimulus to elicit a distant response. Changes in response may indicate injury along any part of the sensory or motor pathway.
- Evoked responses are adversely affected by anesthetics in the following order: VEP > SSEP/MEP > BAEP.
- Volatile anesthetic agents suppress evoked potentials most and propofol less so; opiates, ketamine, and etomidate are minimally suppressive or neutral.
- Physiologic alterations such as hypotension, anemia, hypoxia, or hypothermia may affect evoked responses and result in inaccurate interpretation.

FURTHER READING

Banoub M, Tetzlaff J, Schubert A: Pharmacologic and physiologic influences affecting sensory evoked potentials. Implications for perioperative monitoring. Anesthesiology 2003; 99:716-737.

Harper C: Intraoperative cranial nerve monitoring. Muscle Nerve 2004; 29:339-351.

Holland N: Intraoperative electromyography. J Clin Neurophysiol 2002; 19:444-453.

Legatt A: Mechanisms of intraoperative brainstem auditory evoked potential changes. J Clin Neurophysiol 2002; 19:396-408.

Lotto M, Banoub M, Schubert A: Effects of anesthetic agents and physiologic changes on intraoperative motor evoked potentials. J Neurosurg Anesthesiol 2004; 16:32-42.

Sloan T, Heyer E: Anesthesia for intraoperative neurophysiologic monitoring of the spinal cord. J Clin Neurophysiol 2002; 19:430-443.

44

Chapter 45

Electroencephalography and Cerebral Function Monitoring

Lawrence Litt

BASIC FEATURES OF THE ELECTROENCEPHALOGRAM

The electric activity of the brain comes from axon currents, with larger amplitudes occurring if several long, parallel axons conduct simultaneously. Neuronal activity is detectable as voltage differences between electrodes, which are usually placed on the scalp or on the brain surface during surgery. The voltage differences generated by brain activity are very small, typically 20 to 200 µV. In contrast, electrical signals generated by muscle activity are approximately 1000 times larger. The simplest system for detecting brain activity consists of three electrodes, with the voltage between two of the electrodes measuring *one channel* of activity and the third electrode being "the reference electrode." Differential amplifiers use the reference electrode to provide *common mode rejection*, which is subtraction of the voltage changes common to all three electrodes.

Electrical tracings of detected brain voltage over time make up the *electroencephalogram*, analogous to tracings of voltage from the heart in the electrocardiogram. A formal electroencephalogram, like a formal electrocardiogram, consists of a set of voltage tracings from specific electrodes at designated scalp locations. The ensemble of electrodes used in a study, together with their placement sites, is known as the study's *montage*. There are 20 scalp electroencephalographic (EEG) locations in the *International 10-20 Electrode Placement Protocol*, shown in Figure 45-1. These locations are designated by letter-number combinations that refer to cerebral regions (e.g., frontal, parietal) and distances from the sagittal sinus. Even numbers are used for locations on the right side of the head, odd numbers for locations on the left. Low numbers are for locations close to the midline, high numbers for those more lateral. Many more electrode locations are defined in the numbering system than are used in a recording session. A written or digital record can be made of the voltage between any two scalp electrodes, which is called an *EEG channel*. Although modern EEG systems can

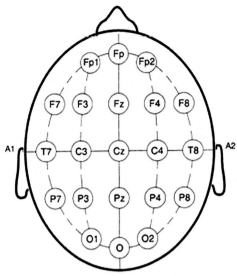

Figure 45-1 Scalp locations for electrode placement in the International 10-20 Protocol. (Reprinted with permission from Billard V: "Surveillance" de la profondeur de l'anesthésie. Conférences d'actualisation 1997. Paris, Elsevier, 1997, pp 17-32. Available at http://www.sfar.org/sfar_actu/ca97/html/ca97_002/97_02.htm.)

handle more than 128 channels of data, intraoperative monitoring typically involves montages aimed at recording fewer than 8 channels, sometimes only 2 or 4.

Frequency analysis of brain electrical signals reveals that on the scalp one detects signals in the range of 0.5 to 30 Hz, with delta waves being defined by the frequency range 0.5 to 4 Hz, theta waves by the range 4 to 7 Hz, alpha waves by the range 8 to 13 Hz, beta waves by the range 13 to 30 Hz, and gamma waves by values above 30 Hz. Alpha waves are characteristic of quiet wakefulness. Lower-amplitude beta waves are correlated with intense mental activity. Theta and delta waves accompany drowsiness and slow-wave sleep.

Neurosurgeons sometimes place electrodes directly on the surface of the cortex, thereby leading to tracings known as the *electrocorticogram*. Electrodes that are directly in contact with the cerebral cortex provide very clean brain electrical signals that are free of muscle signal contamination and scalp and bone attenuation. However, neither scalp nor cortex electrodes can detect brain electrical signals generated deeper in the brain. As explained later, sophisticated mathematical analyses of cortical voltage can be used to infer important information about deep brain electrical activity. There is no set montage for intraoperative electrocorticographic (EcoG) recordings because surgical access is variable and quite limited. Special electrode grids or electrodes are used to determine voltage in the surgical area.

INTRAOPERATIVE USE OF ELECTROENCEPHALOGRAPHIC MONITORING

EEG monitoring during epilepsy surgery is used to detect preseizure (*epileptiform*) or *seizure* activity so that pharmacologic treatment can be instituted immediately. A *seizure* is defined as uncontrolled brain electrical activity, which in turn causes motor convulsions, minor physical signs, thought disturbances, or a combination of these. *Nonconvulsive seizures* can occur without tonic-clonic muscle movements and can

45

be detected only with EEG monitoring. Similarly, tonic-clonic muscle shaking can occur without a seizure being present, particularly in slightly hypothermic patients.

During brain surgery, neurosurgeons typically use direct electrical stimulation of the cortex to identify muscle and speech areas. Repeated stimulation can kindle a seizure by causing numerous *afterdischarges* (ADs; also called *afterpotentials*). Neurologists with expertise in EEG monitoring are often present during surgery to advise the neurosurgeon and anesthesiologist of such epileptiform activity. When ADs are detected, the surgeon stops stimulating and waits to see whether the ADs will terminate by themselves, which is usually the case. If the termination is not sufficiently fast or if the ADs seem to be more frequent or spreading out from the stimulation point, the neurosurgeon might use a fine spray of very cold saline onto the cortex. If this does not stop the ADs, the anesthesiologist usually intravenously injects a small dose of a short-acting anticonvulsant such as thiopental or propofol. The precise protocol, which can vary from patient to patient, should have previously been worked out between the anesthesiologist and neurosurgeon. Sometimes a very low intravenous dose of midazolam is used to reduce or eliminate ADs.

In epilepsy surgery, EcoG monitoring is used by neurologists to identify *ictal activity* (i.e., tracings that denote the presence of a seizure) to provide information to the surgeon about its localization before excising the responsible brain regions. It is only in anesthetized patients that one deliberately triggers intraoperative seizures, often via an intravenous injection of proconvulsant anesthetics such as etomidate or methohexital, which are known to activate epileptic foci. Chronic epilepsy patients often have interictal EEG abnormalities (i.e., abnormalities in EEG tracings obtained between seizures). Interictal abnormalities may or may not be epileptiform and can occur at any time before or after a seizure. It is normal to use EcoG monitoring intraoperatively to look for ictal or interictal patterns after excision of the brain tissue believed to be responsible for the seizures.

ELECTROENCEPHALOGRAPHY-BASED MONITORING FOR DRUG TITRATION OF ANESTHETIC DEPTH AND AVOIDANCE OF AWARENESS

Anesthesia monitors of brain activity use three electrodes that are usually mounted in a frontal region. Two electrodes provide a differential amplifier with the voltage difference between their locations (i.e., with one channel), whereas the third electrode provides an obligatory reference signal. Some monitors can simultaneously process signals from both sides of the head, thereby using six electrodes for a total of two channels. A typical set of raw voltage tracings versus time is shown in Figure 45-2.

Brain monitors digitally record voltage tracings for fixed times known as *epochs*, typically seconds. Microprocessors in the monitors are used to process the tracings at the end of each epoch and display the analyzed data on a time scale of seconds.

Qualitative differences are apparent as shown in the tracing in Figure 45-2. When compared with the tracing for deep anesthesia, the tracing for the awake state is at a lower amplitude with more oscillations per time interval. The number of oscillations per time interval is defined as the *frequency* of oscillations. A tracing that runs for a fixed time interval can be considered the sum of waves at many frequencies. Engineers find it useful to focus on the frequency composition of an epoch's voltage tracing, which usually involves one or more types of *Fourier analysis*. As mentioned earlier, muscle tissue also generates detectable voltage signals, and their epoch tracings constitute the *electromyogram*, with most of the power being in frequencies above approximately 25 Hz. Thus, extraocular and scalp muscles can contribute background voltage to the

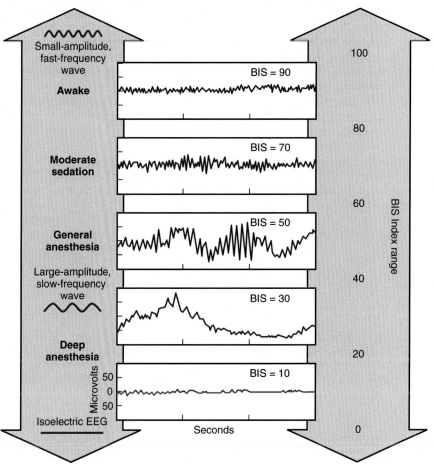

Figure 45-2 General pattern of electroencephalographic (EEG) changes observed during increasing doses of anesthesia. As the anesthetic effect increases, EEG frequency typically slows and results in transition through frequency-based classes: beta → alpha → theta → delta. (Reprinted with permission from Kelley SD: Monitoring Consciousness during Anesthesia and Sedation—A Clinician's Guide to the Bispectral Index. Boston, Aspect Medical Systems, 2005, p 2-2.)

electroencephalogram. Although this can add to EEG background "noise," it can be useful to assess anesthetic depth on the basis that people often frown strongly when they are in pain, and the resultant scalp muscle activity will increase.

BISPECTRAL ANALYSIS

There is much one can do with the Fourier information obtained from EEG signal analysis. Inspiration for the development of one type of brain monitor was based on analysis of the bispectral index (BIS), a computational approach *(bispectra analysis)* approach that permits the calculation of a mathematically complex index of wave synchrony known as interfrequency phase coherence. Two waves of the same frequency are "in phase" with each other when their maxima and minima occur simultaneously. If, for example, persistent knee pain causes brain electrical activity in epoch after epoch, the same phase relationships among waves of different frequencies occur in areas of the brain associated with pain. When such repeated phase relationships persist, BIS analysis produces an *interfrequency phase coherence* of 100%. If a brain is having consistent signal repetitions, be it from pain, thinking, or other sensations, one must be concerned that the anesthetic effects are not dominant and the brain in question may not be adequately anesthetized. The above concepts outline the basis for BIS monitoring.

Because of numerous practicalities, it did not make sense to simply take the pure mathematical formulas that are involved in BIS analysis, apply them to a digital representation of detected waves, and then calculate the coherence. Various artifacts, such as the aforementioned electromyographic (EMG) signals, had to be eliminated. Additional EEG patterns also needed special detection and attention, such as "burst suppression," in which a small number of voltage peaks is followed by a period of electrical silence. Thus, the BIS monitor had to include empirical approaches based on known human EEG responses. When all is taken into account electronically, the BIS monitor produces a single number between 0 and 100, with 100 corresponding to consciousness or near consciousness and 30 corresponding to deep anesthesia.

ENTROPY ANALYSIS

Entropy monitoring is another approach to brain monitoring that is based on frequency and amplitude information in the electroencephalogram. Like the BIS monitor, the entropy brain monitor by Datex (GE Healthcare Technologies, PO Box 900, FIN-00031 GE, Finland; www.gehealthcare.com) begins by obtaining the Fourier information in an epoch. Thereafter, computations determine the plot of EEG power versus frequency, which is then divided into N bins, with each bin given a probability value p_i that is used for calculating spectral and response entropy:

Spectral entropy—where analyzed frequencies are in the range of 0.8 to 32 Hz, thereby emphasizing pure brain electrical signals.

Response entropy—where analyzed frequencies are in the range of 0.8 to 47 Hz, with the frequency region being above 32 Hz, including EMG components from scalp and frontal muscle activity. Frowning, which often occurs clinically as a manifestation of pain or light anesthesia, is an example of such monitoring.

As is the case with the BIS monitor, a number between 0 and 100 is calculated for response entropy, whereas 91 is the maximum value for spectral entropy. The entropy index approximately characterizes the extent to which the frequency composition appears to be highly nonrandom (low values, deep anesthesia) or highly random (high values, awake or light anesthesia). When compared with the BIS approach, the entropy approach has an algorithm that is in the public domain, and it uses fewer prefixed numerical parameters, as well as no study population, thus in principle permitting patients to serve as their own controls.

AWARENESS

Many patients want to hear that brain electrical activity is frequently monitored to help avoid "awareness during anesthesia," an adverse complication that is among those most unwanted. However, such awareness is an extremely rare phenomenon ($\approx$0.02%) outside certain surgical situations such as emergency trauma cases and cesarean section.

Although some practitioners find brain monitoring reassuring, many others, as well as professional societies, believe that brain monitoring is not essential. A recent review of the matter by the American Society of Anesthesiologists concluded that intraoperative brain monitoring by anesthesiologists should be viewed as one tool that is used in concert with other tools, such as the electrocardiogram and blood pressure monitor, to help ensure an "anesthetic depth" sufficient to avoid inappropriate patient responses, such as movement on incision or hypertension on stimulation.

CONCLUSION

In a large patient population there are gaussian characteristics in all stimulus-response data. Therefore, the usual sensitivity-specificity criteria must be carefully evaluated to determine whether a brain-monitoring index can be used as a dependable diagnostic test. Electrophysiologic monitors provide supplementary information that adds to clinical impressions and basic monitoring. Clinical decisions must always include the latter and should not be based solely on a brain-monitoring index.

KEY POINTS

- Neuron activity produces voltage differences between different places on the brain surface or scalp.
- The electroencephalogram is a collection of voltage-time tracings obtained from 10 or 20 electrodes at specific locations on the scalp.
- An electrocorticogram is obtained by placing electrodes on the surface of the cerebral cortex intraoperatively for recording.
- Intense, uncontrolled brain electrical activity that alters brain function is called a seizure.
- Intraoperative EcoG recordings help identify the origin of the seizures and their relationship to cortically mapped regions that control speech and motor activity.
- Modern digital signal processing and a reduced scalp montage have been used to derive indices that correlate with "depth of anesthesia."

FURTHER READING

American Society of Anesthesiologists Task Force on Intraoperative Awareness. Practice advisory for intraoperative awareness and brain function monitoring: A report by the American Society of Anesthesiologists Task Force on Intraoperative Awareness. Anesthesiology 2006; 104:847-864.

Kelley SD (ed): Monitoring Consciousness during Anesthesia and Sedation—A Clinician's Guide to the Bispectral Index. Boston, Aspect Medical Systems, 2005.

Messner M, Beese U, Romstock J, et al: The bispectral index declines during neuromuscular block in fully awake persons. Anesth Analg 2003; 97:488-491.

Nunez PL, Srinivasan R: Electric Fields of the Brain—The Neurophysics of EEG, 2nd ed. New York, Oxford University Press, 2005.

Rampil IJ: A primer for EEG signal processing in anesthesia. Anesthesiology 1998; 89:980-1002.

Viertio-Oja H, Maja V, Sarkela M, et al: Description of the entropy algorithm as applied in the Datex-Ohmeda S/5 Entropy Module. Acta Anaesthesiol Scand 2004; 48:154-161.

45

Chapter 46

Transcranial Doppler Ultrasonography and Other Measures of Cerebral Blood Flow

Jane Sturgess • Basil Matta

VI

PRINCIPLES OF TRANSCRANIAL DOPPLER ULTRASONOGRAPHY

Transcranial Doppler (TCD) ultrasonography is a noninvasive real-time monitor that provides *indirect* information about cerebral blood flow (CBF). It calculates red cell flow velocity (FV) from the shift in frequency spectra of the Doppler signal (Fig. 46-1) and can be used both intraoperatively and in the intensive care unit. Changes in FV correlate closely with changes in CBF, provided that the angle of insonation (the angle between the axis of the vessel and the ultrasound beam) and the diameter of the vessel insonated remain constant (Table 46-1).

FV can be measured by insonating the anterior, middle, or posterior cerebral arteries. These vessels are accessed by the transtemporal route through the thin bone above the zygomatic arch. The transorbital approach allows access to the carotid siphon and the suboccipital route to the basilar and vertebral arteries. The middle cerebral artery (MCA) is most commonly insonated because it is simple to detect and allows easy probe fixation, thereby providing a constant insonation angle. It can be used in adult and pediatric patients.

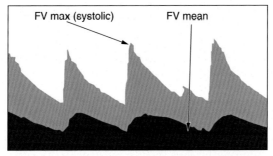

MAXIMAL AND MEAN VELOCITY ENVELOPE

FV max (systolic)   FV mean

Figure 46-1   Transcranial Doppler waveform envelope and spectral outline. FV, flow velocity.

Table 46-1   **Factors to Ensure That Changes in Flow Velocity Reflect Cerebral Blood Flow**
Minimize changes in arterial carbon dioxide tension and blood pressure
Insonate conductance vessels
Fix the probe in position
Provide steady-state anesthesia

FACTORS AFFECTING FLOW VELOCITY

CBF velocity varies with age, gender, and hematocrit.

- Age: FV in the MCA is lowest at birth (24 cm/sec), peaks at the age of 4 to 6 years (100 cm/sec), and thereafter decreases steadily to about 40 cm/sec during the seventh decade of life.
- Gender: Hemispheric CBF velocity is 3% to 5% higher in females, possibly because of a lower hematocrit and slightly higher arterial CO_2 tension.
- Hematocrit: FV is also increased in hemodilutional states.

TRANSCRANIAL DOPPLER MEASUREMENTS AND DERIVED VALUES

A number of measured and derived values are obtained from most commercially available TCD monitors (see Fig. 46-1):

- FV_{mean}—a weighted mean velocity that takes into consideration the different velocities of the formed elements in the isonated blood vessel. This is the most physiologic and is the best correlate with actual CBF.
- Waveform pulsatility—describes the shape of the envelope (maximal shift) of the Doppler spectrum from peak systolic flow to end-diastolic flow with each cardiac cycle. The waveform is determined by the arterial blood pressure waveform, the viscoelastic properties of the cerebral vascular bed, and blood rheology. In the absence of stenosis or vasospasm and changes in arterial blood pressure or blood rheology, the pulsatility of the waveform reflects distal cerebrovascular

resistance. This resistance is usually quantified by the *pulsatility index*: PI or Gosling index = $(FV_{systmic} - FV_{diastolic})/FV_{mean}$. Normal PI ranges from 0.6 to 1.1 with no significant side-to-side or cerebral interarterial differences.

TRANSCRANIAL DOPPLER ULTRASONOGRAPHY AS A RESEARCH TOOL

Cerebral Autoregulation

Both static and dynamic autoregulation can be tested with TCD ultrasonography. The static rate of autoregulation or the index of autoregulation (IOR) is the ratio of percent change in estimated cerebral vascular resistance (CVRe) to percent change in mean blood pressure. An IOR of 1 implies perfect autoregulation, and an IOR of zero denotes complete disruption of autoregulation.

Dynamic autoregulation (dRoR) is tested by measuring the recovery in FV after a rapid transient decrease in perfusion pressure induced, for example, by deflation of large inflated thigh cuffs or carotid compression. dRoR describes the rate of restoration of FV (%/sec) with respect to the drop in perfusion pressure, in other words the rate of change in cerebral vascular resistance, or "the fast process." Normal dRoR is 20%/sec (i.e., dynamic autoregulation is complete within approximately 5 seconds).

TRANSCRANIAL DOPPLER ULTRASONOGRAPHY IN ANESTHESIA AND INTENSIVE CARE

Carotid Artery Disease

TCD ultrasonography allows assessment of cerebral vascular reserve by examining CO_2 reactivity, detection of emboli, monitoring of cerebral perfusion during cross-clamping of the carotid artery, and testing of cerebral autoregulation.

Cerebral ischemia during clamping of the internal carotid artery (ICA) is probably mild if 16% to 40%, and severe if 0% to 15% of the preclamping value. If FV_{MCA} is greater than 40% of the preclamping value, cerebral ischemia is considered to be absent.

Subarachnoid Hemorrhage

TCD ultrasonography is an unreliable measure of CBF in patients with subarachnoid hemorrhage (SAH) because of vasospasm-associated changes in vessel diameter. However, it is useful for detecting vasospasm, which is considered to be present when FV_{MCA} is greater than 120 cm/sec or the ratio between FV_{MCA} and FV_{ICA} (the Lindegaard ratio) exceeds 3.

A baseline TCD examination may be performed at or after angiography/surgery and repeated between days 3 and 10. This will help detect vasospasm before the onset of symptoms and allow early intervention.

Closed Head Injury

After traumatic brain injury, TCD monitoring can be used to observe changes in FV and waveform pulsatility and to test cerebral vascular reserve. In addition, by continuous recording of FV_{MCA}, the autoregulatory "threshold" or "break point" (the cerebral perfusion pressure [CPP] at which autoregulation fails) can be easily detected. This provides a target CPP value for treatment.

VI

TCD imaging can also be used to diagnose and treat cerebral vasospasm via the same criteria as patients with SAH. Increased FV in combination with high jugular venous bulb saturation ($Sjvo_2$) values and an FV_{MCA}/FV_{ICA} ratio less than 2 indicates hyperemia, whereas high FV in the presence of low or normal $Sjvo_2$ values and an FV_{MCA}/FV_{ICA} ratio higher than 3 suggests cerebral vasospasm.

Stroke

In acute ischemic stroke, TCD ultrasonography can help identify the source of emboli, cerebral arterial occlusion, recanalization, and the risk of hemorrhagic transformation of large-volume ischemic lesions. It is also possible to identify patients at risk for further ischemic episodes by repeated TCD examinations.

OTHER METHODS OF MONITORING CEREBRAL BLOOD FLOW

Laser Doppler Flowmetry

Laser Doppler flowmetry allows continuous real-time measurement of local microcirculatory blood flow. A 0.5- to 1-mm-diameter fiberoptic laser probe is placed in contact with or within brain tissue and conducts reflected light back to a photodetector within the flowmeter sensor. The signal is processed to give the blood flow. Although laser Doppler flowmetry is considered an excellent technique for continuous and real-time measurement of regional CBF and for assessment of relative regional CBF changes, the main drawbacks of this technique are that it is invasive, is not a quantitative measure of CBF, measures CBF in a small brain volume (1 to 2 mm^3), and is prone to artifacts produced by patient movement or probe displacement, which limits its clinical applicability.

Thermal Diffusion Flowmetry

The thermal conductivity of cerebral cortical tissue varies proportionally with CBF, and measurement of thermal diffusion at the cortical surface can be used for determination of CBF. The monitor consists of two small thermistors, one of which is heated. Insertion of a thermal diffusion probe on surface of the brain allows CBF to be calculated from the temperature difference between the plates. Thermal diffusion flowmetry has the potential for bedside monitoring of cerebral perfusion at the tissue level, but it is invasive and more clinical trials are needed to validate its use.

Imaging Techniques

A number of techniques are available to assess CBF.

Xenon 133 Washout Technique

Regional decay in radioactivity after intracarotid or intra-aortic injection of ^{133}Xe is measured by scintillation counters positioned over the head. The slope of the washout curve is proportional to regional CBF. The curve is biexponential, the fast and slow components possibly representing blood flow in gray and white matter. This method estimates predominantly cortical blood flow. However, extracranial contamination may affect the results.

46

299

Tomographic Techniques

Dynamic computed tomography (CT) quantifies the washout of inhaled xenon or intravenous radioiodinated contrast agents to measure regional CBF.

Positron emission tomography (PET) provides images of flow throughout the brain and enables assessment of regional variations and the CBF response to increased stimulation/metabolism. PET also provides information about cerebral blood volume, oxygen extraction, and the cerebral metabolic rate of oxygen ($CMRO_2$). However, the equipment is expensive and technically demanding.

Single-photon emission computed tomography produces qualitative images of blood flow across all areas of the brain by using γ-emitting technetium 99. One or more areas can then be compared at a particular moment in time.

Functional magnetic resonance imaging (fMRI) uses MRI to map changes in brain hemodynamics in response to brain neural activity. An intravenous paramagnetic contrast agent or decreases in regional deoxyhemoglobin levels can produce tomographic images of regional CBF.

KEY POINTS

- CBF can be measured directly with invasive techniques such as laser Doppler ultrasound or thermal diffusion flow probes, indirectly with noninvasive methods such as transcranial Doppler flowmetry, or with imaging techniques.
- The most common bedside method of assessing changes in CBF in real time is by measuring changes in flow velocity with TCD ultrasonography.
- TCD examination can be used to assess cerebral vascular reactivity and autoregulatory reserve and may be used as an estimation of CPP.
- High FV indicates vasospasm or hyperemia. Vasospasm is present if the ratio between FV_{MCA} and FV_{ICA} exceeds 3.
- Other applications of TCD ultrasonography include carotid surgery, SAH, severe head injury, and stroke.
- TCD examination may be used to assess changes in CBF in patients with secondary causes of raised intracranial pressure.

FURTHER READING

Aaslid R (ed): Transcranial Doppler Sonography. New York, Springer, 1986.

Alexandrov AV, Joseph M: Transcranial Doppler: An overview of its clinical applications. Internet Journal of Emergency and Intensive Care Medicine 2000; 4(1).

Newell DW, Aaslid R: Transcranial Doppler. New York, Raven, 1992.

Prabhu AM, Matta BF: Transcranial Doppler ultrasonography. In Matta BF, Menon DK, Turner JM (eds): Textbook of Neuroanaesthesia and Critical Care. London, Greenwich Medical Media, 2000.

Section VII
Miscellaneous

Chapter 47

Guillain-Barré Syndrome and Myasthenia Gravis

Nicholas Hirsch

Guillain-Barré Syndrome	Myasthenia Gravis
Pathophysiology	Pathophysiology
Clinical Features	Clinical Features
Diagnosis	Diagnosis
Management	Treatment
Prognosis	Anesthetic Considerations

GUILLAIN-BARRÉ SYNDROME

Guillain-Barré syndrome (GBS) is a term applied to a group of acute inflammatory polyneuropathies characterized by progressive (usually ascending) neuropathic weakness and areflexia; with the decline of poliomyelitis, it is the most common cause of neuromuscular paralysis in the Western world. Respiratory muscle failure requiring mechanical ventilation that may be prolonged will develop in approximately 30% of patients with GBS.

The incidence of GBS is 1 to 3 per 100,000 population, and it has a bimodal age distribution (peak age ranges of 15 to 35 years and 50 to 70 years). Males are affected more than females. GBS is commonly preceded by an often trivial infection of the upper respiratory or gastrointestinal tract. Both bacterial and viral agents have been implicated as triggers. An association of GBS with vaccinations (including influenza vaccine), lymphoma, and surgery is recognized but less well characterized.

Pathophysiology

Though not fully elucidated, evidence suggests that the demyelination that characterizes GBS is a result of antibodies directed at Schwann cells that lead to destruction of the myelin sheath.

Clinical Features

Neurologic Findings

Patients typically have weakness of the limbs and a glove and stocking distribution of paresthesias. The weakness is more prominent in the proximal muscles, and the legs are more frequently affected than the arms (and earlier). The muscle weakness reaches its nadir within 1 week in 75% of patients and by 4 weeks in 98% of individuals.

Table 47-1 Diagnostic Criteria for Guillain-Barré Syndrome

Essential Features	Supporting Features
Progressive weakness of >1 limb because of neuropathy Areflexia Duration of progression <4 weeks	**Clinical Features** Weakness usually progressive Sensory signs mild Cranial nerve involvement Autonomic involvement **Investigations** Cerebrospinal fluid—elevated protein (>0.55 g/dL) after the first week White cell count—<10 mononuclear leukocytes/mL Neurophysiology—includes low-amplitude or absent sensory action potentials and absent F waves

Areflexia is invariable a few days after the appearance of symptoms. Pain, especially in the back, thighs, and shoulders, is a common feature. The cranial nerves (especially the facial and bulbar nerves) are affected in up to 75% of patients. Cranial nerve involvement is prominent in the Miller Fisher syndrome, a subtype of GBS manifested as rapidly evolving areflexia, ophthalmoplegia, and ataxia; frequently there is only mild limb involvement.

Respiratory Findings

Respiratory muscle failure requiring ventilation occurs in about 30% of patients. Bulbar weakness predisposing to pulmonary aspiration may necessitate tracheal intubation for airway protection. Predictive factors, apart from a reduced or rapidly decreasing forced vital capacity (FVC), suggesting that mechanical ventilation will be necessary include a period of less than 7 days from the onset of GBS to hospital admission, an inability to raise the head off the bed and to stand, and a poor cough.

Autonomic Findings

Sinus tachycardia occurs in 75% of patients and usually resolves within a few days. More dangerous are bradyarrhythmias, which may occur with often trivial vagal stimulation (e.g., during tracheal suction). Other autonomic features include postural hypotension, excessive sweating, and less commonly, urinary symptoms, including polyuria or retention.

Diagnosis

The diagnosis of GBS is based on clinical features, neurophysiologic studies, and examination of cerebrospinal fluid.

Table 47-1 lists the essential and supporting criteria necessary for considering the diagnosis of GBS. Differential diagnoses are listed in Table 47-2.

Management

Management of GBS consists of supportive treatment and specific therapy.

Table 47-2 Differential Diagnosis of Guillain-Barré Syndrome

Myasthenia gravis—fatigable weakness present
Botulism—purely motor involvement with descending weakness
Heavy metal poisoning—confusion and psychosis often present
Poliomyelitis—purely motor involvement
Transverse myelitis—sensory level present
Shellfish poisoning—usually resolves in 24 hours
Basilar artery occlusion—usually asymmetric limb involvement

Supportive Treatment

Good general medical and nursing care is the mainstay of treatment. Patients must be carefully monitored during the acute and progressive phases, and early tracheal intubation and mechanical ventilation should be instituted if vital capacity falls below 60% of predicted. If bulbar weakness coexists, intubation should be carried out earlier. Tracheostomy should be performed early if it becomes obvious that a prolonged period of mechanical ventilation will be needed. This affords greater patient comfort and ease of tracheal suction and allows the patient to be managed without sedation.

Careful monitoring of cardiovascular function should be instituted and persistent tachycardia and hypertension treated with the lowest necessary dose of a β-adrenergic blocker. Severe episodes of bradycardia may require temporary or permanent cardiac pacing.

Enteral feeding should be started as soon as possible; however, ileus is common in the acute stages of GBS and may require the use of prokinetic agents such as meto-clopramide. Rarely, parenteral nutrition may be needed.

Regular turning of a patient with GBS is essential to prevent pressure sores; passive physiotherapy and the use of limb splints help prevent tendon shortening and contractures.

Thromboembolic complications remain a major cause of morbidity and mortality in this group of patients; they should be placed on a regimen of prophylactic antico-agulation.

Pain is almost invariable in patients with GBS, especially at night. Although regular nonsteroidal analgesic agents may be effective, stronger medications may be necessary. Meptazinol is a useful agent and provides good analgesia without the constipating effects of other opioid agents. In addition, the neurogenic pain experienced may respond to amitriptyline or gabapentin.

Patients with severe GBS requiring prolonged mechanical ventilation often feel depressed, so support from patients who have recovered from the illness is often helpful. Antidepressant therapy may be required.

Specific Therapy

Specific therapy for GBS consists of high-dose intravenous immune globulin (IVIG) or plasma exchange. Trials have shown that IVIG (400 mg/kg daily for 5 days) is as effective as plasma exchange (five exchanges over a period of 5 to 8 days). Both treatments decrease recovery times (e.g., time to walk unaided, time spent on mechanical ventilation) if given early in the course of the disease. A further trial has shown that there is no advantage to combining the treatments. In general, IVIG is considered by most authorities to be the treatment of choice because it is easier to administer than plasma exchange and has fewer complications than the latter (e.g. sepsis).

Corticosteroids have been shown to have no role in the treatment of GBS.

47

Table 47-3 Forms of Myasthenia Gravis

Acquired myasthenia gravis	
Neonatal myasthenia gravis	Occurs in 10% to 30% of babies born to mothers with acquired myasthenia gravis as a result of placental transfer of acetylcholine receptor antibodies; respiratory support may be needed for 1-4 weeks
Congenital myasthenia gravis	Rare group of nonimmunologic neuromuscular junction disorders (presynaptic, synaptic, or postsynaptic) causing fatigable weakness from infancy
Drug-induced myasthenia gravis	Usually slow onset. Penicillamine is the most common culprit. It generally disappears on withdrawal of the drug

Prognosis

The mortality associated with severe GBS varies between 2% and 13%, with lower rates occurring in centers that are expert at dealing with the condition.

Approximately 85% of patients make a full recovery within 1 year. However, patients who have a rapidly progressive course, are older than 60 years, require mechanical ventilation for more than 1 month, or have neurophysiologic results suggesting axonal loss often recover incompletely.

MYASTHENIA GRAVIS

Myasthenia gravis (MG) is an autoimmune condition in which IgG autoantibodies interact with postsynaptic acetylcholine receptors (AChRs) at the nicotinic neuromuscular junction (NMJ). A number of forms of MG exist, each with different pathologic mechanisms (Table 47-3). MG has a prevalence of 1 in 10,000 and a bimodal distribution; it predominantly affects young women (aged 20 to 30 years) and older men (aged 60 to 70 years).

Pathophysiology

Anti-AChR antibodies reduce the number of functional postsynaptic AChRs at the NMJ by blocking attachment of acetylcholine molecules, by increasing degradation of the receptors, and by inducing complement-induced damage to the NMJ. The result is a decrease in AChR density; on average, patients with MG have 30% of the normal number of AChRs.

Although the origin of the autoimmune process remains uncertain, the thymus gland has been implicated as a possible generator of the immune process. Seventy-five percent of patients with MG have an abnormality of the gland (hyperplasia in 85%, thymoma in 15%), and removal of the thymus results in improvement of symptoms in the majority of patients.

Clinical Features

The reduced AChR density results in decreased generation of action potentials at the postsynaptic junction and failure of initiation of muscle fiber contraction. When such failure occurs over the whole muscle, it is manifested clinically as weakness—the cardinal

Table 47-4   **Classification of Myasthenia Gravis**

I	Ocular symptoms and signs only
IIA	Generalized mild muscle weakness responding well to therapy
IIB	Generalized mild muscle weakness responding less well to therapy
III	Acute fulminating manifestation and/or respiratory dysfunction
IV	Crisis requiring mechanical ventilation

Table 47-5   **Conditions Associated with Myasthenia Gravis**

Thyroid disease
Systemic lupus erythematosus
Rheumatoid disease
Pemphigus vulgaris
Ulcerative colitis
Pernicious anemia

feature of MG. In addition, the muscular weakness increases as the muscle is exercised, a phenomenon known as fatigability. In 15% of patients the disease is confined to the extrinsic muscles of the eye (ocular MG), and diplopia and ptosis are the most common findings. However, in the majority of cases, MG is generalized and affects the eye, facial, bulbar, and limb muscles. Although respiratory muscle weakness is often mild, respiratory failure requiring mechanical ventilation may occur. Classification of MG is based on the distribution of weakness and its response to medication (Table 47-4).

MG is associated with a number of other autoimmune conditions, as listed in Table 47-5.

Diagnosis

Diagnosis of MG relies on a careful history, physical examination, pharmacologic testing with edrophonium, electromyography, and detection of anti-AChR antibodies.

Edrophonium (Tensilon) is a short-acting acetylcholinesterase inhibitor that increases the duration of the presence of acetylcholine at the NMJ and therefore promotes neuromuscular transmission and a transient marked improvement in muscle power. Unfortunately, the test lacks sensitivity and specificity.

The most commonly used electromyographic test is recording of compound muscle action potentials (CMAPs) after repetitive (2 to 5 Hz) stimulation of the motor nerve. In MG, this results in a progressive decrease (>10%) in CMAPs—a finding called decrement or fade. The electromyographic findings suggest failure of the NMJ but are not specific for MG.

Detection of anti-AChR antibodies confirms the diagnosis of MG. However, the antibody is not present in approximately 10% of patients with MG.

Treatment

Standard management of MG includes the use of acetylcholinesterase inhibitors, immunosuppression, and thymectomy. Additionally, short-term improvement of myasthenic weakness may be achieved by plasma exchange and high-dose IVIG.

Acetylcholinesterase Inhibitors

This group of drugs enhances neuromuscular transmission by delaying the degradation of acetylcholine at the NMJ. Pyridostigmine remains the most popular choice in the United Kingdom, whereas neostigmine is popular in the United States. Over time, tachyphylaxis develops and most will therefore require immunosuppression during the course of their disease.

Immunosuppressive Therapy

Corticosteroids are the mainstay of treatment of MG. After MG symptoms have been controlled, the dose of prednisolone is gradually decreased to the lowest alternate-day regimen to minimize complications. Addition of the immunosuppressant azathioprine (1 to 2 mg/kg/day), which acts by suppressing helper T-cell activity, allows further reduction of the maintenance dose of corticosteroid. Cyclosporine may be used as an alternative immunosuppressant agent to corticosteroids, and its action in stabilizing MG is more rapid; however, high cost and nephrotoxicity may limit its use.

Thymectomy

Thymectomy is indicated for most patients between the ages of puberty and 60 years and for those with a thymoma. Although most patients derive benefit from thymectomy, the beneficial effects may take up to 2 years to be fully realized.

Plasma Exchange and High-Dose Immunoglobulin Therapy

Plasma exchange produces short-term improvement in myasthenic weakness and is reserved for patients with myasthenic crisis or those requiring improvement in symptoms before undergoing thymectomy.

Indications for IVIG therapy are similar to those for plasma exchange. IVIG tends to be favored over the latter because it is easier to administer, is less labor intensive, and has fewer complications.

Avoidance of Certain Drugs

A number of drugs exacerbate MG and should be avoided (Table 47-6).

Anesthetic Considerations

Anesthetic management depends on the severity of MG and the nature of the surgery to be performed. Local and regional anesthesia should be used when possible. If general anesthesia is necessary, careful preoperative assessment and meticulous perioperative care must be adhered to.

Preoperative Care

Patients undergoing major surgery (including thymectomy) should be admitted 24 to 48 hours before surgery to allow detailed assessment of respiratory and bulbar function, as well as to allow a thorough review of their medication. If severe weakness is present, a preoperative course of plasma exchange or high-dose IVIG should be considered.

Respiratory function is most reproducibly assessed by serial measurements of FVC. Factors associated with the need for prolonged mechanical ventilation after surgery include an FVC less than 2.9 L, a history of chronic lung disease, a long history (>6 years) of MG, and grade III MG.

The preoperative assessment must also consider associated autoimmune conditions. Thyroid disease (hyperthyroidism, hypothyroidism, or nontoxic goiter) coexists in 15% of patients with MG and needs to be identified.

Table 47-6   Drugs Known to Exacerbate Myasthenia Gravis

Aminoglycoside antibacterial agents
Polymyxin antibacterial agents
Quinidine
Quinolone antibacterial agents, especially ciprofloxacin
β-Adrenergic receptor blocking drugs
Calcium channel blocking drugs
Procainamide
Magnesium sulfate

Sedative premedication is usually avoided if there is any evidence of respiratory compromise. An antisialagogue such as glycopyrronium is useful in reducing secretions. Patients should continue corticosteroid therapy as normal and should receive additional hydrocortisone on the day of surgery. Traditionally, acetylcholinesterase inhibitors are withheld on the day of surgery; myasthenic patients generally have a decreased requirement for these drugs in the postoperative period. Furthermore, they may prolong the action of suxamethonium and could possibly increase the requirement for nondepolarizing neuromuscular blocking drugs.

Induction and Maintenance of Anesthesia

The minimal mandatory monitoring should be supplemented by invasive pressure monitoring in patients undergoing median sternotomy for thymectomy. Neuromuscular transmission should be monitored throughout the perioperative period.

After preoxygenation, anesthesia is induced with thiopental or propofol. Tracheal intubation is usually achieved by deepening anesthesia with a volatile anesthetic agent. Patients with MG show increased sensitivity to the neuromuscular blocking effects of these agents. Because of the reduced number of AChRs, patients are relatively resistant to suxamethonium; however, if higher doses are used, they are often accompanied by the development of a dual block, which is indistinguishable from a nondepolarizing-type block.

In contrast, patients with MG are extremely sensitive to the effects of nondepolarizing neuromuscular blocking agents. These have a faster onset and a more prolonged action in MG. The dose required depends on the severity of the MG and the affinity of the agent for the AChR. Atracurium or vecuronium are the agents of choice and should be used at 50-60% of their normal dose. Despite their mode of metabolism, most authorities reverse the neuromuscullar blockade at the end of the procedure.

Postoperative Management

In general, patients with well-controlled MG preoperatively can have their tracheas safely extubated at the end of the procedure. However, patients undergoing transsternal thymectomy often benefit from a short period of postoperative mechanical ventilation. This allows effective analgesia in the immediate postoperative period; a combination of nonsteroidal anti-inflammatory agents and opioid analgesia is usually effective. Thoracic extradural analgesia may also be used. Whichever regimen is chosen, patients must be nursed in a high-dependency area in which careful monitoring of respiratory function can be guaranteed. Acetylcholinesterase inhibitor therapy is usually restarted in the postoperative period, and the dose increased as the patient starts to mobilize.

47

KEY POINTS

- Guillain-Barré syndrome is an acute infective polyneuropathy that classically results in ascending neuropathic weakness and areflexia.
- It is the most common cause of neuromuscular paralysis in the Western world, and patients may require prolonged periods of mechanical ventilation.
- The diagnosis is reached by history, physical examination, and the finding of characteristic abnormalities in cerebrospinal fluid and on neurophysiologic testing.
- Treatment is largely supportive, but high-dose IVIG or plasma exchange accelerates recovery.
- Although the majority of patients makes a complete recovery, those with axonal loss may be left with considerable neurologic disability.
- Myasthenia gravis is an autoimmune disease in which IgG autoantibodies decrease acetylcholine receptor density at the postsynaptic site of the neuromuscular junction.
- The cardinal feature of myasthenia gravis is fatigable weakness of voluntary muscles.
- Myasthenia gravis is associated with other autoimmune conditions.
- Patients with myasthenia gravis show relative resistance to suxamethonium and are extremely sensitive to the effects of nondepolarizing neuromuscular blocking drugs.
- Myasthenic patients undergoing major surgery may require a period of postoperative mechanical ventilation.

FURTHER READING

Hirsch NP: The neuromuscular junction in health and disease. Br J Anaesth 2007; 99:132-138.
Hughes RAC, Cornblath DR. Guillain-Barré Syndrome. Lancet 2005; 366:1653-1666.
Hughes RA, Raphaël JC, Swan AV, van Doorn PA: Intravenous immunoglobulin for Guillain-Barré syndrome. Cochrane Database Syst Rev 2004; 1: CD002063.
Krucylak PE, Naunheim KS: Preoperative preparation and anaesthetic management of patients with myasthenia gravis. Semin Thorac Cardiovasc Surg 1999; 11:47-53.
Ng KKP, Howard RS, Fish D, et al: Management and outcome of severe Guillain-Barré syndrome. Q J Med 1995; 88:243-250.
Sharshar T, Chevret S, Bourdain F, Raphaël JC: Early predictors of mechanical ventilation in Guillain-Barré syndrome. French Cooperative Group on Plasma Exchange in Guillain-Barré Syndrome. Crit Care Med 2003; 31:278-283.
Vincent A, Palace J, Hilton-Jones D: Myasthenia gravis. Lancet 2001; 357:2122-2128.

Chapter 48

Neuroanesthesia in Pregnancy

Mark A. Rosen

Intracranial Tumors	Hyperventilation
Subarachnoid Hemorrhage	Osmotic Diuretics
Anesthetic Management	Induced Hypotension or Hypertension
Induction of Anesthesia	Hypothermia
Maintenance of Anesthesia	**Fetal Monitoring**

Neurologic diseases, including primary or metastatic brain tumors, acute brain injury, and subarachnoid hemorrhage (SAH), constitute a major source of nonobstetric morbidity and mortality during pregnancy. SAH accounts for between 5% and 12% of all maternal deaths and is the third most common nonobstetric cause of maternal mortality.

INTRACRANIAL TUMORS

Pregnancy may precipitate or exacerbate the clinical symptoms of tumors by hormonally induced acceleration of tumor growth, edema, blood vessel engorgement, or immunotolerance. The increased estrogens and chorionic gonadotropin levels of pregnancy appear to lower the seizure threshold. Clinical diagnosis of neurologic conditions is frequently delayed in pregnant women because neurologic symptoms may be mistaken for those secondary to the gravid state.

When possible, neurosurgical intervention is usually deferred until after delivery. However, indications for surgery depend on tumor location and histology, and the clinical course of the tumor may be aggravated by pregnancy, thus necessitating surgery for improved maternal and fetal outcome. In most cases, pregnancy may continue under close supervision until the baby is reasonably mature.

SUBARACHNOID HEMORRHAGE

The most common non–pregnancy-related causes of SAH are ruptured intracranial arterial aneurysms and arteriovenous malformations (AVMs). Once the diagnosis of SAH is made, management should be based on neurosurgical rather than obstetric considerations. Because the morbidity and mortality associated with recurrent aneurysmal bleeding are significant, surgical or endovascular management of ruptured aneurysms in a gravid patient is generally recommended and has been successfully performed at all stages of pregnancy. Pregnant women with an unruptured AVM and those who are

48

stable after hemorrhage can often be safely allowed to reach term gestation, followed by elective postpartum excision of the AVM. In some cases, a combined cesarean section followed by clipping or excision of the neurovascular lesion is performed.

Before surgery, most patients undergo neurointerventional radiologic procedures and require anesthesia care. The potential risk for radiation-induced fetal abnormalities is highly dependent on fetal age at the time of exposure; neurons are at particular risk during neuroblast proliferation and cortical migration (weeks 8 through 15). However, exposure of the abdomen and pelvis as a result of direct cranial irradiation is extremely limited, particularly with appropriate shielding.

ANESTHETIC MANAGEMENT

Anesthetic management during pregnancy must be designed to avoid fetal asphyxia, teratogenicity, and induction of preterm labor. Hormonal changes and mechanical effects of the gravid uterus induce changes in practically every organ system. Neuroanesthetic care of pregnant women must balance treatment modalities commonly used during neurosurgery to decrease intracranial pressure or reduce the risk of aneurysmal rupture with potential adverse effects as a result of changes in maternal-fetal physiology.

Premedication should be tailored to reflect the patient's medical and neurologic status. Patients should be given medication to reduce gastric acidity, be positioned to avoid aortocaval compression, and have anesthesia induced with full-stomach precautions.

Induction of Anesthesia

Pregnant women past the first trimester and women with a history of significant gastric reflux are at risk for possible regurgitation and aspiration. For these patients, rapid-sequence intravenous induction with succinylcholine and endotracheal intubation should be performed. For patients in whom intubation may be difficult (abnormal airway, morbid obesity, etc.), awake fiberoptic intubation may be the most appropriate method for securing the airway. Hypertensive responses must be anticipated and attenuated by the administration of β-blockers, lidocaine, nitroprusside, nitroglycerin, opioids, or some combination of agents.

Maintenance of Anesthesia

Inhalational, balanced, and total intravenous anesthetic techniques have all been used successfully for maintenance of anesthesia. No modern anesthetic agent has been shown to have teratogenic effects, although many prefer to avoid the use of nitrous oxide in the first trimester, mostly on a theoretical basis.

Hyperventilation

The use of hyperventilation is limited in pregnant patients. Pregnancy induces a compensated respiratory alkalosis that results in a normal maternal $PaCO_2$ of 32 mm Hg and a pH of 7.40 to 7.45. Increasing maternal alkalosis constricts pH-sensitive umbilical vessels, thereby decreasing umbilical blood flow, and induces a leftward shift in the oxyhemoglobin dissociation curve, which increases the affinity of maternal hemoglobin for oxygen and thus decreases placental transfer of oxygen to the fetal circulation. The hypocapnia produced by excessive positive pressure ventilation increases mean intrathoracic pressure, decreases venous return, and reduces cardiac output, which causes decreased uterine blood flow. These mechanisms can result in fetal hypoxia and acidosis, and therefore the use of hyperventilation should theoretically be avoided. However, mild hyperventilation is probably safe. The fetal heart rate should be monitored for adverse effects and the use of hyperventilation limited in extent and duration to the minimum required. $PaCO_2$ values appreciably greater than 32 mm Hg represent hypercapnia, which increases cerebral blood flow and produces respiratory acidosis in the fetus.

Osmotic Diuretics

Mannitol can adversely affect the fetus by inducing maternal dehydration, which can result in maternal hypotension, uterine hypoperfusion, and fetal injury. Mannitol crosses the placenta to a variable extent and can accumulate in the fetus. Free water shifts from the fetus to the mother after mannitol infusion, thereby increasing fetal osmolality and plasma sodium, decreasing fetal blood volume, total body water, and extracellular fluid volume, and possibly causing severe fetal dehydration. However, low doses of mannitol have been administered without adverse fetal outcome but should be used with caution and high doses should be avoided.

Furosemide crosses the placenta and may induce dose-dependent fetal diuresis, partially mediated by increases in fetal vascular pressure. It has been used in parturients without adverse maternal or fetal effects and may provide an alternate to mannitol for some procedures.

Induced Hypotension or Hypertension

Deliberate hypotension has been used. Low concentrations of halogenated agents are not associated with significant reductions in uterine blood flow because of concomitant decreases in uterine vascular resistance. However, high concentrations can produce significant hypotension leading to decreased uterine blood flow and subsequent fetal asphyxia.

Sodium nitroprusside rapidly crosses the placenta, and with long exposure, its metabolites can be problematic for the fetus by causing a concentration-dependent reduction in fetal arterial perfusion pressure. Although sodium nitroprusside has been used in gravid patients, its administration should be limited to small doses for limited periods. Nitroglycerin has been successfully used without adverse fetal or neonatal effects.

There are significant risks to the fetus with the use of deliberate hypotension in a pregnant patient. When necessary to induce hypotension in pregnant patients, blood pressure reduction should be limited in depth and duration to the minimum required and the fetal heart rate monitored. Maternal arterial pH should be measured frequently to avoid the risk of severe fetal or maternal compromise.

Vasopressors may be necessary during periods of cerebral arterial occlusion with the use of temporary proximal clips. Although ephedrine had been the vasopressor of choice during pregnancy, phenylephrine is now widely used, but its safety has not been determined under these circumstances.

Hypothermia

Hypothermia does not appear to increase the risk of fetal morbidity. Although uterine vascular resistance increases and uteroplacental blood flow decreases during hypothermia, oxygen transfer is unaffected. If maternal respiratory acidosis is prevented, the gas and acid-base contents of fetal blood will parallel those of the mother. The fetus also becomes hypothermic, its metabolic needs proportionately decrease, and the fetal heart rate parallels the decrease in maternal heart rate during cooling and increases again during rewarming.

48

FETAL MONITORING

Whenever possible, fetal and uterine monitors should be used for patients in their second and third trimesters of pregnancy. If the uterine fundus is above the level of the umbilicus, an external tocodynamometer is usually effective for monitoring uterine activity. Doppler monitoring is particularly useful because changes in heart rate may signal an abnormality in maternal ventilation, uterine perfusion, or fetal well-being. Anesthetic agents that readily transverse the placenta diminish the normal beat-to-beat variability of the fetal heart rate. However, when patterns of bradycardia emerge, they may indicate a fetal response to maternal hypotension or hypoxia. Maternal systolic blood pressure of less than 100 mm Hg may be associated with pathologic fetal bradycardia, which can begin a few minutes after the onset of maternal hypotension and may be preceded by transient mild tachycardia. Therefore, close observation of maternal blood pressure and prompt treatment of hypotension and hypoxia are essential if the fetus is to have the best chance of surviving with an intact nervous system. If persistent signs of fetal distress occur that are not readily reversed by standard interventions (increased oxygenation, change in maternal position, blood pressure changes, etc.), the neurosurgical procedure should be temporarily suspended while an emergency cesarean section is performed if the fetus is at a viable gestational age.

KEY POINTS

- Neurologic diseases are a major source of nonobstetric morbidity and mortality during pregnancy, and the decision to operate should be primarily neurosurgical rather than obstetric.
- Anesthetic management during pregnancy must be designed to avoid fetal asphyxia, teratogenicity, and induction of preterm labor while being mindful of maternal physiologic changes during pregnancy.
- Rapid-sequence induction of anesthesia with succinylcholine is recommended, along with administration of agents to attenuate the hypertensive response to laryngoscopy and tracheal intubation.
- No modern anesthetic agent has been shown to have teratogenic effects; inhalational, balanced, or total intravenous techniques can be used safely.
- Hyperventilation, osmotic diuresis, and deliberate hypotensive techniques should be used with caution and limitations, whereas moderate hypothermia is safe.

FURTHER READING

Allen G, Farling P, McAtamney D: Anesthetic management of the pregnant patient for endovascular coiling of an unruptured intracranial aneurysm. Neurocrit Care 2006; 4:18-20.
Kittner SJ, Stern BJ, Feeser BR, et al: Pregnancy and the risk of stroke. N Engl J Med 1996; 335:768-774.
Mas JL, Lamy C: Stroke in pregnancy and the puerperium. J Neurol 1998; 245:305-313.
Piotin M, De Souza Filho CBA, Kothimbakam R, et al: Endovascular treatment of acutely ruptured intracranial aneurysms in pregnancy. Am J Obstet Gynecol 2001; 185:1261-1262.
Powner DJ, Bernstein IM: Extended somatic support for pregnant women after brain death. Crit Care Med 2003; 31:1241-1249.
Rosen MA: Management of anesthesia for the pregnant surgical patient. Anesthesiology 1999; 91:1159-1163.
Trevedi RA, Kirkpatrick PJ: Arteriovenous malformations of the cerebral circulation that rupture in pregnancy. J Obstet Gynecol 2003; 23:484-489.

Section VIII
Appendices

Appendix 1

Clinical Information Resources

Keith J. Ruskin

PubMed

Electronic Journals and Databases

Privacy and Security

Conclusions

Clinical information from textbooks, specialty websites, and the latest journal articles is available to any clinician on CDs, on DVDs, or through the Internet. In addition to diverse new medical resources, the choice of portable computers has grown to include laptop computers, hand-held computers, and Blackberries, each of which has become small, faster, and easier to use. This chapter provides an update on clinical information resources, hand-held computers, and information security.

PUBMED

PubMed (www.pubmed.gov) provides on-line searches of every journal indexed by the National Library of Medicine. The government of the United States provides this service free of charge. More than 15 million articles have been indexed in medical journals since the 1950s. PubMed abstracts most articles except editorials, letters to the editor, and reviews. If the article is available on-line, the reference will include a link to it. PubMed is free, and many hospitals and medical schools provide on-line access to the full text of journal articles through institutional subscriptions. Some health care institutions offer literature searches and on-line journals through Ovid (www.ovid.com), ScienceDirect (www.sciencedirect.com), or HighWire Press (http://highwire.stanford.edu). These fee-based services provide much of the information contained in PubMed, social sciences journals, and other medical resources. The HighWire Press website is easily searchable and also has a useful inventory, with free articles offered from their more than 1000 journals.

MEDLINE, the on-line version of Index Medicus, provides the information used by PubMed, Ovid, and other search engines. MEDLINE contains more than 15 million references, which may cause some searches to return thousands of articles, many of which have nothing to do with the desired topic. PubMed offers search tags that allow the context of a given keyword to be specified. Tags are enclosed in square brackets. For example, typing in Ruskin [au] will return any article in which Ruskin is an author. Adding English [la] to a search phrase will return only articles that are written in English. A search for malignant hyperthermia [majr] will return only articles in which malignant hyperthermia is a major topic. The tag [pt] refers to publication type. Boolean operators are always capitalized and include "AND,"

"OR," and "NOT." A search for subarachnoid hemorrhage AND English [la] AND review [pt] will return review articles on subarachnoid hemorrhage that have been written in English. An easy-to-read tutorial is available on the website that will have most new users conducting fast, productive literature searches in less than an hour. PubMed Clinical Queries allows a busy clinician to do a highly focused literature search. Clinical Queries searches return articles pertaining to a specific clinical study category. They can also return systematic reviews and medical genetics citations. The tutorial offers tips on how to use the subject, author, publication type, and other information to limit results to just a few highly relevant articles. The "limits" tab on the PubMed home page offers useful check boxes to help narrow one's search.

ELECTRONIC JOURNALS AND DATABASES

Most medical journals and major textbooks now offer web and print versions. Most publishers offer free access to on-line journals for subscribers and charge non-subscribers a fee for individual articles. Many anesthesia societies include a journal subscription in the membership fee. *Anesthesiology* (www.anesthesiology.org) and *Anesthesia and Analgesia* (www.anesthesia-analgesia.org) are available on the World Wide Web to members of the American Society of Anesthesiologists (www.asahq .org) and International Anesthesia Research Society (www.iars.org). The *Journal of Neurosurgical Anesthesiology* (www.jnsa.com) is available to subscribers. The majority of medical journals now also offer all their content free after 12 months. In addition, all major journals offer free e-mailed tables of contents with links to free abstracts.

There are many specialty and disease-related societies with useful webpages. The Society of Neurosurgical Anesthesia & Critical Care (www.snacc.org) hosts a very useful bibliography that is regularly updated. It is organized by subject but is not searchable. There is also an outline of required knowledge in neuroanesthesia adapted from the American Board of Anesthesiologists guidelines. Washington University hosts a website devoted to cerebrovascular clinical trials that also details stroke scales and other useful links (http://www.strokecenter.org/trials/). The tumor section of the American Association of Neurological Surgeons (AANS) has a page with much useful information about brain tumors (http://www.tumorsection.org/patient/info .htm), and the AANS has some additional useful educational links (http://www.aans .org/education/).

MDConsult (www.mdconsult.com) is a fee-based service that offers access to textbooks, journal articles, and Clinics of North America. A new service, MDC Mobile, automatically downloads tables of contents, abstracts, and journal articles that contain selected keywords to a hand-held computer for later review. Some hospitals and most medical schools have purchased "institutional subscriptions" that allow anesthesia providers, employees, and students to access journal articles and other resources. More information about how to gain access to institutional subscriptions is usually available from the medical library.

PRIVACY AND SECURITY

Everyone should be concerned about the security of his or her computers and information. Unauthorized access to health information can have devastating consequences for physicians and their patients. Unintentional release of information about disease processes, medication use, or visits to health care providers can result in stigmatization, difficulty obtaining credit or employment, or disruption of family relationships. Most importantly, unintended release of information can result in a breach of trust between the patient and physician. In response to these concerns, the European Union, United States, Australia, Japan, and others have enacted stringent regulations that cover the sharing and protection of health information. Most of the requirements for storage and transmission of health care information in the United States are covered under the Health Insurance Portability and Accountability Act of 1996 (HIPAA). Any physician who uses a computer in a patient care setting should use precautions to maintain the security of patient information and ensure that it complies with institutional policies.

Attacks on personal computers in the form of viruses, keystroke loggers, and "phishing" are a growing threat. Viruses are small programs attached to e-mail messages or disguised as useful programs that once activated can destroy information or simply slow the computer down as they send copies of themselves to thousands of other computers. Viruses may also turn the computer into a zombie so that it can be remotely controlled. Such computers are then turned into pornography websites, made to pose as financial websites to collect credit card information, used to distribute unsolicited commercial e-mail, and so forth. Unfortunately, the only sign that a computer may be infected is that the Internet connection seems much slower than it did before.

Adware and spyware are programs that are usually installed along with other, marginally useful software such as a screen saver or file-sharing programs. Once installed, these programs monitor computer use and report back to a central site. They may generate "pop-up" windows with advertisements or redirect Web searches to a preferred site. They also cause the infected computer to slow down and may make it unstable and cause it to crash and lose valuable information. A keystroke logger is a variant of spyware that is usually distributed as an e-mail attachment. This program automatically installs itself and then waits for the victim to log into a bank or credit card site, at which point all identifying information is relayed to the scammers.

The most common method used by criminals to get credit card or bank account information is called *phishing*. This scam involves sending an e-mail message that usually alleges that the recipient's bank account has been corrupted and then directs the computer to a realistic webpage with a login screen. As soon as the ATM card number and PIN are entered, the criminals begin to withdraw money from the bank account. Needless to say, all suspicious messages should be deleted immediately and the financial institution contacted by telephone if fraud is suspected.

Fortunately, a few simple precautions, combined with common sense, can minimize the risk of information theft or damage. All access to websites, especially those of financial institutions, must be protected by a carefully chosen password, which should ideally consist of a series of letters, numerals, and punctuation marks. A good password is easy for its owner to remember but should be difficult for anyone else to guess. Passwords should never be given to anyone else, sent by e-mail, or posted on a webpage. Remote access to home computers that may not have the latest security updates should be allowed only when necessary.

Hardware and software tools decrease the probability that a computer can be infected by a virus, be compromised by a hacker, or become a "zombie." Antivirus programs are an essential tool that should be installed on every computer. It is important to update the programs frequently because new viruses are released every day. Most of these programs also protect against keystroke loggers and Trojan horses. Software or hardware firewalls prevent unauthorized programs from using an Internet connection and thus protect against spyware or adware.

CONCLUSIONS

A wealth of information is available to any clinician with access to a computer. On-line literature searches and journal articles, continuing medical education, and clinical guidelines are just a few of the many resources available and will make any anesthesia provider more effective (Tables 1 and 2). Simple precautions, combined with common sense, will help protect the security of patient information and minimize the risk of infection with a computer virus (Table 3).

Table 1	Internet Resources for Neurosurgical Anesthesiologists	
BrainInfo	http://www.braininfo.org	Information about brain structures. Type the name of the structure for pictures and information
NeuronDB	http://senselab.med.yale.edu/ neurondb/default.asp	Information about neuron physiology, including locations and types
Journal of Neuro- surgical Anesthesi- ology	www.jnsa.com	A peer-reviewed journal devoted to neurosurgical anesthesiology
Society for Neuro- surgical Anesthesia and Critical Care	www.snacc.org	U.S. Neurosurgical Anesthesia Society
Whole Brain Atlas	http://www.med.harvard .edu/AANLIB/home.html	A neuroimaging primer with CT, MRI, and 3-dimensional images of the brain
Stroke registry	http://www.strokecenter .org/trials	Inventory of ongoing cerebrovascular trials and useful resources
Brain Tumors	http://www.tumorsection .org/patient/info.htm	A website devoted to brain tumors, including definitions and treatment
American Association of Neurological Surgeons	http://www.aans.org/ education/	Contains useful links, including a link to Neurosurgical Forum
Cochrane website	www.cochrane.org	Free summaries of Cochrane Systematic Reviews; Evidence Based Medi- cine (EBM) methods, definitions, etc.
HighWire Press	http://highwire.stanford.edu	HighWire Press hosts >1000 journals with many now offering free content
Anesthesia and Analgesia neuroanesthesia articles	http://www.anesthesia- analgesia.org/cgi/collection/ neuroanesthesia	A collection of neuroane- sthesia articles published in Anesthesia and Analgesia, with free access after 12 months
Neurosurgery Online	http://www.neurosurgery- online.com	Useful neurosurgical articles with beautiful illustrations
Brain Trauma Foun- dation guidelines	http://www2.braintrauma .org/guidelines/index.php	Guidelines with indications of the level of evidence for all aspects of head trauma management
Neurosciences search engine	http://www.neuroguide.com/	Extensive links to all aspects of the neurosciences
Reilly and Bullock (eds): Neurotrauma	http://www.edc.gsph.pitt.edu/ neurotrauma/thebook/ book.html	An authoritative on-line textbook

Table 2 Medical Software for Hand-Held Computers

Ectopic Brain	pbrain.hypermart.net	Palm resources for clinical practice
Epocrates Rx	www.epocrates.com	A compendium of drug information, laboratory values, and other information, automatically updated every time that the hand-held computer is synced
Mobile PDR	www.pdr.net	A free drug compendium
PdaMD	www.pdamd.com	PDAs, medical software, and reviews written for physicians
Skyscape	www.skyscape.com	Medical software for hand-held computers
Handango	www.handango.com	Thousands of Palm and PocketPC applications

Table 3 Security Software

Ad-Aware	www.lavasoft.de	Detects and removes most adware and spyware. Both free and paid versions available
Cloudmark SafetyBar	www.cloudmark.com	A very good spam filter and e-mail fraud detector. Works only with Microsoft Outlook
McAfee	www.mcafee.com	Antivirus software and spam blocker
Spy Sweeper	www.webroot.com	Rated the best antispyware program by *PC Magazine*
Spybot Search and Destroy	www.spybot.info	A free antispyware program. Best used as a secondary defense

1

Appendix 2

Case Scenarios

James E. Caldwell

Supratentorial Lesion

Head Trauma

Subarachnoid Hemorrhage

Cervical Spine Injury

SUPRATENTORIAL LESION

Case Summary

A 43-year-old, otherwise healthy woman was evaluated for tonic-clonic seizure. Computed tomography (CT) showed a large enhancing lesion in the right frontal lobe suggestive of glioma with a 2-mm midline shift. She had no focal neurologic signs but had a headache, which improved. Four days after a seizure she underwent craniotomy for biopsy and probable resection. Her medications were phenytoin, 300 mg once daily before sleep, and dexamethasone, 4 mg every 6 hours. Her weight was 81 kg, she had no history of allergies, and airway examination suggested that there will not probably be any problem with tracheal intubation.

Anesthesia was conducted as follows: premedication with midazolam, 2 mg intravenously in the preoperative area; application of standard American Society of Anesthesiologists (ASA) monitors; induction of anesthesia with remifentanil, 2 µg/kg, and propofol, 2 mg/kg; intubation facilitated with rocuronium, 50 mg; and insertion of a 7.0-mm cuffed endotracheal tube without difficulty. The patient was positioned facing the anesthesia team with a bolster under her right side, and her head was secured to the table with a Mayfield frame. Anesthesia was maintained with infusions of remifentanil, 0.1 to 0.25 µg/kg/min, and propofol, 50 to 100 µg/kg/min, and inhalation of sevoflurane, 0.5 end-tidal minimal alveolar concentration (MAC). A radial artery catheter and second intravenous line were inserted. Neuromuscular blockade was maintained throughout with rocuronium. The surgeon requested ceftriaxone, 1 g, mannitol, 1 g/kg, and dexamethasone, 10 mg.

Discussion

Problem List

- New onset of seizures
- Intraparenchymal brain tumor
- Increased intracranial pressure (ICP) symptomatically improved with dexamethasone

Clinical Findings

New-onset seizure is a common manifestation of brain tumors, and these lesions often occur in the middle decades of life. In most patients, symptoms are controlled preoperatively with anticonvulsants and dexamethasone. Lesions in the frontal lobe may have no focal symptoms, but tumors in other areas or when ICP is raised can be manifested as weakness; vision, speech, or balance difficulty; headache; or nausea and vomiting. Acute neurologic deterioration may occur if there is a sudden increase in swelling around the tumor, bleeding, or necrosis.

Management

Preoperative preparation for a patient in stable neurologic condition involves a complete history and physical and, if necessary, optimization of comorbid conditions. Preoperative administration of a benzodiazepine is acceptable because these patients are understandably very anxious. Caution is advised inasmuch as the sedative effect of the benzodiazepine is occasionally greater than anticipated and the patient can become somnolent with increased $Paco_2$ and ICP. Patients who are already neurologically obtunded should not be premedicated.

Many possible combinations of anesthetic drugs could be used for this type of surgery. There is no evidence from clinical trials to support better outcomes with any particular combination of drugs. Suitable alternatives include total intravenous anesthesia with propofol and remifentanil or fentanyl or a low-dose vapor (<1 MAC) with opioid. In this case a combination of remifentanil with low-dose propofol and low-dose sevoflurane was used in the hope of obtaining some benefit from all three. Neuromuscular blockade is indicated for most straightforward craniotomy procedures such as this, and intermediate-acting drugs should be the first choice. Patients taking anticonvulsants (particularly phenytoin) for a week or more may have a very high requirement for muscle relaxant drugs. This is most marked for the steroidal drugs rocuronium, vecuronium, or pancuronium but is also significant for atracurium and cisatracurium.

More important than the choice of anesthetic drugs is understanding the goals of anesthetic management, which are cardiovascular stability to maintain cerebral perfusion, manipulation of brain volume to facilitate the surgical approach, and rapid emergence from anesthesia to facilitate early neurologic examination. In the absence of indications to the contrary, blood pressure should be kept within the patient's normal range and isotonic fluids administered as needed. If there is significant blood loss, a hematocrit of 30% is a reasonable transfusion trigger.

The presence of a space-occupying lesion usually means that measures to decrease brain volume are indicated to facilitate surgical exposure, for example, to relieve pressure under the dura before it is incised. Standard interventions are mild to moderate hyperventilation, administration of mannitol, and reverse Trendelenburg positioning. These interventions should always be performed after communication and discussion with the neurosurgical team. If these interventions are not effective, the surgeon may elect to drain cerebrospinal fluid directly. Finally, whatever drugs are used for anesthesia, the intent should be to have the patient emerge from anesthesia in a rapid and peaceful manner. Coughing on the endotracheal tube or its effects should be minimized, for example, with a head-up position, opioid, or lidocaine. Supplementary doses of antiemetics may be required intraoperatively, especially if the procedure is prolonged.

Specialized Procedures

Tumors in areas of the brain with specific motor or speech functions will require modification of anesthetic management. Identification of motor areas by stimulation of the motor cortex specifically requires that the patient not be paralyzed during the procedure. Tumors in or near speech areas will require speech mapping, which necessitates that the patient be awake for atleast a significant portion of the procedure. Discussion of these cases is outside the scope of this section.

HEAD TRAUMA

Case Summary

An 18-year-old man was struck on the head with a baseball bat and brought to the emergency department by ambulance. On admission his Glasgow Coma Scale (GCS) score was 8, his oxygen saturation was 89% on room air, and he was wearing a hard plastic neck collar. Immediate anesthesia consultation was sought, and the patient's airway was controlled with oxygenation, neuromuscular blockade, tracheal intubation, ventilation to normoxia, and $Paco_2$ in the low normal range.

CT showed severe contusions in the right hemisphere and no skull fracture or cervical spine injury. Once the patient was transferred to the neurosurgical intensive care unit (ICU), a ventriculostomy catheter was placed and a radial artery catheter inserted. His ICP was 25 mm Hg, so 20% mannitol, 2 mL/kg intravenously, was infused, which reduced ICP to 20 mm Hg.

Discussion

Problem List

- Comatose patient
- Elevated ICP
- Intracranial mass

Principles of Care

When faced with head-injured patients in a critical situation such as this, the guiding principle is to treat the greatest threat to life (airway, breathing, circulation [ABCs]) and avoid doing further harm, such as by inducing severe hypotension or further injuring the cervical spine. This patient has an isolated head injury, but many will be seen with multiple trauma. In such patients, clinical suspicion of and examination for concomitant injuries such as a ruptured spleen and bone fractures must be performed. In patients with multiple trauma, aggressive resuscitation and maintenance of hemodynamics and pulmonary function are of paramount importance.

Controlling the Airway

In this patient both the hypoxia and GCS score of 8 are indications for immediate control of the airway with tracheal intubation, followed by mechanical ventilation. It is imperative that the airway be secured as swiftly as possible, usually by direct laryngoscopy. The nasal route should be avoided if a basal skull fracture is suspected. The use of a short-acting neuromuscular blocker such as succinylcholine is usually required to optimize intubation conditions. The transient rise in ICP as a result of muscle fasciculation has not been shown to be detrimental to outcome, and the risks associated with a difficult intubation outweigh those of a depolarizing muscle relaxant.

Concomitant cervical spine injury may be present in patients with a severe head injury (GCS score ≤8), and the tracheal intubation technique must take account of this possibility. To facilitate laryngoscopy and intubation, the anterior part of the neck collar should be removed. Manual in-line immobilization should be performed before the collar is removed. This procedure involves an assistant (from the side or behind) holding the mastoid processes and occiput to minimize neck movement during laryngoscopy. The aim is to stabilize the neck by counteracting the forces of laryngoscopy; active traction should not be applied.

Mainstays of Management

After tracheal intubation, initial goals of ventilation are normoxia and $Paco_2$ in the low normal range (35 to 38 mm Hg [4.5 to 5.0 kPa]). Hypoxia with a saturation of less than 90% is associated with a worsened outcome. Hyperventilation to 30 mm Hg (4 kPa) is indicated only if focal neurologic signs (e.g., dilating pupil) are evident or ICP is sustained above 25 mm Hg because it can exacerbate cerebral ischemia. This patient's ICP of 25 mm Hg responded to mannitol and, without signs of herniation, did not justify hyperventilation.

Hypotension (systolic blood pressure <90 mm Hg) is an independent predictor of outcome in brain injury, and vigorous maintenance of blood pressure is indicated; isotonic fluids with the addition of a vasopressor if required should be instituted. The Brain Trauma Foundation guidelines suggest maintaining cerebral perfusion pressure around 60 mm Hg with a range between 50 and 70 mm Hg.

Evidence suggests that outcome is worse in brain injury with hyperglycemia, so blood sugar should be maintained within the normal range. Hyperthermia increases the cerebral metabolic rate and blood flow and exacerbates cerebral ischemia. Elevated temperature should be returned to normal levels by surface cooling.

Other Therapeutic Modalities

The simplest is elevation of the head to decrease venous pressure. Angles of elevation of 10 to 30 degrees have been proposed. Seizures are very detrimental and should be actively suppressed, although there is no evidence of benefit for prophylactic anticonvulsant therapy. Sedation and neuromuscular blockade are used when ICP remains elevated, and barbiturate coma may be induced if ICP is refractory to all other medical therapies. Surgical decompression by craniectomy with or without lobectomy or excision of contusions is reserved for situations in which brain swelling cannot be otherwise controlled.

Fluids

Hypertonic saline has several potential beneficial effects: it is useful as an expander of intravascular volume and as an osmotic agent. Consequently, it can decrease cerebral edema and improve regional cerebral blood flow. There is ongoing debate regarding colloid versus crystalloid as the preferred fluid, with no clear data in favor of either. Hypotonic fluids should be avoided.

SUBARACHNOID HEMORRHAGE

Case Summary

A 56-year-old woman with a history of untreated hypertension woke up with a severe headache the morning after being at a party where she consumed a large amount of alcohol. She became drowsy and confused but not hemiparetic and was taken to the emergency department by her family. A CT scan showed a grade 3 subarachnoid hemorrhage (SAH) in the area of her anterior communicating artery.

She was admitted to the ICU with a GCS score of 10 to 11 and given labetalol, morphine, and nimodipine. The next morning she underwent cerebral angiography under anesthesia, and an anterior communicating artery aneurysm was coiled under anesthesia by the neurointerventional radiologist. Three days later she experienced deteriorating neurologic function, and severe vasospasm was treated by repeat angiography, angioplasty of the affected vessels, and intra-arterial injection of verapamil. Hydrocephalus developed and was initially treated with an external ventricular drain, which was then converted to a ventriculoperitoneal (VP) shunt 2 weeks after the initial bleeding. She was discharged home a week after the VP shunt was placed.

Discussion

Problem List

Subarachnoid hemorrhage
Vasospasm
Hydrocephalus

Overview

Risk factors for SAH include female gender, hypertension, and binge drinking. Other putative risk factors are a smoking history and nonwhite ethnicity. Her clinical state classified her as grade 3 under the Hunt-Hess system. Early intervention is important because the risk for rebleeding is 4% in the first 24 hours and greater than 1% per day for the first 2 weeks.

Initial Management

She received very conservative management in the ICU. It would have been preferable to have placed an intra-arterial catheter, possibly a central venous line, and urinary catheter, plus administer an H_2 blocker. Her neurologic status did not warrant tracheal intubation.

Treatment Options

Although this patient had her anterior circulation aneurysm treated by endovascular coiling, the other main option would have been to have the aneurysm clipped surgically. There is now good evidence that 2-year outcomes are superior with endovascular coiling versus surgical clipping, although longer-term data are not complete.

Anesthetic Management for Angiography

If the patient were just going to undergo diagnostic angiography without treatment, careful sedation might be sufficient but is often difficult in confused patients. However, the objective was to treat the aneurysm, which required general endotracheal anesthesia. This guarantees no patient movement at critical moments and apnea for improved image quality. Specific management principles focus on tight control of hemodynamics. Severe hypertension might provoke aneurysmal rebleeding. Severe hypotension will worsen the cerebral ischemia that frequently accompanies SAH. Preinduction intra-arterial pressure monitoring is recommended.

Vasospasm

The patient's neurologic deterioration at 3 days was very suggestive of vasospasm, and this was confirmed by four-vessel cerebral angiography. Transcranial Doppler ultrasonography may have been useful, although it is more predictive of vasospasm in the middle cerebral artery territory. Other potential diagnostic modalities are CT angiography, magnetic resonance imaging (MRI), and radionuclide imaging, but definitive treatment requires angiography.

Hemodynamic augmentation (hypertension, hypervolemia, hemodilution), or triple-H therapy, was the only therapy for a long time. Although this modality in its various forms can reverse the symptoms of ischemia, it is associated with significant complications such as pulmonary edema and myocardial infarction. Intraluminal balloon angioplasty is effective for isolated spasm of proximal vessels in the circle of Willis, and intra-arterial infusion of vasodilators (such as verapamil or papaverine) can be used for more distal or diffuse spasm.

Final Disposition

This patient's course was fairly typical. She avoided possible outcomes that can accompany SAH, such as seizures, myocardial ischemia, congestive heart failure, acute lung injury, gastric erosions, and cerebral salt wasting.

CERVICAL SPINE INJURY

Case Summary

A 62-year-old man arrived in the emergency department after a motor vehicle accident while on his way home from dinner at a restaurant. He had multiple injuries, including a femoral fracture, and had a rapidly expanding abdomen, blood pressure of 80/50, and heart rate of 121. He complained of neck pain. His neck was immobilized with a hard collar, sandbags, and tape across his forehead.

A cross-table lateral radiograph showed no cervical spine injury. Because of the urgent need to proceed to exploratory laparotomy, there was no time for a further radiologic work-up. He weighed 97 kg, and his airway examination was MP 2, with a four-fingerbreadth thyromental distance.

He underwent rapid-sequence induction of anesthesia with tracheal intubation via direct laryngoscopy and cricoid pressure. Only the front of the collar was removed, and manual in-line stabilization was performed. At laparotomy he had a ruptured spleen and a liver laceration.

Discussion

Problem List

- Hypotension
- Ruptured abdominal organ
- Fractured femur
- Potential cervical spine injury
- Potential difficult airway

Risk of Significant Cervical Spine Injury and Radiology Work-up

This patient is at significant risk for having a neck injury in that he was involved in an apparently high-speed auto accident and is complaining of neck pain. In the ideal world, a significant and potentially unstable neck injury would be ruled out before the patient's airway was manipulated. The regimen recommended for diagnosing and defining a neck injury is a three-view spine series (lateral, anteroposterior, and odontoid) with supplemental high-resolution CT for poorly visualized or suspicious areas. With this regimen, the risk of a false-negative result is very low. There is little place for MRI in the initial management of cervical spine injury. In this emergency clinical scenario, such an extensive work-up was not possible.

Airway Management

This patient's spine was immobilized in the ideal manner with a hard collar, sand-bags, and forehead tape. For airway management, only the front of the collar can be removed, and other immobilization measures must be maintained. The degree to which the cervical spine moves is greatest with maneuvers such as chin lift and jaw thrust and is less during laryngoscopy and intubation.

No technique for intubation is superior to or recommended over any other. Most clinicians, when asked, are of the opinion that awake fiberoptic intubation is the method of choice, but interestingly, most also state they are inexperienced with the technique, especially in emergency situations. The consensus is to use the technique most appropriate for the urgency of airway control and with which the clinician is most skilled. Techniques both reported and approved include direct laryngoscopy, rigid intubating laryngoscopes such as the Bullard, intubating laryngeal mask airways (with and without esophageal occlusion capability), lightwand, fiberoptic bronchoscopy, and cricothyrotomy.

Secondary Injury

Secondary injury can occur after the initial trauma and may be associated with clinical interventions. The greatest risk factor is failure to suspect an underlying neck injury and not providing adequate immobilization. The spine should be immobilized in a neutral position for that patient. For example, with preexisting spinal deformity, the neutral position is the chronic position of the deformity, and this should be the position of immobilization.

There have been no reports of secondary injury attributable to airway management and tracheal intubation in which neck immobilization and manual in-line stabilization were used. Hypotension may exacerbate a cord injury already present and should be treated aggressively. Other causes of secondary injury are vertebral artery injury and an ascending myelopathy, which may be produced by cord edema and inflammation or an apoptotic process resulting from the initial injury.

Index

Page numbers followed by "f" refer to illustrations; page numbers followed by "t" refer to table. Page number followed by "b" refer to boxes.

A

ACA. *See* Anterior cerebral artery
Acetaminophen
  postanesthesia care unit and, 205
  spinal surgery and, 155
Acetylcholinesterase inhibitors, myasthenia gravis and, 308
Acoustic neuroma, 119
Acromegaly, 144
ACT. *See* Activated clotting time
Activated clotting time (ACT), 175
α_2-adrenergic agonists, 61
  awake craniotomy and, 133
  clonidine, 59
  dexmedetomidine, 59
Adrenocorticotropic hormone-secreting tumors, 144
Adrenoreceptor antagonists, 62
  esmolol, 62
  labetalol, 62
Airway, management of
  in awake craniotomy, 133
  cervical spine diseases and, 160, 162, 164
  head injury and resuscitation, 217
  intracranial hemorrhage and, 231
  pediatric neurotrauma and, 197
  in pituitary surgery, 147
  postanesthesia care unit and, 203
    complications, 204
  spinal cord injury and, 213
  in spinal cord surgery, 156
American Spinal Injury Association (ASIA), 212
Amino acids, cellular metabolism and, 33
γ-aminobutyric acid (GABA$_A$), 51, 125
Amitriptyline, spinal surgery and, 155
AMPLE, 152
Amygdala, 11, 12f
Analgesia
  head injury and, 225
  opioids and, 60
Anesthesia. *See also* Postanesthesia care unit
  arteriovenous malformations and, 116
  autonomic dysreflexia and, 215
  brainstem auditory evoked potentials and, 286
  carotid endarterectomy surgery and, 168
    general, 168
    regional, 169, 169f, 170f, 171f

Anesthesia, *(Continued)*
  cerebral blood flow and, 24
    inhalational agents in, 24
    intravenous agents in, 24
  cerebral ischemia and, 43
    barbiturates, 43
    desflurane, 44
    etomidate, 44
    halothane, 44
    isoflurane, 44
    ketamine, 44
    propofol, 44
    sevoflurane, 44
  electromyography and, 284
  electrophysiologic effects of, epilepsy surgery and, 128
  in infants/children
    anomalies/physiologic status of, 186
    craniofacial reconstruction, 188
    intravenous access in, 186
    intravenous fluids in, 186, 187t
    intubation, 190t
    meningomyelocele repair, 187
    monitoring of, 186
    neurologic assessment of, 185
    preoperative evaluation in, 185
    ventriculoperitoneal shunt placement, 188
  inhaled, effects of, 56
    cerebral blood flow and, 24
    desflurane, 57
    isoflurane, 57
    nitrous oxide, 57
    sevoflurane, 58
    supratentorial surgery and, 108
  intravenous
    benzodiazepines, 53
    etomidate, 53
    ketamine, 53
    propofol, 52
    thiopental, 52
    total, 54
  motor evoked potentials and, 288, 288t
  myasthenia gravis and, 308
    anesthesia induction, 309
    anesthesia maintenance, 309
    postoperative management, 309
    preoperative care, 308

Cardiovascular system
  complications in, postanesthesia care
    unit and, 204
  opioids and, 59
  spinal cord injury and, 212, 214
Carotid artery disease, transcranial Doppler
  ultrasonography and, 298
Carotid endarterectomy (CEA)
  near-infrared spectroscopy and, 275
  surgery for
    anesthetic technique in, 168
    cerebral perfusion monitoring, 167
    cross-clamping during, 167
    postoperative considerations in, 170
    preoperative management, 168
    technique of, 167
Carotid stenosis, neuroradiology and, 177
Catheter, location of, in microdialysis, 280, 280t
Caudate nucleus, 11, 12f
CBF. See Cerebral blood flow
CEA. See Carotid endarterectomy
Cellular metabolism, mechanisms of, 32
  amino acids, 33
  glucose, 32
  ketone bodies, 33
  lactate, 33
  organic acids, 33
Central diabetes insipidus, 242
Central nervous system (CNS), regions of, 3, 4f
Central venous pressure (CVP), fluid
  management and, 237
Cerebellum, 11
Cerebral aneurysms. See Subarachnoid
  hemorrhage
Cerebral autoregulation
  in pediatric neurotrauma, 193
  transcranial Doppler ultrasonography
    and, 298
Cerebral blood flow (CBF)
  anesthetic agents, effects of, 24
    inhalational agents in, 24
    intravenous agents in, 24
  cerebral ischemia and, 36, 37f
  global control of, 21
    arterial carbon dioxide tension in, 23, 23f
    arterial oxygen tension/content in, 23, 23f
    autoregulation in, 22, 22f
    flow-metabolism coupling in, 21
  hematocrit and, 24
  measurement of, 25
  in pediatric neurotrauma, 193
  regional control of, 24
    metabolic factors in, 24, 25t
    neural factors in, 24
  temperature changes and, 24
  transcranial Doppler ultrasonography and
    in anesthesia, 298
    carotid artery disease and, 298
    cerebral autoregulation, 298
    closed head injury and, 298
    derived values, 297
    imaging techniques in, 299
    intensive care and, 298

Cerebral blood flow (CBF), (Continued)
    laser Doppler flowmetry, 299
    measurements, 297
    as research tool, 298
    stroke and, 299
    subarachnoid hemorrhage and, 298
    thermal diffusion flowmetry, 299
    tomographic, 300
    Xenon 133 washout, 299
Cerebral blood volume, increase in, intracranial
  pressure and, 28
Cerebral circulation
  arterial blood supply in, 13
  blood-brain barrier in, 17
  microcirculation in, 17
  venous drainage in, 16, 16f
Cerebral cortex, 6
Cerebral function, monitoring of, with
  electroencephalography
  anesthetic depth drug titration, 292, 293f
  avoidance of awareness, 292
  intraoperative use of, 291
Cerebral hemodynamics, opioids and, 60
Cerebral ischemia
  anesthetic influence on, 43
    barbiturates, 43
    desflurane, 44
    etomidate, 44
    halothane, 44
    isoflurane, 44
    ketamine, 44
    propofol, 44
    sevoflurane, 44
  cerebral blood flow and, 36, 37f
  neuronal death after, 41f
  pathophysiologic mechanisms in, 38
    apoptosis, 39
    excitotoxicity, 38, 38f
    inflammation, 40, 40f
    nitric oxide, 39
    tissue acidosis, 39
  physiologic parameters and, 45
    arterial carbon dioxide tension, 46
    blood glucose, 46
    body temperature, 45
    cerebral perfusion pressure, 45
    seizure prophylaxis, 47
Cerebral metabolic rate, in pediatric
  neurotrauma, 193
Cerebral metabolism
  flow-metabolism coupling in, 34, 34f
  mechanisms of, 32
    amino acids, 33
    glucose, 32
    ketone bodies, 33
    lactate, 33
    organic acids, 33
  suppression of, head injury and, 225
Cerebral perfusion, monitoring of, carotid
  endarterectomy surgery and, 167
Cerebral perfusion pressure (CPP)
  cerebral ischemia and, 45
  head injury and, 224

Cerebral perfusion pressure (CPP), *(Continued)*
  in intracranial pressure monitoring, 261, 263f
  propofol and, 52
Cerebral salt wasting (CSW), 241, 242t
Cerebral salt wasting syndrome (CSWS), 148
Cerebrospinal fluid (CSF), 3
  intracranial pressure and, 28
Cerebrovascular pressure reactivity, in intracranial
    pressure monitoring, 261, 262f, 263f
Cerebrum, 6
Cervical instability, 162, 163t
  airway management and, 162
Cervical spine
  diseases of
    airway management in, 160, 162, 164
    flexible fiberoptic intubation and, 164
    instability, 162, 163t
    occipito-atlanto-axial complex, 160, 161f
    stenosis, 162
  pediatric neurotrauma and, 194
    immobilization and, 196
Cervical stenosis, 162
Chiari malformations, 119-120
Children, anesthesia in
  anomalies/physiologic status of, 186
  craniofacial reconstruction, 188
  intravenous access in, 186
  intravenous fluids in, 186, 187t
  intubation, 190t
  meningomyelocele repair, 188
  monitoring of, 186
  neurologic assessment of, 185
  preoperative evaluation in, 185
  ventriculoperitoneal shunt placement, 188
Circle of Willis, 14f, 16
Circulation, head injury and resuscitation, 218
Citric acid cycle, 33
Clonidine, 59
CNS. *See* Central nervous system
Codeine, postanesthesia care unit and, 205
Coma, evaluation of, in brainstem death, 253
Common carotid artery, 13
Common mode rejection, 290
Computed tomography (CT)
  anesthesia and sedation, 179
  cerebral blood flow and, 300
  intracranial hypertension and, 29, 30
Contusions, hemorrhagic, 151
Corneal (blink) reflex, 10-11, 253-254
Cortical mapping, in awake craniotomy, 132
Corticosteroids, Guillain-Barré
    syndrome and, 305
Corticotrophs, 142t
CPP. *See* Cerebral perfusion pressure
Cranial nerves, functions of, 10t
Craniofacial reconstruction, anesthesia in, 188
  for single-suture synostosis, 188
  synostosis, complex, 188
Craniotomy, for posterior fossa lesions
  arrhythmias in, 121
  emergence of, 121
  extubation after, 122t
  induction in, 121

Craniotomy, for posterior fossa
    lesions, *(Continued)*
  intracranial hypertension treatment in, 121t
  intraoperative management in, 120
  maintenance in, 121
  patient positioning in, 121
  preoperative evaluation in, 120, 120t
Craniotomy, awake
  airway control in, 133
  complications of, 134t
  cortical mapping in, 132
  indications for, 131, 132t
  intraoperative anesthesia management, 132
  intraoperative problems in, 134
  postoperative care in, 134
  preoperative assessment for, 132
  technique of, 131
Cross-clamping, during carotid endarterectomy
    surgery, 167
CSF. *See* Cerebrospinal fluid
CSW. *See* Cerebral salt wasting
CSWS. *See* Cerebral salt wasting syndrome
CT. *See* Computed tomography
Cushing's syndrome, 146, 146t
Cushing's triad, intracranial pressure and, 29
Cushing's ulcers, intracranial pressure and, 29
CVP. *See* Central venous pressure
Cytochrome *c*, 39

D

DBS. *See* Deep brain stimulation
Death, of brainstem
  adjunctive tests of, 254
  confirmatory tests of, 254
  examination of, 253
    clinical, 253
    coma evaluation, 253
    reversible causes, 253
  historical perspective of, 252
  organ donor management and, 254
  pathophysiology of, 254
  versus whole-brain death, 252
Deep brain stimulation (DBS)
  postanesthesia care unit and, 206
  stereotactic neurosurgery and, 132
Desflurane
  cerebral ischemia and, 44
  epilepsy and, 128
  inhaled anesthetics, effects of, 57
  supratentorial surgery and, 108
Dexamethasone, spinal surgery and, 155
Dexmedetomidine, 59
  awake craniotomy and, 133
  neuroradiology and, 174
  spinal surgery and, 155
  stereotactic surgery and, 134
Diabetes insipidus
  brainstem death and, 255
  central, 242
Diazepam
  epilepsy and, 128
  status epilepticus and, 248

Diencephalon, 8
Diffusion-weighted images, 77
Digital subtraction angiography (DSA), 112
Direct-acting vasodilators, 62
  glyceryl trinitrate, 62
  hydralazine, 62
  sodium nitroprusside, 62
DSA. *See* Digital subtraction angiography
Dystonia, 133

E

ECA. *See* External carotid artery
ECoG. *See* Electrocorticography
Edema, of brain
  cerebral ischemia and, 37
  intracranial pressure and, 28
EDRF. *See* Endothelium-derived relaxant factor
Electrical activity, opioids and, 60
Electrocorticogram, 291
Electrocorticography (ECoG), 127
Electroencephalography, 290, 291f
  awareness, 294
  bispectral analysis, 293
  cerebral function monitoring with
    anesthetic depth drug titration, 292, 293f
    avoidance of awareness, 292
    intraoperative use of, 291
  entropy analysis, 294
Electrolyte(s)
  disorders of
    magnesium, 244
    phosphate, 245
    potassium, 243
    sodium, 240
  disturbance of, intracranial hemorrhage
    and, 233
  postanesthesia care unit and, 203
Electromyography, 283, 284t
  anesthetic considerations in, 284
Endoscopic transsphenoidal hypophysectomy,
  postanesthesia care unit and, 206
Endothelial NOS (eNOS), 39-40
Endothelium-derived relaxant factor
  (EDRF), 24
eNOS. *See* Endothelial NOS
Ephedrine, arrhythmias and, 121
Epidural probes, in intracranial pressure
  monitoring, 260
Epilepsy. *See also* Status epilepticus
  causes of, 26t
  classification of, 126t
  pathophysiology of, 125
  risk factors for, 126t
  surgery for
    anesthetic agents electrophysiologic
      effects, 128
    anesthetic technique, 128, 129t
    indications for, 126
    intraoperative management in, 127
    postoperative care in, 129
    preoperative assessment in, 126
  therapy for, 126, 127t

Esmolol, 62
Ethosuximide, 64
  antiepileptic therapy and, 127t
Etomidate
  cerebral blood flow and, 24
  cerebral ischemia and, 44
  epilepsy and, 128
  as intravenous anesthetic, 53
Evoked potentials, 284, 285f
  brainstem auditory, 285, 286f
    anesthetic considerations in, 286
    interpretation of, 285
    typical procedures of, 285
  motor, 287
    anesthetic considerations in, 288, 288t
    response interpretation in, 288
  somatosensory, 286
    anesthetic considerations in, 287, 288t
    procedures of, 286
    response interpretation of, 287
  visual, 284
Excitotoxicity, in cerebral ischemia, 38, 38f
External carotid artery (ECA), 13
Extra-axial mass lesions, intracranial pressure
  and, 28
Extradural hematomas, 80, 80f, 81f, 151
  acute, 152
Extrapyramidal organs, 11
  basal ganglia, 11, 12f
Extrapyramidal signs, 11
Extubation, after craniotomy, for posterior
  fossa lesions, 122t

F

Far lateral neurosurgical procedure, 102
Far lateral suboccipital neurosurgical operative
  approach, 96, 96f
Fentanyl
  anticonvulsants and, 64-65
  awake craniotomy and, 133
  cerebral aneurysms and, 115
  neuroradiology and, 174
  stereotactic surgery and, 134
Fetal monitoring, in neuroanesthesia,
  pregnancy and, 314
Fisher grading system, cerebral aneurysms
  and, 113t
Fixed-head frame stereotactic neurosurgery, 136
FLAIR. *See* Fluid-attenuated inversion recovery
Flexible fiberoptic intubation, cervical spine
  diseases and, 164
Flow velocity (FV), factors affecting, 297
Flow-metabolism coupling
  in cerebral blood flow, 21
  in cerebral metabolism, 34, 34f
Fluid(s)
  head injury and, 224
    resuscitation of, 218
  management of
    administration, 236
    hyperosmolar therapy, 238
    neurologically injured patients and, 237

Hemorrhage, subarachnoid, 82, 83f, 111, 176.
    See also Intracranial hemorrhage
    anesthetic management in, 114
        emergence, 116
        induction, 115
        intraoperative aneurysm rupture, 115
        maintenance, 115
        monitoring, 114
        postoperative care, 116
    diagnosis of, 112
    epidemiology of, 111
    investigations of, 112
    in neuroanesthesia, pregnancy and, 311
    pathophysiology of, 111
    preoperative anesthetic assessment in, 114
    treatment of, 112, 113t
Hemorrhagic contusions, 151
Hepatic enzymes, anticonvulsants and, 65
High-dose immunoglobulin therapy, myasthenia
    gravis and, 308
Hippocampus, 6
Hormonal hypersecretion syndromes, 144
    acromegaly, 144
    Cushing's syndrome, 146, 146t
Hormone
    complications of, in pituitary gland
        surgery, 148
    function preoperative optimization, pituitary
        gland surgery and, 146
        perioperative steroid supplementation, 146
        thyroid function control, 146
Hunt and Hess grading scale, cerebral
    aneurysms and, 113t
Hydralazine, 62
Hyperkalemia, 243, 244f
Hypernatremia, 148, 242
Hyperosmolar therapy
    fluid management and, 238
    head injury and, 225
Hypertension
    deliberate, neuroradiology and, 175
    induced, in neuroanesthesia, pregnancy
        and, 313
    intracranial, radiologic signs of, 29
Hypertonic saline, 63
Hyperventilation, in neuroanesthesia,
    pregnancy and, 312
Hypokalemia, 243, 243f
Hypomagnesemia, 244
Hyponatremia, 148
    management of, 242
Hypophosphatemia, 245
Hypotension
    brainstem death and, 255
    deliberate, neuroradiology and, 175
    induced, in neuroanesthesia, pregnancy
        and, 313
Hypothalamus, 9, 9f
Hypothermia
    head injury and, 226
    in neuroanesthesia, pregnancy and, 313
Hypoxic thresholds, in brain tissue oxygen
    tension, 273

I

ICA. *See* Internal carotid artery
ICAM. *See* Intercellular adhesion molecule
ICP. *See* Intracranial pressure
ICU. *See* Intensive care unit
IJV. *See* Internal jugular vein
Immobilization, spinal cord injury and, 213
Immunosuppressive therapy, myasthenia
    gravis and, 308
Inducible NOS (iNOS), 39-40
Infants, anesthesia in
    anomalies/physiologic status of, 186
    craniofacial reconstruction, 188
    intravenous access in, 186
    intravenous fluids in, 186, 187t
    intubation, 190t
    meningomyelocele repair, 188
    monitoring of, 186
    neurologic assessment of, 185
    preoperative evaluation in, 185
    ventriculoperitoneal shunt placement, 188
Inflammation, cerebral ischemia and, 40, 40f
Infratentorial compartment, 9
    brainstem, 9
    cerebellum, 11
Inhaled anesthetics
    cerebral blood flow and, 24
    effects of, 56
        desflurane, 57
        isoflurane, 57
        nitrous oxide, 57
        sevoflurane, 58
    supratentorial surgery and, 108
iNOS. *See* Inducible NOS
INR. *See* Interventional neuroradiology
Intensive care unit (ICU). *See* Postanesthesia
    care unit
Intercellular adhesion molecule (ICAM), 40
Interhemispheric neurosurgical operative
    approach, 91, 91f, 99
Internal carotid artery (ICA), 13. *See also* Carotid
    endarterectomy
Internal jugular vein (IJV), 13
International 10-20 Electrode Placement
    Protocol, 291f
Interventional neuroradiology (INR).
    See Neuroradiology
Intra-axial mass lesions, intracranial pressure
    and, 28
Intracerebral hematomas, 151, 152
Intracranial aneurysm, neuroradiology and, 176
Intracranial compartment
    hypertension of, radiologic signs of, 29-30
    neurosurgical operative approach by, 88t
    pressure of
        pressure-volume relationship, 26-27
        raised, clinical features of, 29
        raised, pathophysiologic mechanisms/causes
            of, 28
Intracranial hemorrhage
    diagnosis of, 229
    electrolyte disturbances, 233
    findings in, 229

Magnetic resonance imaging sequences, 77
Mannitol, 63
  hyperosmolar therapy and, 238
  venous air embolism and, 121
MAP. *See* Mean arterial pressure
Mass effect, 143, 144
MCA. *See* Middle cerebral artery
Mean arterial pressure (MAP), 45
Meningioma, 85, 119
Meningomyelocele repair, anesthesia in, 188
Meperidine, spinal cord injury and, 216
MEPs. *See* Motor evoked potentials
Metabolic factors. *See also* Cellular metabolism
  Cerebral metabolism
  in cerebral blood flow, 24, 25t
Metastases. *See also* Tumor(s)
  intracranial tumors and, 85
Methohexital, epilepsy and, 128
MG. *See* Myasthenia gravis
Microcirculation, in cerebral circulation, 17
Microdialysis
  in acute head injury, 224
  catheter location in, 280, 280t
  clinical applications of, 280, 281f
  limitations of, 281
  markers, 279
    glucose, 279
    glutamate, 279
    glycerol, 279
    lactate, 279
    pyruvate, 279
  principles of, 277, 278f
  recovery, 278
  research applications of, 281
Microtransducers, in intracranial pressure
  monitoring, 259
Midazolam
  neuroradiology and, 174
  refractory status epilepticus and, 250-251
  status epilepticus and, 248
  stereotactic surgery and, 134
Middle cerebral artery (MCA), 13-15, 14f
Midline suboccipital neurosurgical operative
  approach, 94, 94f
Monro-Kellie doctrine, 27
Morphine
  anticonvulsants and, 64-65
  postanesthesia care unit and, 205
Motor evoked potentials (MEPs), 287
  anesthetic considerations in, 288, 288t
  response interpretation in, 288
MRI. *See* Magnetic resonance imaging
Muscle relaxants. *See* Neuromuscular blockers
Myasthenia gravis (MG), 306, 306t
  anesthetic considerations in, 308
    anesthesia induction, 309
    anesthesia maintenance, 309
    postoperative management, 309
    preoperative care, 308
  diagnosis of, 307
  features of, 306, 307t
  pathophysiology of, 306
  treatment of, 307

Myasthenia gravis (MG), *(Continued)*
  acetylcholinesterase inhibitors, 308
  drug avoidance in, 308, 309t
  high-dose immunoglobulin therapy, 308
  immunosuppressive therapy, 308
  plasma exchange, 308
  thymectomy, 308
Myocardial dysfunction, in subarachnoid
  hemorrhage-related cardiac abnormalities, 231
Myocardial injury, in subarachnoid
  hemorrhage-related cardiac abnormalities, 231

N

NADPH. *See* Nicotinamide adenine dinucleotide
  phosphate
Naloxone, 61
Nausea and vomiting
  intracranial pressure and, 29
  opioids and, 60-61
  postanesthesia care unit and, 206, 206t
Near-infrared spectroscopy (NIRS), 273
  in acute head injury, 224
  advantages of, 275
  clinical applications in, 274
    carotid endarterectomy, 275
    neurovascular procedures, 275
    traumatic brain injury, 275
  disadvantages of, 275
  equipment in, 274, 275f
  principles of, 273
Neocerebellum, 11
Neocortices, 6
Nervous system
  complications in, postanesthesia care unit
    and, 204
  spinal cord injury and, 211
Neural factors, in cerebral blood flow, 24
Neuroanesthesia, in pregnancy
  anesthesia induction, 312
  anesthesia maintenance, 312
  anesthetic management, 312
  fetal monitoring, 314
  hypertension, induced, 313
  hyperventilation, 312
  hypotension, induced, 313
  hypothermia, 313
  intracranial tumors, 311
  osmotic diuretics, 313
  subarachnoid hemorrhage, 311
Neuroendoscopy, postanesthesia care unit and, 206
Neuroimaging, concepts of
  intracranial pressure, raised, 84, 84f, 85f
  intracranial tumors, 84
  magnetic resonance imaging sequences, 77
  spinal trauma, 78, 78t, 79f
  subarachnoid hemorrhage, 82, 83f
  trauma, intracranial appearances in, 78, 79t,
    80f, 81f, 82f
Neuroimaging, outside operating room,
  anesthesia and sedation
  computed tomography, 179
  gamma camera imaging, 179

Printed in the United States
By Bookmasters